Why Am I Sick ?

And
What To Do
About It

1st Edition
2008

Why Am I Sick ?

And
What To Do
About It

Dr. Robert Zee

First Edition – May 2008

Published by
BookSurge
7290 B Investment Dr.
Charleston, SC 29418

To order this publication online, go to www.rue309.com and click on the **Publications** button.

ISBN: 1-4196-9384-0
EAN: 9781419693847

Siúil go doras agus éalaigh liom

Disclaimers

Medical and health information is not medical advice. The content of this book provides information about health and certain health conditions. The information contained herein is presented for educational purposes only, and is not intended to be a substitute for professional medical advice, diagnosis, or treatment. We highly recommend that everyone seek the care of a natural health care provider or holistic medical doctor for proper application of this material to any specific situation. Never disregard professional medical advice or delay in seeking appropriate care because of something presented in this book, any other publication, or website.

No statement in this book has been evaluated by the Food and Drug Administration. Any product mentioned or described in this book is not intended to diagnose, treat, cure, or prevent any disease.

Everyone should consult with a health care professional before starting any diet, or supplementation program, and before taking or ceasing to take any medication. Consulting with a health care professional before starting any exercise program is also important. For anyone who has or suspects that they have a health problem, who may be pregnant, has not exercised in a while, or in a high risk group for exercise complications, a complete physical examination may be recommended by the attending health care provider.

Contents

Introduction

It is safe to assume that hundreds of years ago only the strong and healthy survived. Most people who lived during that era were in excellent physical condition and in good health. They attained health as a result of their daily activities, diet, and lifestyle, which was quite different from the people living in today's society. Modern medical care facilities, hospitals, nursing homes, medical imaging centers, and the corner pharmacy were all nonexistent during that time. Yet, people were not plagued by the diseases of modern day society. In a sense, they were much more happy, very strong, and very healthy.

Before modern times, the source of all health was found from the foods eaten. Certain individuals in nearly every society had special knowledge of the healing properties of certain foods and specific plants. This knowledge was passed down from generation to generation, and anyone entrusted with the secrets invested many years learning from the master. The wisdom and knowledge of these ancient remedies were highly valued, and those who understood their uses were sought out by many people suffering from various diseases and illness. Medicinal applications of the herbs and herbal extracts used in healing were developed independently by many cultures over a period of thousands of years. The Chinese have a long history in using herbal remedies to heal diseases. The Chinese also developed acupuncture, a method of healing by which the stimulation of the meridians of the body restored the function of the systems of the body. Ayurveda, developed in India, incorporates into the philosophy of healing the treatment of the whole person, the body, mind, and spirit. Ayurveda operates under the principle that anything of vegetable, animal, or mineral origin has some medicinal value. The Earth-centered methods of the Native American system of healing also included the use of many herbs. Energy healing techniques, or healing methods of and through the spirit, were developed by many ancient cultures, and are still practiced today. Jesus healed just by speaking the word.

Modern medicine comes along on the scene, and with it so does the discovery of many new diseases and illnesses. More new diseases are being discovered every year, with apparently no end in sight. Modern technology gives us vision into the previously unseen world, uncovering the minute details at every level of both new diseases and old. Scanning electron microscopes let us see antibody-antigen complexes imbedded in tissue structures. Magnetic Resonance Imaging (MRI) scanners give us a look inside the body without exploratory surgery. Computer Aided Tomography (CAT) scanners give us true three dimensional images of the body. Positron Emission Tomography (PET) scanners enable early detection of tumors. Advanced blood analysis not only tells us what has gone wrong, but often where as well. New technology arrives every year to aid in the discovery of yet more diseases. Were these new diseases here all along, or could they be a product of modern day civilization? Could these diseases and disorders that plague society today have gone undetected for centuries? Are the newly discovered diseases actually new diseases, or are they perhaps a symptom or part of another underlying disease?

When a new disease comes along, the proposed cure is often not too far behind. Biomedical engineers working in state of the art technological laboratories invent new drugs to counteract the newly found disease or condition. The advertisements soon hit the airways and we hear "Is work-related stress causing you pain? Can't take it any more? Ask your doctor about Jobocaine." Jobocaine, this month's new and promising medication, is just the magical cure for which everyone has been waiting. A short time later, the supposed cure is found to cause serious health problems, such as liver failure, heart attacks or strokes. The class action lawsuit is quickly organized by attorneys, who run television and magazine advertisements, searching for people and families who may have been injured by taking the miracle cure. While the class action law suit is heard in court, hearings are conducted by some federal agency, where attorneys from both sides, who have no understanding whatever about biochemistry, argue as if they actually know something. Pretending to be experts, their only goal is extracting money out of the pharmaceutical companies, and a token settlement may eventually make its way to the injured parties several years later. It does not take a genius to figure out that something might be wrong with this system. Nevertheless, history repeats itself, and next month yet another miracle cure hits the market.

Even with all the modern day testing equipment and protocols providing valuable diagnostic information, the skill of the doctor and his or her clinical experience is still the most valuable asset in the treatment of disease. The doctor who has a willingness to devote time and thought to the case will be much more effective than the doctor who orders test after test, hoping to stumble upon the correct diagnosis. A doctor who is skilled in analytical thinking does not have to resort to pulling out the prescription pad and trying medication after medication, which amounts to nothing more than trial and error, until a cure is found. Intuition of the doctor also plays a role in diagnosis and treatment, but is becoming less and less common in modern medicine. The art of the diagnosis and treatment of disease is quickly becoming a lost art.

What we have is a knotted up and twisted health care system. Knots are tied by pharmaceutical companies, the professional organizations of doctors, insurance companies, governmental organizations, lawmakers, and unfortunately the doctor as well. With each passing day, yet a new knot is tied, transforming what used to be a simple system of health care into an unnecessarily complicated mess. Unfortunately, it is most often the patient who is tied up by all the knots.

The time has come to unravel the medical and health care knots. While this can be done with great ease, what makes it complicated is the innundation of propaganda from sources whose main goal is driven by corporate profit. What makes it even more complicated is the belief that the solution to every medical problem lie in either a pill, or a surgical procedure to cut out a particular body part that happens to be giving the patient a problem. Daniel J. Boorstin, an American historian, professor, attorney, and writer is quoted as saying "The greatest obstacle to discovery is not ignorance – it is the illusion of knowledge." If we apply his wisdom and approach the subject of health care with the proverbial blank sheet of paper or the clean slate, we are more likely to find the real answers to the questions that are of concern.

I have attempted to make this text understandable to both the reader with some medical knowledge and the reader with no medical knowledge. This method of presentation would provide the most benefit regarding the subject matter discussed. We just as easily could write a text that reads similarly to the following:

> The patient presents with mental fatigue accompanied with transient disorientation, anxiety, palpitations, anorexia, and irritability. For redirection of Qi energy, K-27, Shufu stimulation, should be considered. Adjunct phototherapy may prove beneficial. HPA dysfunction cannot be ruled out, clinical correlation is suggested. Lifestyle changes should accompany therapy for maximal benefit. Counseling may prove beneficial.

Taking this approach would result in a useless text for the general population, and would be just about as understandable as the Federal Tax Code. We could just as easily say that the patient is suffering from chronic depression, which is accompanied by several physical symptoms, and provide a few treatment suggestions and lifestyle changes. This is the approach I have decided to take. Certain instances, however, will arise where we must look at the inner workings of the body at a detailed level to gain a proper understanding of what is actually going on. The discussions of the immune system, meridians, and digestive system are such examples.

Ravi Zacharias, a noted theologian and philosopher, is the host of a radio show entitled "Let My People Think," the title suggesting a take off on the statement of Moses "Let my people go." The host of this show is one of the most brilliant philosophers of modern times. Rather than demanding that his students listen to him and believe and follow blindly, the host encourages intellectual thinking, reasoning, and analysis, thus encouraging the students to come to their own realization of the truth. This book is a prescription for just that type of thinking. It is not a list of foods to eat, activities to participate in, or supplements to take to achieve health. Optimal health requires more than just a specialized diet or taking a supplement. If we approach any health care problem with the intent of discovering how and why the problem began, we stand a much better chance of discovering the cure.

Nearly every healing method has a philosophy associated with it. The associated philosophy is passed on from one generation of healers to the next, but no one ever really stops to examine and question what is being passed on. Philosophical differences are responsible for the never-ending rift between conventional allopathic medicine and the natural healing methods. Any philosophy is up for revision when modern scientific advances offer new information. If philosophy is carved in stone, any advancement becomes difficult, if not impossible. Philosophy, which is found to conflict with tradition, will result in arguments using both the ego and emotion rather than sound principles. When philosophy is found to conflict with science, we have heresy. When opinion overrules sound philosophy, we have stupidity. Financial interests ruling over philosophy will result in a philosophy that is quickly transformed into dogma. Discard the philosophy altogether and anarchy follows. The purpose of philosophy is to prevent nonsense from entering any paradigm. This can only be accomplished if the philosophy is sound, adhered to, followed, and periodically examined and revised if necessary. Sound philosophy stands on its own foundation.

The diseases and syndromes discussed in this book have the common characteristic in that they originate from multiple causes. Additionally, the diseases discussed are primarily treated by the medical profession in a way that suppresses symptoms rather than treat the root cause. The goal of the illustrations presented is to encourage getting off the road of symptom suppression and onto the road of eliminating the real cause of the disease. Most important, however, is identifying the root causes and making sure the disease or problem does not happen again.

If I had to pass a book onto the next generation, it would be a book that would encourage everyone to understand their body and their relation to the environment in which they live. It would encourage health from natural perspective, a concept that appears entirely lost in today's society. The book would not be a list of dos and don'ts, or a book of rules, but would rather emphasize wellness and prevention. Should a health problem ever occur, solving the problem at the root level is the preferred path, not treating whatever is wrong by either eliminating or covering up symptoms. The improper application of medical knowledge and information that the current generation is using is what initially got this society in an unhealthy state. Propagate the misinformation to the next generation and the problems will only get worse. Instead, I would encourage a new way of thinking. This new way of thinking would incorporate both the valuable, older forgotten knowledge and the tried and true methods of healing which have been around for millennia, combined with any applicable modern scientific advances. The book would be of a philosophical basis, and, as a result, a foundational approach would be developed which would be applicable to the subject of health and wellness. Consideration would be given to the discussion of certain disease processes only to serve as examples to illustrate the application of a more realistic approach to health.

No attempt has been made to conform to the demands of the arena of political correctness. Political correctness changes from era to era, and is nothing more than verbal gymnastics applied in such a way of either using or avoiding certain terms associated with the presentation of sensitive subject matter. Political correctness, in the realm of medical care, is often seen in the labeling and naming of certain disorders. By labeling disorders, we then label people. For example, bipolar disorder, once called Manic-Depressive disorder, may be labeled as a mental disorder, psychological disturbance, psychological disorder, disorder of the mind, among many other terms. While all these terms are accurately reflecting the description of the disorder, whichever one is currently the politically correct term on any given date is anyone's guess.

Likewise, no attempt has been made to appease any certain group of the healing profession. Every healing profession has their defined scope of practice. Within the scope of practice, areas of patient care are found in which a particular profession may be regarded as clearly superior, and yet other areas in which the profession fails miserably. When a specific condition is treated, cured, and the patient resumes a normal life, the treatment offered, and the profession offering that treatment, falls into the superior category for that particular disease. If, however, the patient is treated year after year for the same disease, and the disease continues to worsen, the treatment offered is clearly inferior, and the profession offering that treatment clearly does not have the answer. Logic would dictate that if a condition is treated for many years, and is progressively getting worse, another treatment may be in order.

Why Am I Sick? And What To Do About It

Chapter 1
The Problem

Just what should a man or woman know in order to be "in the know" about health? Is there some inside information kept secret by some special elite, some special knowledge, or some secret formula that most health professionals either do not know or will not tell? If there is some special knowledge, where is it contained? If some secret formula exists, what is it, who has it, and how much does it cost? Can it even be bought?

With the arrival of advanced medical technology, society as a whole should be getting healthier. On the contrary, the overall health of the general population is declining. Advanced imaging techniques, billions of dollars of pharmaceutical research, new and improved medications, and advanced surgical procedures, all of which promise a healthier society, appear to have left the health of millions in ruins. In the wake of the modern medical paradigm failure, these millions are left on the never-ending path searching for the precious keys to health, striving to obtain the elusive keys that always seem just out of reach.

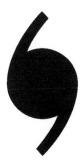

The standard-brand healing methods, whether it is traditional allopathic medicine (your medical doctor), chiropractic, psychology, acupuncture, massage, naturopathy, herbalists, reflexology, or homeopathy, are all traditionally sought when a health problem arises. The health problem is

Why Am I Sick? And What To Do About It

7

usually accompanied by some symptom, pain being the most common complaint. We are taught from a very early age that, when a symptom appears, whether it is pain, a runny nose, or anything that makes us feel uncomfortable, we are now sick. When we are sick, we visit the doctor, and we expect something to be given to us, either a prescription, a treatment, or some advice to eliminate the symptoms and make us feel better. In most disease processes, however, the symptom is the last thing to appear. The disease process has been going on for quite a long time, most likely on several levels, long before the first symptom even became evident. This puts the modern health care system in the position of operating in the realm of damage control, rather than in the prevention of disease. Rarely, if ever, does a patient enter the health care office saying "I am young, healthy and strong, teach me how to stay that way," or "do you offer any courses in wellness?" Should that scenario ever happen, the doctor would most likely think of it as quite odd, wondering why someone with no health complaint is in the office. The doctor would probably be thinking that the patient is playing a joke or something.

With some exceptions not too easily found, the health practitioner, who is supposed to be a well-versed expert in healing and health, is harboring his or her own unhealthy state. Secretly on his or her quest after hours for the same elusive path to health that everyone else is, the health practitioner can often be found searching the internet or medical journals for the solution to their own health problems. Their own notions of good health do not seem to fit in with what they learned in school, or with an environment that is changing so rapidly that much of what one learns today is either obsolete or completely contradicted tomorrow. The medical doctor, with years of education, medical training, and many hours of continuing education classes, has even murkier water to see through in his or her search for the truth. This water has been made murky by misinformation, bad philosophy, and the defective medical paradigm. If the learned medical professional has difficulty in finding the real answers, how much more difficult, then, is it for the nonprofessional?

With the arrival of the internet, enormous amounts of information are at everyone's fingertips. An enormous amount of incorrect and bad information is just as readily available. This is, in a way, very dangerous, enabling the public to diagnose disease through symptoms alone. With no objective or analytical evidence to support the diagnosis, the diagnosis is not very much more than a guess. If someone diagnoses him or herself wrong, they are now treating themselves for a disease that they do not have. In treating a disease that is not present, the treatment will likely cause a problem where originally no problem even existed. This method of treating disease is not much different from walking into a pharmacy and picking a random drug from the shelf and taking the pills found in the bottle. If this sounds scary, consider the fact that millions of people are doing this every day. Adding to this is the complication that everyone in cyberspace is touting a cure for this or that, and not a day goes by that some new promising cure arrives on the scene. As the promise of vibrant health usually goes, the secret magical cure often ends up being some special seed found only deep in the Amazon jungle. The miraculous seed is only made available to those who join the associated multi-level marketing program and go to the weekly cheerleading sessions. Even then, everyone must promise that they will tell all their friends and neighbors about the product.

The internet not only allows us the opportunity to diagnose, or possibly misdiagnose, our own diseases, but also to purchase pharmaceuticals from pharmacies in foreign countries, without a prescription, directly over the internet. Online pharmacies in foreign countries offer medications at greatly reduced prices, making the drugs attractive to persons who are either uninsured, or under insured. The safety of these drugs has been under question, with one controversy being whether the drugs are authentic or counterfeit. This, however, is only the tip of the iceberg. Drugs manufactured in foreign countries are also available for sale on the internet, many of which have not been subjected to any clinical trials or studies. These days, would anyone really feel safe taking an antibiotic manufactured in China? That name brand antibiotic purchased from Canada might just be a Chinese knock off counterfeited in a pill press bearing a famous name brand. When we go to this extreme desperately seeking the cure for a disease or a pill, backtracking might be wise to discover the true cause of the disease. When the true cause is found, health can be restored at the root cause level. Undertaking the search for the true cause of disease takes more time than the endless process of only treating symptoms, but in the end the reward will be much greater.

We must be aware of the fact that the disease process begins long before a symptom ever appears. In treating only symptoms, we are treating a disease from the wrong perspective. Should the symptom disappear because of the treatment, we think that all is well and that the disease has been cured. All we have done by treating the symptom, however, is to hide the disease, allowing further damage to occur undetected. When we stop treating the symptoms, the symptoms are thought to have somehow magically reappeared, and we think the disease has returned, or has "come out of remission," to use a popular medical phrase. The truth is that the disease was never cured in the first place. Tracing the disease process back to its origin, and discovering when and why the disease began, will reveal the appropriate treatment to reverse the course of the disease. When the root cause of the disease is finally identified and appropriately treated, the disease is then, and only then, truly healed. This is the only true way to restore health.

As if treating symptoms is not bad enough, worse yet is the notion that modern medical system is conspiring to keep everyone sick. And why not? In doing so, they create a captive market for their products and services, guaranteeing for themselves and others in the industry a large future profit. Of prime concern to upper level management is the business aspect of health care. Selling promising cures for disease occurs at huge profit margins, which is required to pay dividends to demanding stockholders and huge bonuses to corporate executives. And why stop there? The conspiracy theory would logically extend to selling products that actually cause a decline in health. The side effects, after effects, and problems caused by the treatment create a market for even more cures for the problems caused by the so-called cure. When profits drop, new disorders and diseases are invented, creating a new category of people who are now defined to be sick and therefore in need of treatment. Equally disturbing is that non-medical cures have been known for certain diseases for many years, but are largely ignored by the medical profession today. When an enormous cash flow is associated with a certain disease, such as cancer, little, if any, motivation can be found for finding a cure. While this seems absurd and unthinkable, in some cases it is not far from the truth.

In medicine, we are constantly trying to eliminate the possibility of medical mistakes. More powerful technology, more specific tests, better imaging techniques, increased efficiency of communication, and better safety precautions are all put in place so that no one can make a mistake. This, of course, requires more extensive documentation and greater coordination of care. Recent legislation regarding patient privacy, licensing board requirements, insurance company guidelines, and more complex procedures for maintaining and distribution of medical records creates administrative nightmares. The sheer amount of paper work involved in keeping the patient chart in order has seemingly become more important than what the chart actually contains. Evolution of the health care system has recently turned it into a complicated network of documentation, communication, and medical billing. As if that is not bad enough, two or three administrative employees are required for every doctor just to keep the paperwork moving. The patient chart is inspected closely by the doctor to make sure the forms are in proper order and double checked by the staff. Before the chart is filed and billed, it is rechecked in case of a future audit by an insurance company, the State Board of Examiners, or worse yet, an attorney bringing malpractice charges. In the mean time, no one has any clue what is wrong with the patient, but at least no administrative mistake was made and the documentation is in order.

The health care system has not only evolved into a tremendous communication machine, but has also evolved into a sophisticated conveyor belt for moving the patient from practitioner to practitioner, and from facility to facility. Any belief that the patient may have a condition that might be later construed as a possible malpractice issue will result in a referral issued to a specialty practitioner to shift the responsibility of care, and therefore liability, to someone else. The specialty practitioner is then assigned the responsibility of diagnosing some ill-defined condition, utilizing lab tests, imaging, and any other tests required to identify a disease that may or may not exist. Referrals are often made to avoid liability, and medical tests are often prescribed to avoid malpractice claims rather than for medical necessity. Tests and referrals often require insurance company approval, adding convoluted twists to both the medical documentation machine and the patient conveyor belt. The patient, trapped on the medical conveyor belt, has little or no chance of ever getting off. If nothing is wrong, the patient is allowed off temporally, and given a ticket to get back on the conveyor belt next year for a follow-up examination "just in case something may have changed." Unknown to the patient, however, is that the follow-up visit was probably scheduled for issues of liability or financial profit, and not medical necessity. With all this sophisticated technology to move both information and the patient around, the diagnosis, if any, arrives three months later than it would have if the simpler system of patient care used decades ago was still in operation.

During the process of solving existing problems with the newly developed technology, what we have done, in essence, have created newer, more complicated problems. Any new technology creates new problems that have never existed before the technology came into existence. The problem solvers must keep working harder and harder, faster and faster, just to stay afloat to remain ahead of the competition. Ironically, problems created by technology must be solved with even more technology. The new technology must be purchased, put into operation, and connected to other technology using wires and connections that require an engineer to understand. When the new technology is finally installed and running, it is already obsolete and must be replaced by even newer technology using the newest hardware and updated software. The question is, then, whether technological advances have actually made any progress at all. The medical field ends up spending disproportionately more time playing with the new and advanced technological toys, and disproportionately less time actually working with the patient. Taking an objective view, the project of conquering disease with all this new technology appears more and more of an impossibility, a mirage of sorts, in which technological innovations are a way to get to an unobtainable destination even faster. In other words, we have gotten nowhere very quickly, and have done it faster than we could have if we did not have the technology.

Even with all this new technology, the experience of the patient has not changed much since the last generation, and, if anything, this experience has gotten much worse. To the patient, it almost seems like the doctor speaks some foreign language, and what transpires during the five or ten minute office visit raises even more questions than were answered. Unimpressed by level of the examination performed, the patient is given either the name of a test that is supposed to find the problem, or a piece of paper with the name of some chemical that is supposed to cure the problem. Often, the patient also acquires some level of doubt during the office visit, primarily due to his or her perception that the doctor did not truly hear everything they had to say. The modern day office visit to the doctor is analogous to trying to see the world through a peep hole in a door, or through a slit in a fence. The patient often gets the feeling that if they can only get to the other side of the fence, or through some door, the big picture will become evident, and everything will become crystal clear. When everything becomes clear, the path to healing is then evident. Often, however, the reason the patient cannot get any clear and definitive answers from the doctor is because the doctor simply does not have any. When the patient does not get an answer from the doctor, they usually begin to search for the answers on their own, which usually involves exploring the possibility of any number of alternative treatments.

In the mean time, while the patient is on their own search for the answer, the doctor may have ordered even more tests to "rule out" a particular disease. To rule something out is a statistical and mathematical nightmare, and is literally the dead end street of diagnosis. A potential diagnosis is ruled out when little belief, if any, exists in the possibility that the proposed diagnosis is even remotely correct. This is why the particular disease is being ruled out, and not being ruled in. The process of ruling out disease after disease leaves both the doctor and the patient with a list of diseases that the patient does not have. Even the casual observer will find little value in a list of diseases that the patient does not have. Obtaining the correct diagnosis by the procedure of ruling out is literally hoping to stumble upon the right answer. This can best be illustrated by example. Imagine that a child, who has never been to the beach, finds a sea shell and brings it to their parent and asks what it is. The parent replies, without even looking at the sea shell, "it is not a tomato." The child asks again what it is. With their eyes closed and soaking up the sun, the parent replies "it is probably not a rock." Yet again, the child asks what it is. Remembering last Christmas, the parent replies, "it is not the Roto-Annihilator toy that you lost," to which the child responds "duh." So then, it is not a rock, it is not a tomato, it is not Roto-Annihilator, and so on. One by one, every possibility is ruled out. The processing of ruling something out in conjunction with little or no analysis gets us nowhere very quickly. By using this method, we have tremendous amounts of evidence proving what diseases the patient does not have, yet still have no evidence at all of what disease the patient does have. This exploration of dead ends is exactly what happens all too often in medicine. If the medical doctor has a good idea about what the problem is, they rule something in. If, on the other hand, they have no clue about what the problem is, they start the process of ruling out. It does not take a genius to figure out that time and energy put into finding the problem is more valuable than attempting to discover what is not the problem. When the medical doctor starts ruling out diseases, the doctor should be ruled out and a new doctor should be found.

Confusing matters further are the controversial diagnostic methods and treatments offered by doctors in foreign countries. In industrialized countries, modern medicine dismisses these treatment protocols as quackery without even having an understanding of them, or because the proponents of the treatment do not have the newest and latest technology. Regarding these controversies, a basic rule of modern day society generally applies. This rule is, that for every controversy, two diametrically opposing views will be discovered. These two views can be always reduced to two reasons surrounding the controversy, the real reason and the stated reason. The stated reason is always what will calm the public. Following the money trail, one will always arrive at the real reason. This principle also applies to the attitude of modern medicine regarding any alternative form of health care. The real reason these treatments and forms of health care are dismissed can be found by examining the money trail. Specifically, the shifting of the health care dollar from mainstream medicine to alternative forms of treatment is the real concern of the medical doctors and pharmaceutical companies. This concern primarily involves money, specifically money being spent somewhere other than the services and products offered by the medical profession. Any group with a financial interest in this monetary shift resorts to hiring lobbyists to strong arm legislation supporting their cause. Behind the scenes, they secretly distribute literature and warnings about the alternative treatment, exposing the so-called threat to the patient's health, and reassuring the public that modern medicine is the only proven and effective method of treating the problem. The real concern of the modern medical machine is money, not the controversial treatment. One does not have to look very far to see this mechanism in action. One must also consider the fact that if the so called controversial treatment did not work, why would anyone spend money and time to fight it. Conversely, if a product or alternative form of treatment is found beneficial in the treatment of disease, some organization will attempt to control and regulate it. Modern medicine has a solid track record of attempting to dim the light on every alternative healing method that comes along with a promise of a cure.

The attack of modern medicine on alternative forms of healing can be best illustrated by the continued policy of the American Medical Association (AMA) of attempting to contain and eliminate the chiropractic profession. In a lawsuit filed in 1976, *Wilk v. American Medical Association*, the AMA was alleged to be in violation of the Sherman Anti Trust Act; an injunction was therefore sought barring the AMA from harassing the chiropractic profession. Claiming that associating with chiropractors was unethical for medical doctors, and labeling chiropractic as "an unscientific cult," the AMA was, in 1983, found to have violated the Sherman Act. This issue has been revisited by appeal after appeal, extending into the 1990s. U.S. District Court Judge Susan Getzendanner concluded that the AMA had actively engaged in a "lengthy, systematic, successful and unlawful boycott" of the chiropractic profession. The results of this systematic boycott can still be seen today, primarily evidenced by the continued lack of cooperation between medical doctors and chiropractors. Unfortunately, this lack of cooperation of the medical profession is not limited to only chiropractic, but extends to other branches of the healing arts as well. In the end, it is always the patient who ends up suffering due to this ridiculous turf war between the medical profession and other branches of the healing arts.

The modern medical doctor then, armed with voluminous information about new medications and drugs from the most recent continuing education seminar sponsored by the pharmaceutical companies, has almost no knowledge regarding any alternative treatments. Because of this lack of knowledge, he or she may be quick to dismiss any alternative treatments as "risky," "dangerous," or "unproven." The same list of buzz words somehow shows up repeatedly, and their use is about as predictable as the sunrise whenever some form of alternative treatment is suggested by the patient. It almost appears as if this list of buzz words is circulated through literature and educational material presented to the doctor. This suggests evidence of a propaganda war, and, in a game of this sort, the most aggressive and vocal propagandist is usually the winner. The propaganda war is never limited to those activities that occur in private and at the medical office. An increased presence of pharmaceutical advertisements can be found in alternative health magazines, trying to lure back patients who are on the quest for real answers to health outside the medical arena. None of this propaganda, however, ever seems to stop the patient from seeking alternative care.

Following the long dissertation delivered by the medical doctor to the patient regarding alternative therapies, the infamous words "Let's go ahead and try this" usually ends the conversation. This is perhaps the biggest red flag in medicine, and is actually worse than the protocol of ruling out specific diseases. Health care should not be delivered using a trial and error methodology. Trying something, just to see if it works, suggests a very low confidence level in the treatment. This trial and error methodology is also suggestive of the possibility that the doctor has no clue about what the problem actually is. The suggestion made to the patient of trying something does nothing more than give the doctor more time in hoping to discover what the real problem is. The fact that something is at least being tried is supposed to give the patient the comfort that something is being done to solve the health problem. One undisputable fact, however, is often overlooked; to deliver the proper treatment, it must first be known exactly what is being treated. This is simply common sense, and is a nonnegotiable requirement of the treatment of disease. Randomly prescribing medication in order to find the one that best suppresses the symptoms actually borderlines upon stupidity. We cannot simply rely upon luck or a Magic 8 Ball when treating disease.

The notion that health can be restored or every disease can be cured by ingesting chemical compounds manufactured in a chemistry lab is actually quite absurd. To believe that chemicals can cure a disease requires us also to believe that the reason the disease was allowed to occur in the first place is because of a deficiency in the body of some manufactured chemical. That notion is equally absurd, and is nothing more than ad ridiculum. This absurd principle of a chemical cure is most evident in healing a disease, particularly a chronic disease, or a "syndrome," in which no specifically identifiable cause is known. The healing of a chronic disease or syndrome cannot simply be reduced to a chemical formula. In addition, if the cause of the disease or syndrome cannot be identified, how can the cure be known? What really happens is, in most cases, multiple factors contribute to any chronic disease process. Rather than address each individual issue of the disease at the root cause level, a chemical is prescribed to give the illusion that the disease is being cured. The illusion eventually, over time, becomes a very expensive illusion. Equally expensive, but much more practical, would be to take the time with a practitioner willing to treat the problem at the root cause. Unraveling the cause of a disease at the level at which it originated and subsequently treating it at that level is very time consuming, but, in the end, well worth the effort. The practice of treating only the symptoms will only allow a further unhealthy state to develop, making the real problems even more difficult, and therefore more expensive, to solve in the future.

When a doctor, professor, or researcher comes along and looks at a particular problem from a holistic viewpoint and suggests a more natural route, they are quickly labeled as some sort of Natural Hygiene Oriented Biological Theologian who advocates gathering berries, nuts, and leaves for food. Quack monitoring groups put the practitioner or the methodology used by the practitioner on the hit list, and the propaganda machine goes into high gear to discredit both the messenger and the message. If any substantial truth to the methods is found, particularly if they pose a financial threat to the practice of mainstream medicine, attorneys get involved to suppress the voice of the messenger through threats and lawsuits. Interestingly, the advice given by the natural health care provider has already been proven or eventually will be proven by the very science used to condemn the methodology in question. The problem is that doctors leading quack monitoring groups, propaganda moguls, and attorneys representing the financial powers of the world of medicine do not read the modern medical journals. All the information needed to support the natural health practitioner's message can typically already be found in research published in these peer-reviewed journals, much of it written by researchers in the medical field.

Within health care, clear evidence exists regarding the serious competition for the health care dollar. This competition leads to conflicting opinions offered by health care professionals regarding the appropriate course of action for any particular disease. With every specialty within the healing profession claiming to have the answer, the patients often find themselves in the dark about what the problem really is and what the appropriate treatment should be. In any given situation, examining the track record of the profession in question regarding their treatment of a particular disease or condition is a worthwhile exercise. If the practitioner has nothing more to offer than to relieve symptoms or "maintain the disease," it is perhaps worthwhile to continue searching for the real answers leading to the real cure. If a practitioner has a track record of properly diagnosing the issue at hand, able to explain to the patient what the problem is, has a clear treatment plan, and, most of all, has had success with similar cases, confidence in that practitioner is well justified.

The competition for the health care dollar does not end at the practitioners office. Money flows into research organizations in search of some cure for a disease, and, just as with an investment in the stock market, a certain financial rate of return is expected. Advertising, specifically targeting the emotions, goes into high gear, searching for more potential patients to convert corporate red ink into black ink. Advertising of this type usually addresses those disorders having a highly emotional component. Those suffering from depression, bipolar disorder, genital herpes, excessive weight, eczema, hair loss, and pain are all targeted by the advertising campaign in the search for more patients. This is because these issues, clearly having an emotional component associated with them, also have patients who are seeking in desperation for an answer to their health problem. The distressed patient is more willing to listen to anyone who offers any shred of hope. Furthermore, advertising of this type is usually directed toward those disorders that are subjectively diagnosed, for example depression or bipolar disorder. This often leads to self-diagnosis of the patient's condition. Convinced of having a certain disorder, the patient enters the doctor's office, and walks out with a prescription for a disorder they most likely do not have. Advertising, however, is rarely, if ever, directed toward any disorder that is either diagnosed objectively or does not have an emotional component. Advertisements cannot simply be found targeting patients suffering from Myositis ossificans, Hand-Schuller-Christian syndrome or a phosphofructokinase deficiency.

Albert Einstein is quoted as saying "If we knew what it was we were doing, it would not be called research, would it?" Yet, the medical profession relies upon research to solve every health problem that arises. Examination of medical research, however, often reveals conflicting conclusions regarding an identical hypothesis. For example, one researcher comes to the conclusion that drinking coffee poses a greater risk in contracting a *Helicobacter pylori* infection, and consuming alcohol offers protection against contracting a *Helicobacter pylori* infection. Another researcher, attempting to validate the claims of the first researcher, finds no correlation whatever between alcohol, coffee, and *Helicobacter pylori*. In using the same research methods, both researchers arrive at differing conclusions regarding such a simple issue. At the same time, the old true and tried methods of healing are quickly disposed of due to the purported lack of research proving their efficacy. So, in the twenty first century, it is demanded that we prove acupuncture works, prove the existence of meridians, prove herbs have healing power, prove energy medicine works, prove chiropractic works, prove prayer heals, and even prove that God exists. Modern allopathic medicine has a vague rule and understanding that if no proof exists, then it cannot possibly work. This places everyone who believes and uses these older forms of healing methods in a defensive position by the very researchers of modern medicine who do not know what they, themselves, are doing. Nevertheless, both the doctors who employ the older or natural methods of healing and the patients who use them do not care about this so-called modern research. They know the method they have chosen works, they use it, and, as a result, the patients condition ultimately resolves.

It is exceedingly conceited to believe that God has placed man on the face of the Earth for thousands of years, and, finally, in the latter half of the twentieth century, decided to give man the tools needed to heal the body, and furthermore, limited these tools to only the industrialized nations of the world. The tools have been here on Earth all along, and they are not necessarily found in a hospital, research facility, or some highly technological electronics laboratory somewhere. While the modern tools are valuable in diagnosing certain disorders, they have little real value in long term restoration of health. Restoration of health is most often not dependent on using the latest technology.

To many people, the thought of contracting incurable diseases and permanent conditions is deeply disturbing to contemplate. For one thing, the manifestation of a serious health condition seems unfair, people who have done nothing to deserve it are afflicted while others are seemingly not. Both people fasted, ate properly, prayed, practiced yoga, exercised, rested, did good deeds, went to Church, yet one contracts some syndrome causing a complete disruption of life, and the other is living a life of pure joy and happiness. It seems altogether way too easy when the cure for the problem simply comes along either in the form of a pill or a specialized diet. The pill, more often than never, ends up being nothing more than a cruel illusion. The specialized diet, which appears to be promising at the outset, ends up being nothing more than a mirage. Insight into the true cure can only occur after the medical view regarding the physical representation of a person as a series of biochemical processes is discarded, and replaced with a philosophy to reflect the physical, mental and spiritual aspects of the whole person. When this new philosophy is understood, hope is then, and only then, restored.

A growing apprehension exists, which is becoming increasingly evident, that stressful human existence is contributing to the decline in overall health. In most households, two wage earners are now needed to make the monthly budget balance. The teenagers always seem to need the latest electronic toy, and for a very good reason, because their friends have one. When the toy breaks, no one wants to call the toll-free customer service number for fear of being connected to a customer service representative in India. The daycare center seems to take half your paycheck, and in return your child gets bitten by another child in preschool, brings home yet another ear infection, or breaks an arm during recess. Within the business world, serious competition exists regarding who is going to occupy the top of the corporate ladder. The executive at the top demands 110 percent from each and every employee and will expect nothing less. Keep in mind, no one can give more than 100 percent, that extra 10 percent will eventually manifest itself as disease of the body. All this is for, as a famous singer put it, the struggle for the legal tender. All this seems seriously futile, and yet, when one thinks about it, it appears to be quite odd. For a person to mortgage their personal health to gain the latest model automobile or newest electronic gizmo that will eventually break anyway is simply not worth it.

Chronic stress is becoming more evident in today's society. This is, in part, due to the time pressure exerted on us as a society to be somewhere at a certain time, and at another place shortly afterwards. It appears as if the pressure of planning a schedule down to the microsecond level has become the norm of today's society. If that is not stressful enough, multitasking is introduced to squeeze 25 hours somehow out of the 24 available each day. This is analogous to a plane flying 750 miles per hour at an altitude of 100 feet, trying to navigate through a maze of 110 foot rocks. Nerves are unraveled when we sit in rush hour traffic, or when an unexpected long line at the grocery store delays the next stop on the list of errands to run. As anxiety levels raise, we think that if we can only get to that next destination on the list, all will be well. The same high stress level is inevitably found in that situation or event, just as was found in the previous one. We then find ourselves again just wanting to move to the next scheduled event, as if that will make anything better. When someone is late to the next event because they had a flat tire, everyone looks at them as if they should have foreseen the flat tire and factored that into their schedule. At the end of the day, the dreaded phone call comes adding another thing to tomorrow's already full schedule. This anxiety about the current situation, and just wanting to move on to the next situation to escape from the stress of the current one, is a good indicator of chronic stress.

Stress is not limited to the activities of daily life. Oddly, the very system that we rely upon to cure disease quite often actually causes disease. One way disease is caused is through the stress introduced by the modern medical experience. This is evident in the fact that in the modern medical office visit, the patient is examined, poked, prodded, and stuck in scanning tubes by a bunch of intellectual porcupines, and then often has to wait weeks for any test results. Apart from the fact that the test results are usually available in a day or two, the patient is often unable to get in contact with the very busy doctor to get the report. Test results often lead to follow-up tests being conducted, and in the mean time, the patient cannot seem to get even the simplest of questions answered. When making a call to the doctor's office, the patient is again reminded how busy the doctor is, and the return call always comes when the patient is in the shower. The waiting game and list of unanswered questions cause stress to the patient, and justifiably so. This stress, in itself, can lead to any number of diseases. Finally, after months of tests, the doctor notices that the patient may have some anxiety, and prescribes a pill to calm the patient down. Everyone, except the patient, is oblivious to the fact that the patient's anxiety was caused by the modus operandi of the medical care system. The anxiety and stress end up causing a disease, such as an ulcer, that would not have occurred if it were not for the way in which the health care system operates.

Health and sickness quite predictably follow periodic seasonal patterns. The great yearly downturn in health begins on October 31, but is not readily apparent until a few months later. To kick off the annual down slide of health, all the kids dress up in costumes and go house to house knocking on every door in hopes of bagging the coveted treasure – candy. For the next two weeks, sugar enters their body like a tsunami, paving the way for a *Candida albicans* yeast overgrowth in the intestines, and creating blood sugar swings that resemble an EKG. This results in mood swings and crankiness, and the parents give in by giving the kids even more candy just to quiet them down. Unknowingly to the kids, the parents sneak some of their candy while they are away in school, desperately trying to reduce the private stash so the kids will not gorge themselves on something that is so unhealthy. Then comes the big feast on the fourth Thursday in November. In preparation for the festivities revolving around the large meal, the hosts make their guest lists, buy all sorts of food – vegetables, bread, pies, cakes, wine, and the twenty two pound bird that will be the centerpiece of the celebration. When dinnertime finally arrives, the whole home is filled with more stress than a bad day on Wall Street. The kids are cranky, the wrong team won the big football game, and the one relative with more than one screw lose somehow showed up at dinner anyway despite many desperate attempts to leave him off the guest list, quite by accident of course. For the next few days, the menu is the same, with the words "turkey again" seeming to echo around the house. All the desserts that were left over seem to have disappeared first, and everyone is frantically searching around for something to satisfy their sugar craving. In keeping perfect tradition, the stress level rises higher than Mount Everest as the events turn from eating to shopping. Panic arises as everyone wants to be the first in line to get this year's coveted new toy, Roto-Annihilator, an ugly piece of molded plastic with its head mounted on a turret, a remote control, a computer inside, imported directly from China. With any luck, junior is really not interested in that toy this year and hopefully spare anyone from having to wait in lines or searching the internet to find one. The shopping spree continues for four more weeks, with stress levels rising each day. In anticipation of the next great celebration at the end of December, choir practice for the Christmas caroling adventure is mandatory, never mind the fact that everyone has sung these songs their entire life, and knows them quite well by now. To make things worse, the kids are let out of school as the parents are trying to arrange dinner plans for the big event. Every spare moment is used frantically to find that Roto-Annihilator contraption from China because, at the last minute, junior decided he needed one because Johnny down the street is getting one. Checking every store, Roto-Annihilator cannot be found anywhere, and the Korean knock off, Roto-Flunkkor, simply will not do. After returning from church on Christmas Eve, the parents try to get the kids to sleep, which finally happens at 2:00 A.M., and two hours later the parents finally get to sleep. The kids are then up at 5:30 A.M., tearing open boxes and packages, many of which were wrapped only three hours earlier. Within no time, the living room looks like a dump truck backed up and dropped a load meant for the local toy store. A little time later, the remote control toy aircraft somehow flew itself around inside and shredded everything in sight, including the furniture. No one seems

Why Am I Sick? And What To Do About It

to know how the plane could fly by itself, primarily because no one was around when it happened. Right before the crash landing, the plane's propeller chopped the head off that stupid Roto-Annihilator thing, which, in the future, will prove to be a blessing. The parents try to restore order and clean up the home so it looks presentable when the guests arrive, shoving presents back under the tree and in the corner. As usual, the relative with more than one screw loose arrives late, opens his presents, and wonders why, yet again, he got four brand-new screwdriver sets. For the next week, the kids are off from school, and everyone's emotions are running in high gear. Finally, New Years Eve gets here, and in a day or so everything will be back to normal. The adults all go out and get drunk in order to forget about the last three months, only to repeat the same thing next year. Finally, some semblance order seems to be restored when the holiday season is finally over.

However, that is not the end. For the last three months, everyone has been stressed, and the immune system was being compromised and is now most likely functioning at its yearly low. All the refined carbohydrates, desserts, and foods served during the holiday season, which are not typically served during the rest of the year, has taken their toll on the digestive system and immune system, not to mention the mind. As a result, colds, the flu, and other seasonal maladies seem to run rampant, being passed from person to person. Just as one person in the family gets over it, another one gets something else and passes it around. Nevertheless, soon Spring is on its way, and everyone will begin to feel better. Since Spring is bathing suit time, it is time for everyone to go on a diet, and lose those extra pounds gained over the holiday season. The newly discovered diet and a desperate attempt to lose some weight now put the body into a nutritional deficit mode, and everything eaten turns to fat. Severe lack of energy follows, and what looked to be a promising new year starts off as a disaster.

A type of individual, however, can be found that rarely, if ever, gets sick. Oddly, this type of person also rarely, if ever, seeks the advice of any health care professional. How could excellent health be afforded to this group of people considering the fact they are not even searching for it? What are they doing that the majority of society is not? Equally important, what are they not doing that the majority is constantly doing? Do they have a secret? If so, what is their secret? Why are they not sharing it with others? If we can somehow learn their secret, and apply those principles to our life, will it make us healthier too?

Is there, then, some kind of inner scoop on this astounding and annoyingly complicated thing we call the health care system? Is there some hidden scheme not portrayed to the public, something that never really gets out through the normal channels of communication? We do not hear the truth that is right before us because our modern day civilization does not actively and openly communicate the truth. We do not understand the truth because, in many instances, we have been programed to believe a lie instead. These lies not only contradict the truth in every way imaginable, but those who invented the lie are actively engaged in suppressing the truth as well. This makes the lie subversive, in the sense that it takes a normal course of conservative action, turns it upside down, inside out, complicates it, uses convoluted logic to make it believable, and sells it at a price beyond what anyone can reasonably pay. In a sense, then, what we end up with is a twenty thousand–dollar solution to a fifty–dollar problem. What, then, is this truth hidden from society, and where can it be found? Whom has the truth, and how do we find them?

The truth most can often be found outside the traditional medical system. The inner revolution against the standard health care paradigm has never been undertaken by a society as a whole. If anyone seriously suggests the idea of a health care paradigm change, they will obtain enormous moral support, but very few true followers. Society, though, programs us to play a game of follow the leader, health care being no exception to the rule. Any opposing message will quickly be squelched and various attempts will be made to alienate the messenger. This inner revolution, therefore, has been confined primarily to independently thinking individuals who have lost faith in the medical system, and have undertaken the task themselves. The ones who leap out in the search for the truth will always find it. Eventually, the search will lead the seeker to the inner revolutionaries of the alternative health care system. These are the natural health care providers who practice under various divisions of the health care system. Find the right practitioner, and the true path to health restoration and wellness can be found.

When an inner revolutionary of the health care system is found, the message is always the same. The messenger is often found to have either authored a book, market a line of products that address specific health conditions, offer seminars on finding the path to true health, or operate a practice in which the patients have the same chronic issues the doctor once had. Most often, however, the practitioner is one who has never believed in the modern medical paradigm, but instead has always trusted and believed in the alternative methods that they employ. The message offered by the health care revolutionary is short and clear, *come to the door and escape with me*, which is the offer of the natural health care provider given to the patient to escape from the medical system, get healthy, and start living again. This message has only two requirements. The first requirement is that the patient must to come to the door. The second requirement is to take the offer to escape. Just what, exactly, are we escaping from? What we are escaping from is this nonsense paradigm of a so-called health care system in which pills are incessantly prescribed, and, when no more pills can be found to cover up the symptoms, body parts are extracted one by one, often leaving the patient in even worse shape than if nothing was done at all. The offer to *escape with me* implies that the practitioner has already escaped from the traditional system of medicine proven, in most cases, to be a dismal failure. The choices are very simple, either restore health through natural means, or stay on the path that leads to more serious disease.

Wisdom, then, suggests finding a natural health practitioner as a guide in the quest to correct any health issues that may be present, and is highly advisable for everyone attempting to restore his or her own health. A natural health care provider or holistic doctor has a true understanding about the causes of disease and true cure for disease, and does not quickly reach for the prescription pad to write the name of some pill just to get the patient out of the office. When searching for a natural health practitioner, checking out their credentials is advisable. The doctor should have graduated from an accredited school, passed a board examination, and be licensed to practice. The doctor should be able to prescribe pertinent laboratory tests, or refer the patient to a facility or other health care provider that can run specialized tests if needed. Keep in mind that licensure regulations and scope of practice laws vary from state to state, requiring referral to the appropriate practitioner who will then order the appropriate tests or procedures. Most of all, the practitioner should have a solid track record of success in treating the condition for which care is sought. When such a practitioner is found, they will serve as an invaluable guide on the path to health.

When the patient seeks health care, whether it is through the services offered by a holistic doctor, natural health practitioner, chiropractor, or other practitioner, they naturally expect to get well. Holistic health care practitioners take a different approach than the typical medical doctor in the sense that they will address health from a broad perspective, not only write a prescription and send the patient on their way. When under the care of a natural health or holistic health practitioner, following their advice is imperative. This includes all the advice offered, not only the advice that is convenient, fits into the schedule, or is easy to follow. This is especially important in the reversal of any chronic disease process. To reverse a chronic disease process, certain changes in lifestyle and diet are mandatory. Other aspects of a person's lifestyle may have to be changed as well, and this will vary from person to person. For example, two separate patients suffering with fibromyalgia may be given completely different dietary protocols to follow by the same health practitioner. The difference in the prescribed dietary protocols is based upon the biochemical individuality of each patient. Specifically, since the biochemistry of each individual is subtly different, the health practitioner is addressing these differences in various way to restore specific facets of each patient's health. Lifestyle changes will most likely be recommended, and is also based upon each individual patient's current activities. One patient may be told to exercise, and yet another patient may be told not to exercise at all for a few weeks. With so many variables making up the infinite facets of each individual, it is therefore reasonable to assume that the treatment for a particular disease will vary from person to person.

Two types of care can be found within the health care system. These types are passive care and active care. Passive care includes those activities or procedures done which require little or no effort on the part of the patient. Examples of passive care include taking a pill, getting a chiropractic adjustment, acupuncture, and massage therapy. Active care, on the other hand, involves physical or mental participation of the patient. Physical therapy, exercise, stretching, change in diet, and certain lifestyle changes are some examples of active care. Active care cannot be done for the patient. The patient must do any and all active care activities for themselves. Any treatment program addressing chronic disorders must involve both active care and passive care. Modern medicine primarily offers passive care, requiring virtually no effort of any sort on the part of the patient. Unfortunately, virtually no results are ever obtained with the exclusive use of passive care either. Other types of programs, such as programs that claim exercise is all that is required to restore health, are purely active care. While exercise has many benefits, under certain circumstances, exercise can cause certain conditions to worsen. The holistic approach, however, will have a balance between passive care and active care. When working with a holistic health provider, the balance between active care and passive care will most likely change from month to month, reflecting the progress of the patient.

When a patient seeks the services of the natural or alternative health care professional, the experience will be quite different from the typical trip to the medical doctor. This is because the alternative practitioner does not subscribe to the basic philosophy of modern medicine as practiced in today's society. The holistic doctor will not be interested about every ache and pain, for they are only symptoms of another disorder that must be corrected. The natural health care provider, while documenting any symptoms that may exist, will generally not treat any of the symptoms directly. What the holistic doctor will be interested in, however, is restoring the complete health of the patient, and in doing so, any symptoms associated with the disease process will ultimately be resolved. This is done in many ways. Since patients are individuals, an individualistic approach will be taken.

It is quite sad when someone finds out too late that something could have been done earlier to restore their health. Years of accumulated damage, years of pain, and years of lost enjoyment could have been averted if only the right information or the right health care practitioner were found earlier. One consistent observation is that if nothing is done to reverse the course of a disease process, the patient will get sicker and sicker with each passing year. With the proper information and guidance, however, restoring health can actually be accomplished quite easily. The primary two factors involved are knowledge and determination. The appropriate knowledge must be applied under the proper circumstances in order to produce the desired result. This is the job of the doctor. The determination to apply the advice offered by the doctor is the job of the patient. The doctor-patient team who accomplishes both will obtain positive results. One highly kept secret in health care is that the doctor's favorite patients are those who are enthusiastic and excited about reaching the goal of true health. Reversal of chronic disease, however, takes time, therefore patience is of the utmost importance.

We are in urgent need of a roadmap leading to true health. This roadmap would give us a better understanding of our own existence, how our body works, and our relation to the environment in which we live. The approach and resulting methodologies would be in accord with the physical facts of sound biological knowledge, overcoming any societal programming that initially got us, as a society, in an unhealthy condition. The roadmap would not be a medical text in the usual sense, but it would discuss many things with which various health care paradigms have been concerned. Most important, the roadmap would have to be understandable to the layman, not just the medical professional.

Why Am I Sick? And What To Do About It

All entrance forms in medical offices have a section that states "In case of emergency contact _____." One very astute patient entered 911 onto the form. We certainly can't argue with that, now can we?

Chapter 2
What is Health Anyway?

Before we discuss illness or the cause of an illness, it would be desirable to first look at health, and discover what normal, or ideal health really is. In discovering what health is, we also discover what illness and compromised health really are.

Pick up any dictionary and look up the word health, and a definition similar to the following will undoubtably appear:

Health n. 1: the condition of being sound in body or mind; *especially* freedom from physical disease or pain. 2: Soundness, *especially* of body or mind; freedom from disease or abnormality.

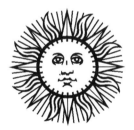

On the surface, the dictionary definition may sound like a reasonably good definition of health. Freedom from disease and soundness of body and mind fits quite well with what we were all taught about health. When examined closely, however, the dictionary definition gives us an inadequate picture of what health really is. Pain, for example, is a very poor indicator of health. Consider the fact that liver cancer, ovarian cancer, or pancreatic cancer all produce no pain or other discernable symptoms until the disease process has progressed to the terminal state. Physical disease is often referenced in the definition of health, again reflecting the belief that the physical body contains all the indicators of true health.

Why Am I Sick? And What To Do About It

25

Reference to a sound mind is usually included in the definition, but almost sounds like an afterthought. The field of psychoneuroimmunology tells us that our thought processes are very strongly linked to the condition of our physical body, specifically our immune system. The mind, therefore, must be included in a proper definition of health. No mention at all is made of the spirit in the definition, perhaps because in today's society any mention of the spirit has religious overtones and is therefore taboo to discuss because someone might get offended. So, the first thing that has to be tossed aside is the dictionary definition of health.

The medical definition of health is commonly cited as:

> *Health is an organism's ability to efficiently respond to challenges (stressors) and effectively restore and sustain a "state of balance," known as homeostasis.*

The medical definition of health clearly addresses the physical body only. This is evidenced primarily by the use of the term homeostasis, which is a term that applies to the physical world, and is a principle of chemistry and physics. The medical definition does not take into consideration either the mind or the spirit. This omission is not surprising at all, since the modern medicine primarily treats disease from the perspective of the physical body only. Furthermore, any mentally related illnesses, such as depression or schizophrenia, are not addressed by this definition. By not including the mind in the definition we in essence say that the schizophrenic patient in the hospital who is taking antipsychotic medications is in good health. Furthermore, we can also say that since the antipsychotic medication is disrupting the schizophrenic's normal homeostasis, and it should therefore not be prescribed. Homeostasis is more applicable to the ideal gas law learned in chemistry class, $pV=nRT$, than it is to health. While homeostasis may be a factor to be considered in health, it is not the final and determining factor. Health cannot simply be reduced to homeostasis.

An very odd and interesting quirk exists in the medical definition of health that is not readily obvious. If a vitamin deficiency occurs, say for example Vitamin C, a person will typically scrounge around for food to eat, which is a natural activity. By eating some citrus fruit, the vitamin deficiency will be satisfied and homeostasis will then be restored. Searching for food and eating it is therefore defined as part of the organism's method to maintain homeostasis. This satisfies the medical definition of health in the sense that homeostasis was restored and the biochemical stress that resulted from the lack of Vitamin C was removed. If a person, however, becomes addicted to a drug, for example heroin or morphine, biochemical changes occur in the body that modify homeostasis. The presence of the drug over time creates a new homeostasis in which the presence of the drug is required to sustain this new homeostasis. Withdrawal from the drug disrupts this homeostasis. The medical definition demands that homeostasis be restored following a challenge, the challenge, in this case, being drug withdrawal. Administering the drug then restores homeostasis. We must conclude, therefore, that drug addiction is within the realm of the medical definition of health.

Since this notion of health being related to purely homeostasis is absurd, the medical definition of health must be dismissed, and tossed aside with the dictionary definition. Oddly, the dictionary definition of health, by including the mind in the definition, is actually better than the medical definition. Health cannot be reduced to simply biochemical homeostasis. This, in itself, is sufficient reason to dismiss the medical definition of health.

The World Health Organization has developed their own definition of health, The World Health Organizations's definition is

> *Health is a state of complete physical, mental and social well-being and not merely the absence of disease or infirmity.*

The World Health Organization's definition of health gives hearty approval to the idea that there is more to health than just the absence of disease. Bringing the concept of well-being beyond that of the physical body and mind, the social aspect of a person's life is introduced as a facet of health. While this might be a little better than the dictionary definition, the World Health Organization's definition fails to address the spiritual aspect of the complete person. The omission of the spiritual aspect of the person may be again as result the fear of approaching a taboo subject, or perhaps to keep in line with political correctness. The World Health Organization's definition of health, therefore, has earned a place with both the dictionary definition and the medical definition of health.

Health, then, needs a definition that encompasses the whole person, not only the physical body, but the mind and spirit as well. An appropriate definition of health would also include that person's relation to not only their social environment, but physical environment as well. When we speak of the whole person, we refer to the physical body, the mind, and the spirit. Our better definition of health, which takes into account all aspects of the person and their surroundings, is found in these words:

> *Health is the perfect harmony of the whole person in body, mind, and spirit, and perfect harmony of that person with respect to their social and physical environment.*

Health, therefore, is attained when harmony is attained in all aspects of an individual's life. Health, then, requires that the body and mind are in harmony, the spirit and mind are in harmony, and the spirit and body, as well, are in harmony with each other. In short, no inner conflict must be found in the person's life. Harmony must also be extended to the persons social environment, in other words, the relationship of the person to other people, whether they are significant others or just mere acquaintances. Harmony with the physical environment must be considered as well, since this is where the vital nutrients that sustain life all originate. Health, then, is an indicator of the state of the body, mind, and spirit.

If health is a harmonious state of the whole person, anything done to disrupt this harmonious state is detrimental to health. The degree of this disruption determines the extent to which the health of the individual will be affected. An unhealthy state is not confined to only the physical body, but always extends to both the mind and spirit as well. How, then, does an unhealthy state of either the body, the mind, or the spirit begin? In reference to the whole person, unhealthy state of the body occurs for one or more of three specific reasons. The three reasons are the same whether we are talking about disease entering from either the body, mind, or spirit. These three reasons, as applied to the physical body, are:

1. *Something enters into the body that should not be in the body,*

2. *Something that should be in the body is not in the body,*

3. *Something enters into the body, but, for some reason, the body can no longer process it correctly.*

The same three statements also hold true regarding the health of both the mind and spirit as well. Therefore, in the three reasons above, remembering the word body in the above reasons refers to the physical body is important. These three reasons also are in harmony with our definition of health. These reasons illustrate what should and should not be allowed to happen to the body to maintain health.

Applying the three principles to mental health also gives us an insight into how an illness affecting the mind may begin. An illness affecting the mind is often purely subjective, with little or no objective evidence, such as laboratory tests, supporting the diagnosis. Depression is one example of an illness of this type. In the case where depression has a social, or non-organic cause, the depression had to have begun as a result of one or more of the three principles. By replacing the word *body* with the word *mind*, we can reword the three principles to gain a better understanding of their application to the mind.

1. *Something enters into the mind that should not be in the mind,*

2. *Something that should be in the mind is not in the mind,*

3. *Something enters into the mind, but, for some reason, the mind can no longer process it correctly.*

The question arises, then, of what should be in the mind. A good start would be seeking proper loving relationships, activities that lead to happiness, friendships, adequate rest, enjoyment in recreation, and doing the things that one wants to do. The question also arises of what should not be in the mind in order to be healthy. Examples of what should not be in the mind are activities that lead a person to withdraw, express hate and anger, pursue vindictive behavior, or to do something against their inner will. Unhealthy thought processes which result in undesirable lifestyle activities will ultimately lead to future negative consequences regarding health. Healthy thought processes, on the other hand, will have positive and beneficial effects on future health.

The third principle, concerning the statement that the mind can no longer process something correctly, is the psychological basis for most mind-related illnesses or conditions that occur due to events that occurred during some persons life. A specific example of this can be found in one case of what is incorrectly termed post traumatic stress syndrome. In this classical example, someone who was once a soldier on the battlefield is walking down the street and hears an automobile engine backfire. The similar sound of the engine backfire to a gun causes the person to relive the stress of the battlefield. This causes the person to respond in a variety of ways consistent with a severely stressful situation. To the person in this situation, the experience is indistinguishable from the events that once occurred on the battlefield. The response of both the body and mind are also indistinguishable from what might have occurred on the battlefield. In this example, the mind should not be concerned with the sound of an engine backfiring, but, because of some prior event, the mind is no longer able to handle this situation correctly. Incorrectly termed post traumatic stress syndrome, this illustration is a clear example of neurological switching, the phenomena responsible for multiplicity. This example is further discussed in the chapter on multiplicity.

The three principles leading to an unhealthy state can also be applied to the spirit. In the case of the spirit, following your inner beliefs, or true self is the primary issue at hand. Violating your inner beliefs paves the path to spiritual disease. Spiritual disharmony, unfortunately, is not widely understood in Western society. As a result of spiritual disharmony, one thing is certain to occur; internal spiritual conflict or disharmony will always eventually manifest as disease of the physical body. The problem is that spiritual disease or conflict cannot be measured by a laboratory test or seen on an MRI. The Superconducting Quantum Interference Device (SQUID), which is a highly sensitive magnetometer, can detect the subtle energies of the meridians, which are classically considered as part of the spirit. Using a device of this type can identify disease affecting the spirit long before its manifestation in the physical body.

Applying the three principles to the spirit will gives us insight into how an illness of either the body or mind is related to the spirit. This relationship, however, will become clearer after studying the chapter on the Body-Mind-Sprit Connection. The spirit, consisting of the soul, chakras, meridians, and aura, is, just like the body and mind, subject to disruption. This disruption is detectable in the subtle changes of the energy of a meridian, chakra, or aura.

By replacing the word *body* with the word *spirit*, and adding the concept of the energy that makes up the spirit, we can reword the three principles to gain a better understanding of their application to the spirit.

1. *Some energy enters into the spirit that should not be in the spirit,*

2. *Some energy that should be in the spirit is not in the spirit,*

3. *Some energy enters into the spirit, but, for some reason, the spirit can no longer process the energy correctly.*

Disease cannot be confined to the physical body, the mind, or the spirit. Any disease affecting one of the three will ultimately affect the other two as well. Disease, furthermore, often cannot be confined to just a single person. Since health requires us to be in harmony with our social environment, disharmony within the social environment affects the health of everyone involved. The proverbial "dysfunctional family" is an example of how disharmony in the social environment affects not only those individuals directly involved, but also to individuals far beyond the immediate dysfunctional family unit. The chronic alcoholic, for example, is exporting his or her disease to their social environment, creating disharmony far beyond the confines of just their own physical body. This situation can, in no way, be construed as healthy for anyone involved.

If we attain good health from harmony with those around us, we must first understand what this type of harmony is relating to our social environment. The concept of perfect harmony with others and with our environment can be illustrated by simply observing nature. When birds fly in a flock, they fly as a group. Sandpipers and Starlings are often observed to follow this pattern. When one turns, they all turn in unison. At other times, particularly while on the ground, they move and act independently. They all watch for danger as they scrounge around for food to eat. If danger arises, when one takes to the air, all follow. When they take to the air again, they all leave at once and move through the air again as if they are one. Fish frequently act much in the same way. When fish move through the water in schools, they appear as if they have a single mind, changing direction almost instantaneously. Fish have no leader, and the resultant movements are a result of being in perfect harmony with the immediate surroundings. When fish are feeding, or outside the school, just like the birds, they act independently. Perfect harmony, then, requires that any of our relationships with others around us be healthy. In this regard, our health and survival, just like the fish and the birds, is often dependent on the health of others who are around us.

When disharmony of any type is allowed to persist for an extended time, chronic disease is often the result. The definition of a chronic disease or ailment is one that has been there for three months or longer. The time factor of a chronic disease is readily obvious to the casual observer, since the root of the word *chronic* is *chron*, which means time. A chronic health problem did not occur overnight, and does not resolve overnight. Contrary to popular beliefs, miracle drugs, magical diets, special acupuncture points, special berry juice, or a chiropractic adjustment with something extra will not cure any chronic disease instantly, if at all. With a chronic disease, two things are for sure. The first is that someone who has a chronic disease or ailment is in need of drastic changes to reverse the course of the disease. The second is if a change is not made, the disease process will continue and progressively worsen over time. Improperly treated, the chronic disease sufferer will have a wide assortment of pills and remedies on the table, with new ones being added each year for yet a new problem that has arisen. While it may not be easy to correct long-standing health problems at the root cause level, it is definitely worth the effort.

In Western medicine, there is a vague rule that states that in order to cure a disease or illness and restore health, a pill or something added to the diet is the course of action. It is repeatedly ingrained into society is that whenever a health problem arises, the solution is found in a pill. The pill is marketed as an "easy out" for a disease, and is often thought of as an instant cure for any problem that may arise. The pill is typically a drug, herb, homeopathic remedy, or some vitamin or mineral supplement. More and more often today, some concentrated or refined food product, when added to the diet, is the proposed solution. This methodology is programmed into society through television advertisements, magazine advertisements, and multi-level marketing groups. Appealing to the emotions, the advertisement promises an instant cure, but fails to deliver satisfactory results or does nothing more than to treat the associated symptoms. The pill seems like an easy fix for the problem, but, if it sounds too good to be true, it most often is. Could it be, however, that removing something from the diet, or eliminating some unnecessary supplement is what provides the cure? For example, if the health issue is caused by a food allergy, removing the offending food is the only real cure.

This modern day pill popping mentality causes another problem to arise which must be dealt with. Primarily a problem of a philosophical origin, this type of thinking should be carefully analyzed, and must not be ignored. The problem is that, by taking some pill day after day, year after year, we are in essence saying that the body is primarily a stupid organism. The philosophy that a cure can be found in a pill also demands the belief that the body lacks any understanding at all of its own internal processes that are going on, and therefore unable to function and regulate itself correctly outside the ingestion of chemicals manufactured in some pill laboratory somewhere. By using the pill, we also must believe that the universe is equally as stupid, if not more so, because in creating the biology that forms such a perfect and harmonious organism, the ability of that organism to maintain its own health has been somehow left out. If that sounds absurd, the only alternative belief is that the solution to true health is found outside the pill. This is, in fact, the case. The body runs on food, not pills manufactured in some chemistry lab. Health and happiness simply cannot be found by ingesting chemicals. The body is not a stupid organism, and is well able to regulate itself and well able to maintain health.

How, then, do we solve these health problems that arise from disharmony from within and disharmony with the environment? Yet another problem comes up because we begin with preconceived beliefs regarding health and ask the relevant questions in the wrong way. When we ask a question regarding health, we expect an answer in terms of what we have been previously taught by the modern medical system. Likewise, when we think of disease, we think of disease also as it is defined by modern medicine. We supposed that health is one thing and disease is another, and that they are separate and distinct. One mistake is in the assumption that all disease is disease, and is distinctly identifiable as disease. In reality, disease and health are as two aspects of the same thing. The point is that disease and health are distinct but inseparable, much like the inside and outside of a basketball. Without the inside of the basketball or the outside of the basketball, no basketball exists. We are taught to believe that every disease must have a cause, that is, some outside germ, event, or other vague "thing" that caused the disease. We are also taught that the disease will, in turn, be the cause of other more serious forms of disease. So how does a cause then lead to an effect? The answer lies in the fact that many diseases are simply an adaption of the body to its environment, and nothing more. To complicate matters further, multiple adaptations to the environment accumulate to the point the body can no longer function properly and efficiently. In essence, these accumulated adaptations have taxed the body's resources beyond any acceptable limit. When adaptation does occur, it is a strong message the body is no longer functioning normally. Where, then, do we cross the line to true disease? Again, this is asking the wrong question. The absurd notion that the state of health and disease are two separate entities is confusing and wrong. Simply put, from the time a person is born to the time they die, the immune system is fighting off some pathogen that was allowed to enter the body from the environment in one way or another. This being the case, if health were found in the absence of a pathogen, no one can ever attain health. Health and disease are two dynamic forces at work, and the real question is whether they are in acceptable equilibrium. If health were found in a peaceful and an noncontentious external environment, again, no one can ever attain true health. Contention and less than peaceful situations will invariably arise in everyone's life, the question is whether they are handled appropriately or not.

Disease is not necessarily bad. Disease stresses and challenges the immune system, which makes the immune system stronger and better equipped to handle future encounters with any pathogens. As an example, in recent times, the H5N1 avian influenza virus (bird flu) has been identified as a possible pandemic threat to society. The vast majority of human deaths caused by the H5N1 bird flu are in persons under the age of forty years. In persons over the age of forty, deaths from this virus are rare, and are confined primarily to those with suppressed immune systems or otherwise deteriorated health. The immune systems of persons over the age of forty appear to be better equipped to handle the H5N1 bird flu than those of persons less than forty. This is presumably due to the greater exposure to various pathogens during their lifetime, resulting in a better developed immune system. As a result, in the patient over the age of forty, the immune system responds quickly and more efficiently, destroying the pathogen before the pathogen kills the patient. In the patient under the age of forty, however, the immune system response is inadequate or too slow to eradicate the disease before the disease kills the patient. The disease of today can, in some cases, be an invaluable asset in the defense of the disease of tomorrow.

Another problem arises when we assume every disease must be specifically identified, categorized, and named. Lists of symptoms, the organs affected, how cellular level functions are affected are all extensively documented by researchers. For some reason, when a disease is discovered or examined, the search for more characteristics of the disease goes into high gear, and the mechanism by which the disease causes harm is well documented. Attention is then given to finding a cure and selling the cure to the people who have been labeled with the named disease. Rheumatoid conditions all fall into this category. Dozens and dozens of separate and distinct rheumatoid disorders are very well documented and categorized, but in reality they are all the same disorder. Even more interesting is the notion that if all rheumatoid disorders are really the same, the corrective measures to reverse the condition should be the same. Evidence, in fact, suggests that this is actually the case.

What governs, then, when we choose to decide to reverse the course of an adaptation or reverse some condition that has allowed to develop in the body? In short, what disease do we treat, and what disease do we choose not to treat? Is it whatever seems advantageous for our survival, our social status, our future, our longevity, or our comfort? Of greater importance, how and at what level so we treat the condition that has been allowed to develop? Treating the symptoms seems to be the favorite course of action of traditional allopathic medicine, and is about effective as filling the cracks in the San Andreas fault to prevent an earthquake. Promoting wellness through proper nutrition, exercise, and lifestyle is the choice of the natural health practitioner, but who has the time these days to live such a perfect life? Who, then, is right, or is there a happy medium?

Today, for example, everyone is worried about cholesterol. High cholesterol, according to the medical doctor, must be lowered or some form of heart disease, or perhaps a stroke, will eventually follow. Not surprisingly, the pharmaceutical companies have developed drugs to treat elevated cholesterol, and these are often prescribed by the medical doctor. Interestingly, the accepted upper limits of serum cholesterol have been adjusted downward by the medical profession over the years, resulting in more people diagnosed with high cholesterol. The natural health practitioner, on the other hand, may give the patient a list of foods to eat, a list of foods to avoid, along with some natural supplements that may help to lower cholesterol levels. An exercise physiologist will suggest that the patient eat a more healthy diet and exercise more. A psychologist may recommend stress reduction activities, because stress has been shown to elevate cholesterol. Who, then, is right? In the usual allopathic paradigm failure, treating high cholesterol is really treating a symptom of a completely different issue. If we examine this issue, and get to the root cause, we will find the true answer, and therefore the real solution. Simply put, the body obtains cholesterol in two ways. The first way of obtaining cholesterol is through the diet, specifically through the foods consumed; the second way is through the body manufacturing it. Cholesterol, however, can be eliminated in only one way – certain beneficial bacteria in the small intestine break the cholesterol down, and it is subsequently eliminated in the feces. If little or no beneficial bacteria are found in the intestine to break down the cholesterol, the cholesterol gets reabsorbed into the blood. This results in the HDL and LDL numbers revealed in blood tests go higher and higher each year. So, high cholesterol is a symptom of the disruption of the bacterial flora of the intestine, not just some random event that seems to occur for no reason at all. Research indicates that a beneficial strain of bacteria known as *Lactobacillus plantarum* is a particular strain that breaks down cholesterol, and therefore an effective treatment in lowering cholesterol. It would logically follow, then, that if drastically decreased levels of *Lactobacillus plantarum* was found in the intestinal tract, cholesterol would be elevated. High cholesterol is an adaptation of the body due to disruption of these bacteria. The bacteria are required to be present in the intestinal tract, and their absence due to improper nutrition, antibiotic usage, or a combination of the two subsequently caused another disruption to occur in the body. Treating any disorder at the appropriate level would be much more advantageous, as opposed to limiting the treatment to symptoms alone. Therefore, the only true solution to the problem of high cholesterol is to restore the proper functioning of the digestive system. This would be accomplished by eliminating any yeast overgrowth in the intestines, and reestablishing the natural bacterial flora normally present in the intestinal tract. Avoiding the dietary cause that allowed the digestive system to get out of balance to begin with must also be addressed, and will require a permanent change in diet. In making these changes, all the dangers associated with high cholesterol will be averted.

Claims are made from time to time that certain foods have a cholesterol lowering effect. Some of these claims are substantiated and other claims are later disproved. Certain other claims of a cholesterol lowering effect off foods may be due to the substitution of one food in the diet for another rather than some inherent property of the food itself. Particular strains of probiotic bacteria have been shown to exist in or on certain foods. *Lactobacillus plantarum* is naturally found in sauerkraut, pickles, some cheeses, brined olives, sourdough, and fermented sausages. The presence of *Lactobacillus plantarum* on these foods would cause these foods to appear to have a cholesterol lowering effect. Causal notice of the foods listed suggests those that are commonly served in Germany or Austria. This would explain, in part, why persons in that area of the world who have what the American medical community would consider a high fat diet, such as sausage and cheese, do not have a high incidence of heart disease. *Lactobacillus plantarum*, in being present in the fresh food, keeps the intestinal tract well equipped to handle any the breakdown of any cholesterol that may be contained in the foods consumed.

The body is perfectly capable of healing itself. The challenge arises in placing the body in the correct and optimal conditions to facilitate healing. If certain foods, drugs, and dietary supplements are being consumed that are causing harm, they must be eliminated from the diet. Likewise, in some cases, foods and dietary supplements which are not being consumed should be consumed, therefore properly supporting health. Yet other dietary supplements may be used for a short time to correct a condition that was allowed to develop, and then discontinued once the condition has resolved. Avoidance of certain dietary habits will be required to prevent any relapse of the condition that was initially allowed to develop.

In medicine, we not only speak of health and disease, but often talk about life expectancy. Life expectancy refers to the number of years a person lives, but it does not take into consideration the quality of those years. A common saying used to describe the decline of health from chronic disease is "dead at 40, buried at 60." While this sounds depressing, it is a very good description of the feelings that people suffering with chronic diseases have. Making matters worse, more symptoms are experienced by the chronic disease sufferer each year, for which more pills are then prescribed. Chronic disease sufferers not only suffer physically, but emotionally, affecting the mind as well. In most cases, however, the disease process does not have to follow the expected course of taking its toll on the body and the mind. The expected course of a disease, incidently, is termed *expected* because if nothing is done to find the real problem and reverse the disease process, all sufferers of the same disease generally follow the same predictable downhill pattern. The expected course, however, is not the only course available. To avoid the expected course of a disease, all it comes down to is finding the problem, fixing it, and making sure the disease process is not allowed to happen again. When this is done, a new course is charted, the course to health.

We also must consider the social aspects of a person's life when we talk about health. The social aspects of a person's life are defined by where they live, who their friends are, their activities, and what they do for a living. A desirable social life includes freedom of expression resulting in a person doing what they really want to do. This goes beyond just being happy at the moment. Often, we refer to someone as a "free spirit." The free spirit is characteristically happy, full of joy and happiness, and doing what they really want to do in life. The same can be said of the eccentric person, who, on the surface, may seem odd and different when compared with others, but is the picture of success in his or her own eyes. When the free spirit or eccentric person arrives at a holiday gathering, everyone knows who they are and secretly wish that somehow, someday, perhaps their own life can be just a little like that too. The free spirit or eccentric simply will not be placed in a box. Many people, however, feel boxed in, tied down, and their lives so restricted that stress related disease is inevitable.

When we look back to our teen years, it is difficult, if not impossible, finding someone who was suffering from any chronic disease process. For the most part, everyone did what they wanted, ate what they wanted, everyone had fun, and everyone was healthy. Freedom of expression was at a lifetime high. If someone wanted to wear shorts and a T-shirt, they did. When we wanted to go to the mall with our friends, somehow we found a way to get there, and laying around listening to music or hanging out at the beach was a cool thing to do. If someone had the desire to have bleached blonde hair, they somehow figured out a way to bleach it, and the fact that their parents did not want them to lighten their hair did not seem to matter in the least. Somehow, at some point in time, all that ended. It has been replaced by a rigid schedule, office politics, the dress for success lifestyle, a mound of never ending credit card debt, not to mention writing a check for a mortgage or rent that literally can suck the life out of a person. Freedom of expression is now on the flip-side, at an all-time low, and a person's life begins to feel boxed in, to the point that everything they do is seemingly regulated and controlled by someone else. Stepping outside the lines is corporate or social suicide, so life becomes more of what someone else thinks and wants from someone rather than what anyone really wants for their own life. This leads to emotional stress and pressure, which ultimately leads to an unhealthy state of the body and mind. The unhealthy state does not happen overnight, but it will eventually happen unless something is drastically changed.

When we talk about health, we must also address the subject of employment. This includes matching a person to a particular profession in which they can express their strengths and creativity in ways that will provide satisfaction to both the employee and employer. Some people excel at artistic creativity, and yet others excel at analytical thinking. The right side of the brain is associated with artistic expression, and the left side is associated with analytical thinking. We often think of people as left-brained or right-brained, but, in reality, a balance is always found to exist between the two. So, whether someone is termed right-brained or left-brained becomes a matter of dominance. If a person is dominant in their right brain, they would be much happier with a profession that requires artistic expression, for example, a profession where they lay out artwork for advertising brochures. Likewise, the person with left brain dominance would step forward and gladly write the budget proposal for the advertising campaign, have all the figures balanced, and stay up all night to do it. Left-brained versus right-brained dominance in the working environment is just one factor that must be taken into consideration if a person is to attain true health. This translates into finding the proper job to express individual desires and strengths, not the one with the shortest commute time or the one with the highest salary.

How then do we solve these social problems associated with health? A problem comes up yet again because we are not brought up to believe that social and employment issues are important factors in health. The preconceived beliefs regarding health usually address the physical body, and that health of the mind is somehow unrelated to physical health. When the term mental health arises, it is often thought of in terms of significant cognitive dysfunction where psychiatric evaluation and treatment are indicated. Mental health, however, is a broad term that applies to everyone, specifically referring to the overall state of the mind. Mental health is impaired whenever chronic emotional stress is found to exist. Acute emotional stress resolves quickly and usually carries little effect in long term health consequences if handled in the proper manner. Chronic emotional stress, however, has serious long term consequences on a person's physical and emotional health. Chronic emotional stress, if left unabated, will eventually lead to disease of the physical body.

One often overlooked factor in health is socioeconomic status, which appears to be a factor only in industrialized countries. For example, current research suggests that acute gastrointestinal illness appears, at least to some degree, associated with lower socioeconomic status, specifically lower income groups. In children, this increased susceptibility to gastrointestinal infections is suspected to be linked to the overall condition of the immune system. In young adults, this increased risk may be due to various behavioral factors. Despite socioeconomic status, one can still obtain harmony of the body, mind, and spirit, leading to better health. In addition, perfect harmony within the physical and social environment is not limited by socioeconomic status.

Just like with physical diseases of the body, a problem arises when we assume every mental issue or disease must be also specifically identified, categorized, and named, along with the never-ending search for the cause and cure. In dealing with issues of the mind, the list of symptoms will comprise many subjective complaints with few objective complaints, accompanied by little, if any, objective criteria, laboratory tests, or examination results to support the diagnosis. In fact, in many cases, diagnosis of the condition is made purely on the basis of the subjective complaints of the patient. The patient history and subjective complaints are closely examined, analyzed, categorized, and finally, the patient is assigned a diagnosis. If the diagnosis falls into a known category for which there is a pill, the patient is then assigned the appropriate pill to take. If the diagnosis falls into a category for which there is no pill, then a pill from another category is assigned because it gives everyone involved the impression that the problem has been at least addressed to some degree. When this occurs, we lose sight of the original problem. The original problem did not arise because of the absence of some man-made chemical in the bloodstream. It logically follows that ingestion of a man-made chemical, then, is not going to anything to fix the real problem at hand. The original problem must be identified by examining the social aspects of a person's life, making some changes, and traveling a path more conducive to overall health. This, however, is a far greater challenge than the typical health practitioner is willing to accept. This places the health care ball back in the patient's court, which is a good place for the ball to be. If the patient serves the ball back to the medical professional, they are likely to get yet another pill in return.

When the patient seeks the advice of a health care professional, it is because they suspect that they have some disease, or that something is wrong with their body. When the health professional reviews the patient's complaint on the patient intake form, it echos the patient's concerns, but, since the patient does not have extensive medical knowledge, the complaint is usually documented as some perceived change in the way the patient is accustomed to feeling. Pain and fatigue are very common examples of documented complaints, but are not much for the diagnostician with which to work. Pain and fatigue, incidently, are, for the most part, next to useless diagnostic criteria with respect to chronic disorders anyway, primarily because they characteristically show up as part of most any disorder. Based upon the complaint, the health professional has their own list of concerns, most of which do not resemble the concerns of the patient. Patients have limited knowledge of the inner working of the body, which is why they sought out the knowledge of the medical professional. The medical professional of even average skill may have an enormous knowledge of the inner workings of the body, but only sees these inner workings, and does not see anything regarding the patient's lifestyle. The medical professional, therefore, cannot comprehend the real scope of the problem. Nothing beyond the contents of the patient's physical body is ever examined, and even then, examination is often limited to a cursory check of the area of complaint. The superior health care professional will look beyond the physical body, examining the spirit, mind, social environment, and physical environment of the patient. In examining the entire person, including the body, mind, and spirit, and giving consideration to both the physical and social environment, the true cause of the problem is much more likely to be found.

Eventually the realization will occur that health is not confined to the physical body. Enlightenment regarding the understanding of true health will be accompanied by the realization that every disease has a unique expression in the body, mind and spirit, not the physical body alone. Mental diseases cannot truly be separated from physical diseases, physical diseases invariably in one way or another affect the mind, and spiritual issues work their way into both the mind and the body quite easily. With this realization, we also can conclude that this categorization ad infinitum of every disease into classes and subclasses is largely a waste of time. If depression and inappropriate anger are caused by a biochemical issue originating from improper nutrition, are we dealing with a physical, mental or spiritual issue? In reality, any disorder has specific manifestations in the body, mind, and the spirit. Categorizing disease and subsequently attributing the disease to a dysfunction of exclusively either the body, mind, or the spirit is a dead end street. This activity of categorization will ultimately lead to focusing treatment on the area of the most symptomatic complaint, which may have nothing to do at all with the real problem. This often excludes any further diagnosis, leaving the real issues completely unaddressed.

Health, then, is perfect harmony of the person in body, mind, and spirit, and perfect harmony of that person in the externally defined relationships within the physical and social environment. The question arises as how to obtain this harmony. One way required to accomplish this is to look internally, and find what creates perfect harmony in the body, mind and spirit. Elimination of any internal conflict and creating perfect internal harmony will therefore lead to better overall health. On the other hand, internal conflict will always lead to disease of the physical body. Harmony and disharmony also apply to the externally defined relationships within the physical and social environment. It is also necessary to examine life externally, and discover what creates perfect harmony with the external world and acquaintances. When these are accomplished, we find ultimate health.

The First Law of Genetics: Choose your parents carefully.

Chapter 3
The Body-Mind-Spirit Connection

If we look at ourselves from a broad perspective, we find that we are much more than a physical body. We are all body, mind, and the spirit, the sum of which is often termed the "whole self" or the "complete person." The body refers to the physical body, the mind refers to a person's thought processes, and the spirit is made up of the soul, chakras, aura and meridians. They are all interrelated, for one cannot exist without the other in this realm.

To understand healing and the nature of illness in the proper framework, having a basic knowledge of what we are healing is highly desirable. This is especially true concerning healing at the spiritual level. Gaining the knowledge of how the body, mind and spirit all harmoniously fit together is invaluable knowledge in understanding the healing process. While not part of traditional medicinal teaching in the West, the information presented here regarding the spirit provides the foundation for all types of healing methods as taught in the East. This information is essential and must be understood adequately to grasp certain relationships of the body-mind-spirit model.

When a person goes to the medical doctor, the doctor is most concerned with examining and treating the physical body. Little attention, if any, is given to the mind or spirit. If a person goes to a psychologist, the psychologist is going to be primarily concerned with that person's thought processes and the inner workings of the mind, and little attention is generally given to the spirit or the physical body. Spiritual healing is quite a bit different. A spiritual healer is one who heals through the spirit, which includes the chakras and meridians, and provides some level of spiritual counseling. With spiritual healing, the attention paid to your physical body or mind depends on the type of healer seen. Once any disease becomes chronic, it must be treated at all three levels, the body, mind and spirit. Choosing the appropriate practitioner(s) in each case is therefore very important.

Before we can fully understand the relationship of the body, mind, and spirit, we must first have a basic understanding of the individual components of each. Classical teachings break the person into the body, mind, and spirit, and further break those components down to smaller components in an attempt to classify structure and function to a very exacting level. Modern teachings recognize the interrelation of these systems at a much deeper level, often concluding that, although thought as separate components, they are all more closely related than originally realized. The field of psychoneuroimmunology, for example, recognizes the interrelationship between the mind, nervous system, and immune system. Psychoneuroimmunology explains why, when someone is diagnosed with a potentially terminal disease and they decide, in their mind, they are going to beat this disease and get well, they ultimately succeed. Psychoneuroimmunology also explains why, when another person is diagnosed with the identical disease, with an attitude of defeat, they succumb to the disease faster than if they otherwise would have by not knowing of the diagnosis. Research has uncovered substantial evidence, primarily at the biochemical level, demonstrating the link between the nervous system and the immune system. Mind over matter is another way to think of psychoneuroimmunology.

Once it is understood that the whole notion of there being particular, separate entities called the body, mind and spirit, we realize that this division is nothing more than systematic division and classification of the whole person. We will also come to the realization that the process of division and classification can continue until a common denominator is finally reached. Each separate entity can be divided further, identifying smaller and logically grouped sub-parts. When all biological subclassifications are exhausted, more science is brought into the picture to continue the process of division and classification at deeper level. The deepest level to which this has been done is at the quantum physics level. The representation of the body, mind and spirit at the quantum physics level reveals nothing less than perfect congruity of the three. At the quantum level, both energy and matter have the same representation. Once this is understood, it is realized that the body, mind, and spirit are clearly indivisible, and the inner workings of the three at the quantum level are in perfect harmony. All matter and energy can be represented at this level, including light, the food we eat, and everything else found in the universe. Taking this one step further, what we have to recognize is that the interconnected system that constitutes the body, the mind and the spirit are, at the quantum level, interconnected with the rest of the universe that surrounds us. This connection with the universe is precisely why the proper definition of health must also include the physical and social environment, and not be limited to the health status of only one individual. Quantum physics clearly supports the premise that health of an individual is directly related to the physical and social environment in which that person lives. This indisputable fact must be taken into consideration by every healing philosophy and methodology that expects to cure any disease.

With all these interconnections involving both the people that are around us and our surroundings, we already have unity with people, nature, and the environment in which we live. We do not have to go to great extremes to find this unity. This unity is not found on some mountain top, in some ancient writing, or in a seminar taught by some guru from a foreign country. This unity is already given to us, but the problem is that we just do not recognize it. The reason we do not recognize it is that we, as a society, are terrified of silence and being alone. There has to be something going on all the time, a headset connected to some electronic gizmo pumping noise into our ears, fingers clicking away on a keyboard sending messages back and forth, all while we are trying to have a conversation with the person on the other end of the phone. We do this because of an inner sense of loneliness, and all this noise, typing, and busyness are just an escape from the silence and loneliness we fear. As a society, we are hopelessly distracted by noise of every sort. In escaping from the silence, we are really escaping from ourselves. In escaping, we place ourselves in disunity with ourselves, those around us, and our environment.

Modern technology that allows us to be in constant communication with others deserves special attention. This technology is especially prevalent with teenagers today. Information flies around at the speed of light, and no one dares miss a message in fear of falling behind on today's agenda or losing their position in the social hierarchy. Taking away the cell phone or the MP3 player from a teenager is about as traumatic as cutting out some internal organ. While this technology appears to have connected people, in actuality, what this technology has done, is to alienate us from each other under the illusion of being connected. As a result, the upcoming society of hyperactive over-achievers is setting a new standard of communication performance and information exchange. The use of this technology eventually makes its way into every facet of life, setting new competitive standards that must be abided by all who wish to participate. Newer technology, when it is available, will be a mandatary addition to the collection of electronics that controls everyone's life. This will ultimately lead to more stress, ultimately resulting in more stress related disease. What we have in essence done, then, is built a society connected by wires, and not by relationships. We have gone to such a great extent to connect our lives using modern technology that we have become literally out of touch with ourselves and those around us.

Relationships between people are not intended to be through an intricate network of wires, radio frequency wireless networks and satellite communications. The notion that any one person's place in the universe is dependent on this thing called connectivity is nothing but a false understanding of human relationships. The more a person tries to search for their place in the universe, the farther away from electronic connections they will ultimately find themselves. When electronic connectivity is all lost due to a disastrous hurricane, massive earthquake, or other natural disaster, true human connections and relationships are then formed. When true connections to other people are realized, the electronic connections begin to seem artificial and plastic. Unfortunately, after the natural disaster is over and life returns to normal, we quickly abandon any true connections formed, and return to the electronic connections that previously ruled our life. When a person deeply contemplates their place in what we call the universe, the more they will discover that their place is defined in terms of relationships with other people, and not defined around any form of technology.

A true understanding of the body, mind and spirit, or the whole person, is not widely found in today's society. What is further lacking is a clear understanding of our relationship to our environment. This relationship with the environment occurs on all three levels, involving the body, mind, and the spirit. Specifically, the physical level as related to the body, the spiritual level as related to our spirit, and the social level as related to our mind, all have a relationship with our environment. Enlightenment is simply harmony of the body, mind and spirit. When we obtain this enlightenment, and become also in harmony with our physical and social environment, we find true health. We will therefore review the body, mind, and spirit to gain a deeper understanding into health.

The Body

The human body is a remarkable creation. The body is simply the physical structure of the human organism. It is what one sees when they look in the mirror. The body can be categorized into its logical parts, which consist of systems, organs, tissues and cells. Systems are made up from organs, organs are made of tissues, and tissues are composed of cells. Human anatomy studies the organs of the human body. Physiology is the study of the body's systems. Histology is the study of the body at the cellular and tissue level. Pathology, incidently, is the study of the human disease process. Biochemistry is the study of the chemical processes of the body that occur at the sub-cellular level.

All of the systems of the body perform a very specific function. A system typically contains multiple organs grouped together in some logical way to accomplish a specific purpose. All systems of the body are closely interrelated with the other systems of the body, communicating with each other through various means. This communication is accomplished by nerves, hormones, neurotransmitters, and various other biochemical compounds, to name just a few. The organs that make up one system are typically shared with other systems of the body. The pancreas, for example, is shared between the digestive system and endocrine system. In our study of healing, we are going to be mostly concerned with the systems of the body rather than the individual organs, tissues, or cells. Of concern also will be the biochemical processes of the body, which is where most disease processes of the body begin. A brief overview of the systems will provide us a better picture of how all the organs and tissues of the body interrelate.

One system we will be very concerned about is the digestive system. The digestive system digests the food eaten, breaking it down into its basic components, and absorbs these components into the bloodstream. The organs of the digestive system are the mouth, salivary glands, esophagus, stomach, liver, gallbladder, pancreas, small and large intestines, rectum, and anus. Everything that eventually becomes part of the physical body has had to pass through the digestive system at one time. The gastrointestinal tract, the major component of the digestive system, is also considered part of the immune system. The bacterial flora that inhabits the gastrointestinal tract, while not classically considered part of the digestive system, plays a vital role in digestion and has a strong influence on the immune system.

The circulatory system pumps and delivers blood to and from the tissues of the body. It is composed of the heart, arteries, veins, capillaries, and blood. Arteries, as a general rule, bring oxygenated blood to the tissues of the body. Veins generally bring oxygen depleted blood back to the heart. The exception to this rule is the pulmonary arteries and veins. The pulmonary arteries bring the oxygen depleted blood to the lungs, and the pulmonary veins bring oxygenated blood back to the heart. Blood passes from arteries to arterioles, and finally to capillaries. It is at the capillary level that nutrients are supplied to the cells. Capillaries drain into veins, which return the blood to the heart. Another function of the circulatory system, in conjunction with other system of the body, is to maintain and normalize body temperature. Immune system components, such as antibodies and leukocytes, circulate in the bloodstream. Blood is technically considered connective tissue.

The endocrine system is classically considered to facilitate communication within the body using hormones produced by the endocrine glands. An endocrine gland secretes these hormones directly into the bloodstream. The endocrine system is composed of the hypothalamus, pituitary, pineal gland, thyroid, parathyroid, adrenal, pancreas, liver, and gonads. Modern research has discovered that the heart, uterus, and parts of the digestive system also have an endocrine function. The term *neuroendocrine system* has come into usage recently, resulting from modern research that has shown that the endocrine system and nervous system are strongly interrelated. The hypothalamus gland, being part neurological tissue and part glandular tissue, provides one of the many physical links between the nervous system and the endocrine system.

The immune system protects the body from harmful outside invaders, such as bacteria, parasites, and viruses. The thymus gland, bone marrow lymph nodes, spleen, tonsils, Peyer's patches (found in the intestines), liver, and appendix all make up the immune system. The workhorse of the immune system, however, are specific proteins, called immunoglobulins, and specialized immune cells, broadly known as either white blood cells or leukocytes, which systematically eliminate anything that poses a threat to the body. Of all the body's systems, the immune system is perhaps the most challenging to comprehend fully.

The lymphatic system is composed of structures involved in the transfer of lymph between tissues and the blood stream. Dividing the lymphatic system from the immune system is quite difficult, so, for the purposes of our discussions, we will consider the lymphatic system and the immune system as one system. The lymphatic system is composed of lymph glands, certain leukocytes, tonsils, adenoids, thymus, spleen, and the appendix. Casual observation will reveal that these components of the lymphatic system significantly overlap the components of the immune system.

The integumentary system is composed of the skin, hair and nails. Creating an effective barrier with the outside world, this system provides the body's first line of defense against environmental pathogens such as harmful bacteria. This makes the integumentary system technically part of the immune system. The skin is technically an organ, and is the largest organ of the body.

The musculoskeletal system is composed of the skeletal muscles, the skeleton, and also includes cartilage and ligaments. A tendon is the fibrous extension of muscle tissue that connects the muscle to the bone and is also included in this system. A ligament connects a bone to another bone. Cartilage forms the articular surfaces of joints. The purpose of the musculoskeletal system is to facilitate movement. Simply put, muscles contract and bones subsequently move. The field of biomechanics studies the relationship between muscles and joints, and how they are related to human movement.

The nervous system consists of the brain, spinal cord and peripheral nerves. Movement, the senses, thought processes, and coordination are all functions involving the nervous system. The nervous system has many divisions associated with it, each division performing a very specific function. The somatic nervous system controls the functions of the body under voluntary control, muscle contraction being a prime example. The autonomic nervous system is divided into two distinct divisions, called the sympathetic and parasympathetic divisions. The autonomic nervous system controls secretions from exocrine and endocrine glands, heart rate, reflex arcs, constriction and dilatation of blood vessels, pupillary constriction and dilation, and smooth muscle control among many other functions.

The reproductive system in the female consists of the ovaries, fallopian tubes, a uterus, a vagina, and Mammary glands. In the male, the reproductive system is composed of the testes, vas deferens, seminal vesicles, prostate, and penis.

The respiratory system contains the organs of breathing, which include the sinus cavities, pharynx, larynx, trachea, bronchi, lungs, and diaphragm. Oxygen and carbon dioxide are exchanged within the alveolar system of the lungs. This exchange occurs by diffusion. Certain metabolic wastes from the circulation are also removed by the lungs, such as volatile compounds. The respiratory system also plays a part in maintaining the pH balance of the body.

The excretory system classically consists of the kidneys, ureters, bladder and urethra. The primary function of this system is to eliminate metabolic waste from the body. The excretory system also plays a major role in the regulation of electrolytes, and, in conjunction with other systems, maintaining the pH balance of the body. Metabolic waste is also eliminated through the pores of the skin.

All systems of the body are closely interrelated. What may appear to be a clear and distinct function is often shared by several systems of the body, each system playing a vital part in the function. Electrolyte balance, and regulation of pH are clear examples of this. Other systems, such as the immune system, reach into every other system of the body. In medicine, we try to clearly divide the systems of the body, but, in reality, no true division can be made. The more one tries to divide the systems of the body, the more they realize that the task cannot truly be accomplished.

At times, this division of the body into systems can obstruct the diagnosis of a particular disorder. When this is the case, stepping back and looking at the body as a whole, or as a complete organism, is imperative. This is particularly true when it comes to chronic diseases. When a chronic disease is diagnosed, the cause will never be confined to only one system. The complaints associated with chronic diseases, however, seem to be confined to only certain systems of the body. In rheumatoid arthritis, for example, symptoms, diagnosis, and treatment are focused primarily on the joints of the body. The real problem, however, is not the joints themselves. The joints are just the most symptomatic part of the body to be affected by the autoimmune process; therefore, they receive the most attention. Since the joints are the primary regions of discomfort, a disease classification encompassing the area of complaint is selected. The rheumatoid disease process, however, has its origins in the digestive system and immune system. In the case of Multiple Sclerosis, another autoimmune disorder, the focus of treatment is placed upon the nervous system. Since Multiple Sclerosis is an immune system issue involving Th1 / Th2 cell balance, the focus should be placed upon restoring and balancing the immune system. Proper restoration of the immune system must also involve a properly working digestive system. Clearly, this methodology of chasing and treating symptoms often misleads both the patient and diagnostician. In treating only the symptomatic part of the body, the real cause of disease is often overlooked, and the real cure is never found.

When a person goes to a medical doctor, the doctor is primarily concerned with the systems of the physical body. A typical examination involves a review of these systems. The general practitioner evaluates the systems, and either renders a diagnosis, or refers the patient to a specialist. A specialist is a doctor who is highly trained and focuses on one specific system of the body. A cardiologist, for example, is an expert in the heart, a gastroenterologist is an expert of the digestive system, and a dermatologist is an expert regarding the skin. In many disorders, however, multiple systems are affected. As a result, the patient is often seeing multiple doctors for different facets of the same condition. In these cases, coordination of care is of utmost importance, but rarely occurs.

When a person chooses a specialty practitioner, in many cases they have already chosen their diagnosis. For example, if a patient who has shortness of breath, a cardiologist will check the heart and do a blood work up, giving particular attention to cardiovascular risk factors. Even if nothing is wrong with the heart, the patient will probably walk out with a prescription to treat something that was found during the examination, perhaps elevated cholesterol. If the patient went to a pulmonologist instead, they would check the lung function, and most likely order an x-ray of the lungs. The patient might even walk out with an allergy medication or some corticosteroid. An otolaryngologist (ear, nose, and throat doctor) will most likely find a problem with the sinuses, or perhaps a deviated nasal septum, causing restricted air flow. The sports medicine specialist will tell the patient that he or she is out of shape and needs to exercise more. The psychiatrist might diagnose the patient's shortness of breath as stress related or possibly associated with a panic attack, and prescribe a suitable medication. No matter whom the patient sees, if the patient is carrying a lot more weight than they should be, their weight will be considered a factor in shortness of breath, and physical deconditioning would be considered part of the cause. Rarely does the medical professional examine the body beyond the system level. Oddly, most diseases have their origins at the cellular or biochemical level, a level generally ignored by the medical profession today. Ignoring the origin of disease is the reason that many diseases are allowed to progress to a very advanced level before they are even detected. In the example of the patient with shortness of breath, the problem at the biochemical level lies in a collection of biochemical processes that occurs in the mitochondria, which is a structure that is found in every cell of the body. This collection of biochemical processes is collectively known as the electron transport chain. In the electron transport chain, electrons are removed from an electron donor and passed on to an electron acceptor, which is Oxygen. For some reason or reasons, sufficient amounts of Oxygen are not getting to the mitochondria. It does not take a Nobel Laureate to realize that shortness of breath can have hundreds of causes. So, in choosing a medical specialist, the patient has placed him or herself in a position that limits the diagnosis to those diseases treated by that specialty.

Any disease process most likely has its origins at the biochemical level. Treating an illness, such as nutritional issues involving vitamin or nutrient deficiencies, is treating the illness at the biochemical level. Long standing biochemical issues ultimately cause cell damage. Exposure to heavy metals is one example of cell damage due to exposure to a toxin. Since tissues are made up of cells, tissues also become damaged as a result of biochemical abnormalities. Decreased function of the organs are to be expected as a result of damage to the tissues of which they are composed. Finally, the systems, which are made up of organs, suffer. Treating any illness at the biochemical level is, therefore, advantageous in every respect. Exclusively treating an illness at a level above the biochemical level is not addressing the true cause of disease. If the biochemistry of the body, however, is restored, the disease process will ultimately reverse. The best equipped physician, regardless of the specialty, will have a solid foundation in biochemistry.

The Mind

The mind refers to the various aspects of intellect and consciousness that make up what we refer to as "I" or "me." Thought, memory, perception, emotion, and imagination all contribute to what we commonly refer to as the mind. Exactly which attributes of human consciousness are considered parts of the mind varies based upon culture, societal beliefs, religion, science and philosophy.

When we think of the mind, the brain naturally comes to mind. Recent advances in imaging give us further knowledge into how the brain works. These advances, however, give us little insight into how the mind works. Modern day image enhancement can even give us a color view of the areas of the brain that are active during a certain experience or a particular thought. While imaging can show us that areas of the brain are involved during a specific activity, it cannot tell us exactly what a thought really is or how the thought originated.

In the body, an enormous number of things are going on at once, many of which we are conscious of, and many of which we are not conscious. The division between what is voluntary and involuntary is made clear by the two divisions of the nervous system, the autonomic nervous system and somatic nervous system. The autonomic nervous system carries out all those things that we are not conscious of, such as the secretions from glands, heart rate, respiration, and digestion. The brainstem, controlling most autonomic functions, is strongly influenced by other regions of the brain, therefore must be considered a component of the mind. The somatic nervous system, on the other hand, controls those things that we are consciously aware of, such as muscular movement. However, this is only part of the picture. Long term memory, short term memory, emotions, moods, though processes, sensory integration, and so on, all relate to the mind. The seat of consciousness in the brain is understood to be the Limbic system. Connecting higher and lower functions of the brain, the Limbic system interjects human emotion with any experience, and therefore must be also considered part of the mind. In defining the mind, what we will ultimately find is the all neurological tissue is in one way or another related. Dividing the components of the nervous system into the categories of being related to the mind or not is a monumental task.

When identifying what the mind is, great advantage will be found in not dividing, categorizing, and dissecting the nervous system endlessly to arrive at the answer. By stating that memory is part of the mind and the autonomic nervous system is not part of the mind would be a grave error. This is evident because certain thoughts can affect the heart rate, which is an autonomic nervous system function. To divide and categorize the parts of the brain as part of the mind or not part of the mind is futile. Any attempt at such an exercise will prove to be a waste of time.

In defining the mind, examining how the transmission of nerve impulses occurs will lead us to the answer. At the cellular level, the nervous system is made up of neurons. These neurons communicate with each other by a process called neurotransmission. During neurotransmission, a nerve is depolarized, and the electrically charged state inside and outside of the neuron membrane changes, thus energizing the nerve. The energy is propagated along the path of the nerve, and, at the end of the nerve known as the synaptic connection, communication occurs directly with other nerves through the action of neurotransmitters. Numerous neurological pathways may be taken, and depending on various factors involved, some desired thought pattern or other action results.

To define the mind is not as hard as it may seem. Simply put, whenever a neurotransmitter is engaged, or a neuron is active, the mind is also engaged and active. In other words, whenever neurotransmission occurs, the mind is actively engaged. Complicating the definition of the mind any further than this is unnecessary.

Someone could justifiably come along and argue that neurotransmitter receptor proteins have been found on monocytes and macrophage cells, and those types of cells are part of the immune system. Specifically, neurokinin-1 receptors have been found on human monocyte and macrophage cells, and respond to substance P, a neurotransmitter involved in both pain transmission and immune function. T-lymphocytes, another type of immune system cell, also have neurological receptor sites on their surface for neurotransmitters. Dopamine, a catecholamine neurotransmitter considered part of the nervous system, has been found to influence growth and proliferation of lymphocytes, an immune system component. To answer this argument regarding neurotransmitter receptors on immune system cells is quite simple. This relationship between the nervous system and immune system provides the basis for the field of psychoneuroimmunology, a field that studies the relationship between the mind, nervous system and immune system. The presence of neurotransmitters and their associated receptor sites on cells considered part of the immune system clearly illustrates one method of how the mind communicates directly with the body. This also lays the foundation of proof at the biochemical level of the body-mind connection.

Likewise, the argument can also be made that the heart has its own nervous system, but it is not part of the mind. This argument assumes that just because we are not aware of, or can easily influence, a particular segment of the nervous system, that segment of the nervous system must be unrelated to the mind. The basal ganglia and cerebellum, which are parts of the brain, are also performing activities that we are not aware of and cannot directly control, but nevertheless are specifically related to conscious actions of the mind. In the case of the basal ganglia and cerebellum, the connection to the mind is easily visualized. In the case of the heart, the connection is not as easily visualized. Simply put, the heart literally has a mind of its own, and is perfectly capable of rhythmically contracting day after day, while communicating directly with the brain. This communication is done through both the Vagus nerve and neurotransmitters, specifically norepinephrine and adrenaline, which are found circulating in the blood. The mind, therefore, is not necessarily synonymous with higher intellect.

Disorders commonly associated with the mind invariably involve some aspect of neurotransmission. Since neurotransmission is accomplished by neurotransmitters and their associated receptor sites, imbalances in neurotransmitters are often implicated as part of the cause of the disorder. In other cases, variations in the receptor sites found on neurons are often discovered in persons with certain types of mental disorders. Medications to treat these disorders target these neurotransmitters and their associated receptor sites. Natural approaches also target these sites, but with precursors to the associated neurotransmitters or herbs that have similar actions to prescription medications. Neurotransmission is implicated in many disorders, such as schizophrenia, bipolar disorder, and depression. Often, the presence of one disorder involving neurotransmission excludes the presence of another disease or disorder. As an example, persons with bipolar disorder are rarely diagnosed with chronic fatigue syndrome, especially during the manic phase.

One problem, which is often overlooked that is associated with the mind, has to deal with this never ending preoccupation with the physical symptoms associated with disease. The brain normally discards much of the sensory information it receives as irrelevant, minor aches and pains included. By constantly focusing on physical symptoms, the mind reinforcing to itself that the symptoms are important and careful attention must be paid to them. The mind then becomes more aware of the symptoms, and, in a way, the body subsequently becomes more sensitized to any unusual feelings that may be experienced. Specifically, the synaptic connections involved in processing the sensory information become more efficient, and become more active. More attention is then given to this normally benign sensory information, and the ordinarily benign sensations will eventually begin to feel very pronounced because the mind has, in essence, been instructed not to discard this innocuous information.

The mind, then, is defined as neurotransmission. In some cases, the result of this neurotransmission can be something as simple as a reflex arc. In other cases, neurotransmission can result in highly intellectual thinking. Problems associated with the mind can be due to either organic causes, thought patterns, or both. In any case, when a problem exists, the root cause must be addressed.

The Spirit

The term *spirit* refers collectively to the soul, meridians, chakras and aura. The spirit is often considered to be what leaves the body when a person dies, and is also considered by some to be the inner essence or true person. Simply put, the soul is the seat of one's existence. Meridians are energy pathways that link your physical body to your spirit. A chakra is a location of high energy found along the meridians of the body. The aura may be thought of as the radiance of the soul, chakras and meridians.

Western medicine has largely ignored the spiritual aspect of the individual when it comes to healing. This is because, in Western healing methods, the spirit is generally poorly understood, and subsequently discounted as unimportant, therefore ignored, in healing. Continued resistance of Westernized medicine to incorporate the spiritual aspect of an individual into health care is detrimental to patient care. Western society also has great resistance in accepting the philosophies associated with Eastern healing methods as part of the health care paradigm. This, in part, is due to the lack of understanding of the spiritual concepts involved in these methods. The great rift is evident when, as a society, we pray fervently in for the sick, but, at the same time, put trust in the medical profession who has no understanding of the spirit in its relation to healing. This is not unlike clinging to a form of Godliness, but denying its power.

The material presented on the spirit and its relation to healing is included here to gain a basic understanding of healing methods that reference them. The basis of the discussion on the chakras, meridians, aura, and soul are taken from classical healing methodologies that incorporate these concepts into the diagnosis and treatment of disease.

The Chakras

Knowledge of the energy centers of the body, known as chakras, will enhance one's understanding of healing of the overall body. This knowledge has been known for thousands of years and is just making its way into Western society. The word *chakra* is a Sanskrit word meaning "wheel." More specifically, a chakra is an "energy wheel," or vortex. A chakra is a center of high ki, also called chi, energy, which is energy flowing through both these centers and the meridians. A chakra is formed at a point of high energy along a meridian. Seven major chakras, numerous minor and lesser chakras are known to exist. The minor and lesser chakras often correspond to acupuncture points, also termed acupoints.

A major chakra is considered to be an energy vortex, where energy exchange occurs with the universe, sometimes termed the Universal Energy Field. This is particularly true for the seven major chakras. Energy flows into the chakra, ultimately finding its way into the meridian system and the nervous system. Energy can also flow out of a chakra, entering the universe where the energy can be sensed by other individuals. Each of the seven major chakras would appear as a circular energy vortex approximately four to five inches in diameter. The chakra extends approximately a distance of 1 inch from the body. This position would be within the first, or etheric, layer of the aura. The chakra tapers as it gets deeper into the body, where it comes to a point at a location very close to the spinal cord. This point is called the root of the chakra. The roots of all chakras are connected through a line of energy within the body, which runs through and parallel to the spinal cord. This line of energy is called a meridian. Many meridians exist in the body, but the one that follows the spinal cord related to the seven major chakras is the body's main meridian. The names of these main meridians are the Du Mai and Ren Mai meridians, and are found along the dorsal (rear) and ventral (front) side of the body respectively.

A normal chakra is one that has energy flowing into it is sometimes called an "open" chakra. Being in an open state is important for a chakra because it increases our spiritual energy flow, which is necessary for good spiritual, emotional and physical health. A person with all open chakras is freely expressing life as they were intended to, expressing appropriate emotions, accepting of life's circumstances, and is unaffected by negative criticism from others.

If energy is not flowing into a chakra, the chakra is termed "shut" or "blocked." Lack of energy flow into the human energy system eventually results in physical disease and emotional issues. On the emotional side, a person with multiple shut chakras has difficulty expressing life freely and has difficulty in relating to life overall. All chronic illnesses have a physical, emotional and spiritual effect on the person, and are always accompanied by one or more shut chakras. Since the chakras are conductors of ki energy, they are extremely important in energy healing techniques. When the chakra is blocked, this ki energy will not flow properly and will hinder all healing efforts, no matter the type of healing methodologies and techniques that are used. A blocked chakra is sometimes called by some an energy block. Energy blocks must be removed before healing can be truly effective.

If energy is leaving the body's energy system, the chakra is open but exuding energy rather than absorbing it. Many texts errantly claim that this is not normal and represents an unhealthy state of the chakra. A chakra that is exuding energy is incorrectly referred to as a blocked or reversed chakra. A normal, healthy chakra is exchanging energy with the universe in both directions. A normal, healthy chakra is a bidirectional pathway, not a one way pathway.

Although we term chakra as "open" or "shut," varying degrees of open and shut exist. Chakras may also be termed hyperactive, or hypoactive. These terms are used to describe the relative energy levels of one chakra to another. The term "chakra balancing" refers to equalizing the energy intake of each chakra so that energetically they are all nearly equal. Open and balanced chakras are an indication of a harmonious spirit.

The term chakra is becoming more popular these days. Healing methods, such as Reiki, in which healing is accomplished through energetic touch, make reference to the chakras quite often. Nurses and other health care professionals have learned these ancient healing methods, and frequently use them in their work. Hospitals are beginning to employ alterative healing specialists to provide adjunct therapy to the medical paradigm. This synergistic step will undoubtably be proven as a great step forward for modern medicine.

Each chakra has specific characteristics associated with it. From a standpoint of the physical body, associated with each chakra are one or more endocrine glands, a nerve plexus or other neurological tissue, and various organs or systems of the body. From a psychological point of view, each chakra has a particular human drive or desire associated with it. In some teachings, each chakra also has a color association. Table 3.1 identifies the location of each of the seven chakras.

Chakra (name)	Location
1st (Root)	Base of the spine
2nd (Sacral)	Between the genital area and navel
3rd (Solar Plexus)	Just above the navel
4th (Heart)	In front of the heart
5th (Throat)	In front of the throat
6th (Third Eye)	Center of the forehead
7th (Crown)	Top of the head

Table 3.1   Chakra Locations

In relation to the mind, each chakra has a specific drive, or desire associated with it. These drives represent the natural human desires. In order from the first to the seventh chakra, these desires are to possess, reproduce, achieve, love, communicate, understand, and finally, to ascend. While not a part of classical and traditional teachings, in modern teaching, a specific color is associated with each chakra. Table 3.2 depicts the color and drive associations of each chakra.

Chakra	Color	Associated Drive
1st (Root)	Red	Material Objects, Monetary Issues
2nd (Sacral)	Orange	Sex Drive, Bodily Issues, Health Issues
3rd (Solar Plexus)	Yellow	Power, Obsessions, Control
4th (Heart)	Green	Love, Intimacy, Forgiveness, Compassion
5th (Throat)	Blue	Communication, Creative Expression
6th (Third Eye)	Indigo	Intellect, Spiritual Insight, Visions
7th (Crown)	Violet	Spirituality

Table 3.2   Emotional Chakra Associations

Each of the first seven chakras are also related to an endocrine gland, organs, and neurological tissue of the body. The relationship between the physical body and each chakra are shown in Table 3.3. When a chakra is found to be weak, or partially shut, examining the systems and organs of the body relating to that chakra would be advantageous. A weak chakra is an indicator of potential disease. Energetic changes are apparent in the chakra long before any symptoms will be present.

Chakra	Associated Organ(s), Glands and Nerve Plexus
1st (Root)	Adrenal glands, Kidneys, Coccygeal plexus
2nd (Sacral)	Prostate, Spleen, Bladder, Uterus, Ovaries, Testes, Sacral plexus
3rd (Solar Plexus)	Liver, Stomach, Spleen, Gallbladder, Pancreas, Solar plexus
4th (Heart)	Heart, Lungs, Parasympathetic nerves, Thymus gland, Cardiac plexus
5th (Throat)	Trachea, Esophagus, Lungs, Thyroid and Parathyroid glands, Brachial plexus
6th (Third Eye)	Cerebellum, Brain stem, Ears, Upper respiratory organs, Eyes, Pituitary gland, Hypothalamus
7th (Crown)	Cerebrum, Pineal gland

Table 3.3   Physical Body Chakra Associations

The Meridians

The meridians may be termed "energy pathways" located throughout the body. Many energetic healing methods have long been known to diagnose disease through the Ki energy flowing through the body's meridians. Ki energy has been discovered independently by many cultures over the years. In India, this energy is known as Prana. In China, this energy is known as Chi. The Russians call it bioplasma. Ki energy is also known as Qi, Odic force, Mana, Orgone, vital energy, and perhaps by a few other names. Eastern medicine teaches that it is the imbalance of this Ki energy in the different meridians that cause disease.

The concept of a meridian can more deeply be explored by examining any of the healing methods that use them. The two most fully documented, researched, and widely accepted systems of healing utilizing the meridian system are acupuncture and Applied Kinesiology. For the purposes of this text, we will look at the meridian from the perspective of both acupuncture and Applied Kinesiology. These healing methods are well documented, accurately described by various authors, and well known in the West as compared to other methods. An in-depth discussion of meridians, however, is beyond the scope of this text. The information in this section is included to gain a better understanding of the meridians and to become more fully aware of the relationship and integration of various healing methods.

Diagnosis through the meridians involves finding the meridians with either excess or depleted energy. In any healing method that references these meridians, treatment is focused on points of high energy, termed acupoints, which are found along these meridians. Aberration of energy flow at these points is known to have a direct relation to the patient's condition. An Applied Kinesiologist uses the body's meridians to diagnose and correct imbalances of both structural and physiological origin. A reflexologist attempts to correct an organ dysfunction through stimulation of the meridians. Oriental meridian therapy, known as acupuncture, corrects an end organ and system dysfunction through stimulation of the appropriate locations found along the meridians. Magnetic healing methods, employing magnets placed on or along a meridian, restores the flow of energy along that meridian. Whatever method is used, the goal is restoration or balance of energy flow through the meridian. With freely flowing and balanced energy flow, health is ultimately restored.

The human body is composed of both energy and matter, matter being a highly dense form of energy. The meridians are networks of energy channels related to the systems and organs of the body. When a steady flow of energy is found in the meridians, we remain in good health. The matter associated with the physical world may be thought of as a high-density form of energy. The ki energy associated with a meridian is a low-density form of energy, often termed spiritual energy. Quantum physics teaches us that matter and energy are indistinguishable, and that subatomic particles are actually "energy ribbons" that can be represented mathematically. The discovery and refinement of the quark theories of modern physics in the early 1980s paved the way for a single unified representation of matter and energy, specifically that matter can be represented as energy in its purest sense. Matter, composed of electrons, protons, neutrons and a whole host of other subatomic particles, can now, according to modern quantum physics, be represented as energy. Health must take into account the unobstructed energetic relationship of the physical body and the spirit. It is primarily through the meridians that this relationship is established.

Energy is associated with the spirit world, but this energy is of a much lesser density than the energy often associated with the physical world. This spiritual energy is the same energy that all matter is composed of, but it is not bound to the laws that modern physics would apply to a subatomic particle. Terms such as the etheric body, mental body or spiritual body all refer to this spiritual energy. In reality, all energy is the same, and all matter is energy.

Characteristically, all tissues of the body have an impedance associated with them. Impedance, a term associated with the physics of electromagnetic energy, is a measure of opposition or resistance to a varying signal. The signal can be either a nerve impulse or the energy flowing in a meridian. Removal of any internal organ, such as the appendix, uterus, or kidney, causes a change in tissue impedance of the surrounding tissues. This can cause the position of a meridian or chakra to move as well, altering the flow of ki. Transplantation of an organ also causes a change in tissue impedance. Energy flowing along a meridian, then, has direct effects on the surrounding tissues. Tissues also have an effect on the flow of energy along a meridian. Energy flowing through any medium that has an impedance associated with it energetically affects that medium.

Meridians typically follow the same paths as nerves, but this is not always the case. The laws of electromagnetism tell us that when energy is transmitted down a pathway, an electromagnetic field is associated with the flow of energy down that pathway. If energy flows through a nerve, the electromagnetic field generated by the energy flow affects any meridian in the general vicinity. Simply put, the energy flowing down a nerve affects the meridian. Likewise, the energy flowing down the path of a meridian will affect any nerve in the general vicinity. This relationship provides the basis of the connection between mind and spirit.

More than 20 meridians are known to exist in the meridian system of acupuncture, some of which are directly related to organ systems and some that are not. These are classically divided into 12 main meridians, two extraordinary channels, and eight other documented meridians. The 12 main meridians of the body are shown in Table 3.4. Extraordinary channels, comprising the Du Mai and Ren Mai meridians, which are the main, or major, meridians of the body, are also included in the table. Although some meridians are named after an organ, the meridians specifically refer to biological functions, and not the physical organ itself. Along these meridians are found more than 600 acupuncture points. Most acupuncture points are areas of high energy on the body surface. Some acupuncture points lie outside a meridian, and these are termed special points. Meridian points can be visualized with a device known as the Superconducting Quantum Interference Device (SQUID), which is a highly sensitive magnetometer. Aberrations in meridional energy flow can also be detected by the Superconducting Quantum Interference Device. A skilled practitioner, however, does not need advanced technology to detect aberrant energy flow in a meridian. A doctor of acupuncture or skilled kinesiologist can detect and correct energy flow effectively without the use of any modern technological innovations.

The energy of meridians also plays a role in growth control, cell migration, and differentiation in embryology. Western medicine has failed to explain adequately cell differentiation using cellular biology alone. The ki energy associated with meridians is likely to be the key element. Ki energy flows through the body of an embryo just as in the adult, and it is this flow of energy that guides development of the body.

The Chinese are unique in the sense that they figure out ways of connecting things, rather than dividing and classifying every part of the body as done by the Western healing methods. In other words, they try to assemble, instead of disassembling, the aspects of the body. Using the process of assembling and connecting, understanding the interrelation of the body, mind, and spirit is easy. The philosophy of assembling and connecting things leads us down the path to understand the connections. Connections within the body, and connections with each other, and with our environment become clear as well. Anyone who attempts to divide and classify the oriental meridian system using the methodologies traditionally used in the West would be undertaking an impossible project. Such an attempt would be futile and a waste of time.

Meridian	Energy	Channel	Peak Activity	Element
Heart	Yin	Arm	11:00–13:00	Fire
Pericardium	Yin	Arm	19:00–21:00	Fire
Lung	Yin	Arm	3:00–5:00	Metal
Spleen	Yin	Leg	9:00–11:00	Earth
Liver	Yin	Leg	1:00–3:00	Wood
Kidney	Yin	Leg	17:00–19:00	Water
Small Intestine	Yang	Arm	13:00–15:00	Fire
San Jiao	Yang	Arm	21:00–23:00	Fire
Large Intestine	Yang	Arm	5:00–7:00	Metal
Stomach	Yang	Leg	7:00–9:00	Earth
Gallbladder	Yang	Leg	23:00–1:00	Wood
Urinary Bladder	Yang	Leg	15:00–17:00	Water
Ren Mai			Midnight	
Du Mai			Midnight	

Table 3.4   The Main Meridians of the Body

Meridians also hold a specific type of energy, and this is reflected in the yin / yang grouping associated with the meridian. In the Oriental way of thinking, yin and yang are thought of as opposing forces. Yin and yang forces are opposite forces always at work. The forces are complimentary and, in a sense, control each another. While the male is classically considered the yang force, and woman as yin, each gender has a balance of both yin and yang forces constantly at work. The Yin Yang symbol, depicted in Figure 3.5, has its origin in Daoism, and portrays the pairs of opposing forces seen throughout the universe. This symbol is intended to depict the changing forces while maintaining balance.

Meridians are found in every region of the body. Each of the twelve main meridians has a major component found in either an arm or a leg. When an acupuncture practitioner is working on a specific organ, the needles are not necessarily placed anywhere near where the location of the physical problem or area of complaint. Many of these needles may be placed in the arm or leg, no where near the symptomatic complaint of the patient. The same holds true for a kinesiologist, acupoints worked on by the doctor may not be anywhere near the region of complaint. A reflexologist primarily works on the terminal meridian points of the hands, feet, and ears.

Chinese medicine pays close attention to yin / yang balance. Beyond addressing the yin / yang balance through the meridians, specific herbs are often used for balancing and the restoration of energy flow. Chinese yin / yang tonifying herbs such as *Herba Cistanche*, *Ganoderma* and *Cordyceps* have been also shown to participate in immunomodulatory activities, possess antioxidant properties and increase production of adenosine triphosphate (ATP). Since adenosine triphosphate is the body's primary energy source, understanding how the proper application of the appropriate herb under the correct circumstances can restore yin / yang balance is easily seen.

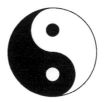

Figure 3.5   Yin - Yang Symbol

In traditional Chinese philosophy, natural classifications fall into one of the five elements of Earth, metal, wood, water, and fire. As with yin and yang, these elements also remain in natural balance. According to Chinese medicine, each meridian is associated with one of these five elements.

In the system of traditional Chinese medicine, a strong belief exists that treating an organ during the particular time of day most appropriate to it is more efficacious. This chronological association recognizes the diurnal variations in the flow of ki energy. The best time to treat an excess of energy is during or shortly before the time of greatest meridian activity, as shown in Table 3.4. Depleted energy is best treated following the energetic peak of the meridian. Other types of Eastern healing methods, such as medical Qi Gong, recognize these daily energetic variations of the meridians, and incorporate such timings into various practices of the art.

In 1964, Dr. George Goodheart, a chiropractor, developed the field of Applied Kinesiology. The original basic premise of Applied Kinesiology was to correct structural imbalances in the body caused by poorly functioning muscles. These improperly functioning muscles allowed the skeletal structure to deviate from normal, causing structural imbalances of not only the spine, but other joints as well. As advances were made, through muscle testing, it was found the patient's structural and neurological state could be determined. If any weakness were found to exist, by using the meridian system, the weakness could be used to map back to the patient's physical organs and systems. In many cases, situations involving biochemical abnormalities and mental health issues could be also diagnosed, and therefore corrected. Specific muscles were discovered to be related to specific organs or bodily systems through the acupuncture meridian network. Applied Kinesiology treatment protocols often include nutritional counseling, chiropractic adjustments, manual stimulation of meridians, acupressure, and exercise. Since its discovery, the field of Applied Kinesiology has grown tremendously, and is today incorporated in various fields of the alternative healing arts.

A major element of Applied Kinesiology, discovered by Dr. Goodheart through the use of neurolymphatic reflexes, is the specific relationships between the body organs and the muscles. This led to the inclusion of Oriental Meridian Therapy, known more commonly as acupuncture, into the practice of Applied Kinesiology. This provided an objective technique to determine the need for neurolymphatic stimulation through muscle testing. The Oriental meridian model reveals that organ function is related to a particular energy meridian. Combining the organ – muscle relationships of Applied Kinesiology with the organ and the meridian relationships of acupuncture gives us a specific relationship between both the muscles and the meridians, and the meridians and the body's organs. With this knowledge, both muscle inhibitions and the related organ dysfunction found through muscle testing can be corrected through meridian therapy.

Changes in the normal meridional energy can precede anatomical changes during pathogenesis (the development of pathology). If an organ exhibits a dysfunction, the dysfunction is reflected as a weakness in the corresponding meridian, possibly multiple meridians. If a muscle proves weak, this weakness may also be detected in a meridian. Chiropractic research has proven, beyond any doubt, that a neurological dysfunction will manifest itself as muscular weaknesses, organ dysfunction, or impaired bodily function in one form or another. This neurological interference also can be detected in a meridian. Consider for a moment that chakras are related to both meridians and the aura. Consider also that chakras are related to bodily organs, glands, and the various facets of a person's mind including personality. With all this in mind, the meridian is clearly at least one link between the body, mind, and spirit. The components of the body, mind and spirit obviously cannot be as easily separated as classically thought. The Chinese are correct in their notion that connecting the concepts relating to the body is easier, as opposed incessant division and classification of the parts.

Balance of the whole person through meridian therapy is the goal of both acupuncture and Applied Kinesiology. These healing methods treat the whole person, not just the parts. Today, we find many advancements and specializations within the field of Applied Kinesiology. The Neural Organization Technique, developed by Carl A. Ferreri, D.C., of New York City, Contact Reflex Analysis, taught by Dick A. Versendaal, D.C., and the Neuro Emotional Technique (NET) developed by Scott Walker, D.C. are just a few examples of techniques promising to take meridian–based healing methods to the next level.

Another major advancement, which occurred during the development of Applied Kinesiology, was Dr. Goodheart's discovery of Therapy Localization. Doctor Goodheart found that a muscle that initially tested to be weak became strong when the patient touched that part of their body where the dysfunction causing the weakness was found. This principle was later shown to identify dysfunctional reflexes, organs and neurological interference. The method of Therapy Localization developed by Dr. Goodheart can also be applied to testing and diagnosis of the condition of the chakras and the meridians. This technique of analysis has been perfected by George Petryk, D.C., of Fort Meyers, Florida. Specifically, a muscle indicator, which initially tested to be strong, will test as weak when the practitioner touches a chakra or acupuncture point that is in need of stimulation. Aberrations in auric energy flow can also be detected by Therapy Localization.

The Soul

The soul is simply the seat of one's existence. In most religious traditions the soul is thought to incorporate the inner essence of each living being. The soul is believed to be, in many cultures and religions, the unification of one's true sense of identity. The soul is usually considered immortal and to exist eternally.

The Aura

The aura is a subtle field of energy radiated from the soul, chakras and meridians. Some believe the aura reflects the moods or thoughts of the person. The aura has multiple layers, and each layer is associated with the corresponding chakra.

If someone becomes aware of the fact that they are an inseparable body, mind and spirit, then thought processes, autonomic functions, immune functions, relationships with others, astral projection and everything else that the person experiences do not just randomly happen. These, and everything else experienced, are done consciously in conjunction with the world around us. At the lowest level, the quantum physics level, or the spiritual level, each person is completely linked and one with their surroundings.

If we are therefore linked to the universe at the lowest energetically described level of physics, when we are in harmony with our surroundings we can expect greater harmony within. When we obtain greater harmony within, we are then able to obtain harmony with our environment. When we obtain this harmony, we then obtain health.

A patient came in suffering from low back pain and, sometime during the examination, asked whether I believed in the body - mind connection. He was unsure of the connection himself, and was seeking the answer. I asked him if his low back pain was annoying him. He responded *"Of course it is."* *"Well, there's your body - mind connection,"* I replied. He left enlightened.

Chapter 4
Nutrition

When we talk about nutrition, we are mainly concerned with food. The terms *diet* and *nutrition*, however, are not synonymous. Diet refers to the choice of foods a person consumes. Nutrition refers to how the foods of the diet supply the needs of the body and react with the body. With a better understanding of nutrition, better choices can be made regarding the diet, ultimately leading to a healthier state of the body.

At any given time, there seems to be a diet that is fashionable to be on. Books are published explaining the diet in detail, the infomercial hits the cable and satellite channels, and special foods are sometimes available in stores or through a mail-order company. Famous celebrities may endorse the diet, and groups of followers form support networks and have get-togethers to share their successes. When the diet falls out of popularity, the authors of these diet books

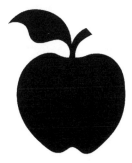

and programs invent a new diet program, publish the book, and travel the country giving new talks. All the followers move on to the new craze, forgetting completely about the old diet. The old book is then left on the shelf, collecting dust, along with several other books on the subject of health and wellness. If the original diet really worked, one would have to wonder why the new diet was necessary at all. Over the decades, hundreds of diets have made it into popularity. Figure 4.1 identifies just a few of these diets.

All these diets have one thing in common – they do not work, and neither will the next diet to arrive on the scene. Chronic dieting simply does not work, and typically will lead to weight gain rather than to weight loss. So, as far as diets go, forget it, drop it, and move on to learning about what does work.

Diets or diet books, which claim to have the key to health or the power to cure disease, should immediately arouse suspicion. For example, a particular diet may claim certain benefits of eating a specific food. The claims may be backed up by sound biochemistry, and the nutritional value of the food may be well documented. Research may even support the benefits of that particular food in healing some particular disease. Controlled research studies may even be published in peer-reviewed journals proving the nutritional and health benefits

The Grapefruit Diet	High Fat Diet
High Protein Diet	Fat Busters Diet
Macrobiotic Diet	Sugar Busters Diet
Anti-Candida Diet	Vegetarian Diet
Fruit Diet	Diet Pill Diet
Vegan Diet	What Would Jesus Eat Diet
Juice Diet	Eat What You Want Diet
Elimination Diet	Alkaline Diet
High Fiber Diet	Seaweed Diet
Raw Food Diet	Anti-Ageing Diet

Figure 4.1   Popular Diets

of the specific food. Jesus may have even eaten the same food. The problem is that if a person has developed either an acquired hypersensitivity, a food intolerance, or allergy to any food in question, it will cause an illness, not cure it. Eating food that causes an allergic reaction is analogous to consuming poison, in the sense that harm is being done to the body. No health benefits at all are found in a consuming a food that will cause an immune system reaction. Testing for IgG mediated food allergies would be of great benefit in identifying these food allergens, and, if found, eliminated from the diet. What is a healthy diet for one person may lead to a major health disaster in another person. Going on a grapefruit diet would be a disaster to anyone who has a citrus allergy. Eating natural whole grain wheat bread will cause serious health issues in someone with Celiac disease. Even if the dieter did not have a food allergy, the diet based around certain foods will cause overexposure to those foods, subsequently setting up an IgG hypersensitivity that did previously did not exist. Consequently, nutrition and diet must be not only based upon biochemical individuality, but also common sense.

With some knowledge and common sense, developing an appropriate diet can be easily accomplished without enrolling in a university and obtaining a PhD in nutrition. Biochemical individuality must always be taken into consideration when choosing foods, and is particularly important in the presence of any chronic disease. Genetic factors also come into play, which often involve genetically missing or defective enzymes affecting the digestion of food. Because of many factors, foods that are healthy for one person may be detrimental to another person's health. The goal, then, is to develop a diet that provides good nutrition to the body, taking into consideration biochemical individuality, genetic factors, and current health status. In adopting a proper and appropriate diet, a variety of health issues can be avoided.

In order for food to be digested properly, the digestive system must be functioning correctly. Foods must also be eaten in the proper amounts, in the correct order, and combined correctly with other foods. Certain foods should be avoided completely because they are no benefit to the body. Highly refined foods, which overload not only the digestive system, but the biochemistry of the whole body, leads the list of foods that should be avoided completely. Other foods contain artificially synthesized chemicals to mimic the taste of fat or sugar. These fat and sugar substitutes have no nutritional value, are detrimental to the body, and should also be avoided completely. Most digestive problems occur because of violating these simple rules. Violate the rules long enough, and the digestive system will fail to function correctly. When the digestive system fails, it is a very serious matter because it will eventually affect every other aspect of health. While this may seem like a lot to learn and keep track of, it is not really as complicated as it sounds.

A properly functioning digestive system is able to digest naturally occurring foods completely and efficiently. Once the food is digested, a healthy digestive system will permit the absorption of the basic food components into the bloodstream, and eliminate the waste regularly and quickly. Not surprisingly, if a person has one digestive system disorder, other problems with the digestive system are often found as well. Digestive system problems will very quickly lead to immune system problems, and once the immune system is compromised a downturn in health is just around the corner. The first step in regaining health, then, is to correct any digestive system disorders that may exist, and, therefore, an entire chapter, entitled Digestive System Restoration, has been devoted to this subject.

The digestive system is not designed to digest the wide variety of foods eaten in the typical modern day meal. Furthermore, the digestive system is not designed to digest tremendous quantities of food at once. Continuously presenting the digestive system with huge quantities and large varieties of food leads only to the incomplete digestion of food. Incompletely digested food contains toxins. If absorbed into the bloodstream, these toxins must be broken down by the liver and eliminated by the kidneys. This toxic waste buildup eventually leads to a host of chronic disorders.

In developing a proper diet, an understanding of the classes of nutrients would be of great benefit. The six basic nutrients of the body are proteins, carbohydrates, fats, vitamins, minerals and water. The function of the digestive system to take food and break the food down into these basic components so they can be assimilated into the body. Fiber, although it has no nutritional value, is considered essential to human nutrition. In gaining an understanding of these basic classes of nutrients, an appropriate diet can easily be developed to supply the nutrients the body needs.

Protein

Protein is composed of sequences of amino acids. Human metabolism uses 20 standard amino acids used in synthesis of protein. Eight of these are essential amino acids, ten are nonessential amino acids and two are known as semi-essential amino acids. Table 4.2 identifies each amino acid and whether they are essential, nonessential, or semi-essential. An amino acid is termed *essentia*l because it is essential that the amino acid be obtained through the diet because the body is unable to synthesize it. Semi-essential amino acids can be synthesized by a normal healthy adult, but not by younger children because the involved metabolic pathways have not yet been fully developed. Nonessential amino acids can be readily synthesized by the body from other amino acids, providing, of course, that sufficient quantities are available for the synthesis. Excess amino acids cannot be stored in any significant quantity by the body. Any excess amino acids are broken down in the liver by the enzyme *amino acid oxidase*, and are converted to glucose and urea. Elimination of any by-products of this breakdown is then carried out by the kidneys.

The digestive system breaks down protein into the individual amino acids of which they are composed. Protein digestion occurs in the stomach. This is done by hydrochloric acid and specialized enzymes, called proteases, such as *pepsin*. The hydrochloric acid provides the necessary medium for the enzymes to break the protein into amino acids. Other forms of acids, such as the carbonic acid or phosphoric acid found in soft drinks, or acetic acid found in vinegar, do not provide the proper acid medium for protein digestion. These other acids, conversely, inhibit protein digestion to some degree. Without the proper medium of hydrochloric acid, protein digestion cannot occur. The use of medications to suppress or neutralize hydrochloric acid is interfering with the digestion of protein.

Amino acids come in two isomeric forms, the *d* form and the *l* form. These letter designations are abbreviations for the terms *dextrorotatory* and *levorotatory* respectively, and are derived based upon whether polarized light is bent to the right or left when transmitted through a solution of the amino acid. Only the *l* form of the amino acid has value in human nutrition. The d form of the amino acid cannot be incorporated into a human protein. The names of amino acids are often written using the isomeric type, for example l-Tryptophan. For the purposes of literature and food supplements sold concerning human nutrition, the isomeric designation is often omitted. Tryptophan, l-Tryptophan, and L-Tryptophan are all therefore analogous in the discussion of human nutrition. One exception to this rule can be found. The amino acid Phenylalanine can be purchased with both the d and l isomers combined in a single supplement. This supplement is called dl-Phenylalanine. Evidence suggests that isomeric form d-phenylalanine inhibits the breakdown of endorphins, which are the body's natural pain killers. While d-Phenylalanine has the property of inhibiting the breakdown of endorphins, as with other d isomers, d-Phenylalanine cannot be incorporated into a human protein. Certain other amino acids that are not required for human nutrition can be purchased in supplement form from health food stores. These amino acids are particularly popular in the bodybuilding circles. One such amino acid is Ornithine, which is not an amino acid called for in the DNA coding of the human body. Ornithine is an intermediate in the urea cycle, and is involved in the elimination of excess nitrogen.

Nonessential	Essential	Semi-essential
Alanine	Isoleucine	Arginine
Asparagine	Leucine	Histidine
Aspartate	Lysine	
Cysteine	Methionine	
Glutamate	Phenylalanine	
Glutamine	Threonine	
Glycine	Tryptophan	
Proline	Valine	
Serine		
Tyrosine		

Table 4.2   Amino Acids

Many sources of protein are available, including plants, animals, and food supplements. Meat, fish, milk, cheese, eggs, and other animal sources of protein are known as complete proteins. The term *complete protein* means that the protein contains all the necessary amino acids required by human metabolism. Vegetables, fruits, grains, beans, nuts, seeds, and other plant foods do not contain all the amino acids required by human metabolism, and are therefore known as *incomplete proteins*. With the proper combining of foods, various sources of incomplete protein can supply all the amino acids required by the body. Vegetarians should be well educated in food combining, otherwise specific amino acid deficiencies can result. Protein, in food supplement form, is often used by bodybuilders or persons with specific nutritional needs that cannot be addressed by a normal diet. Unless a specific nutritional issue is being addressed, such as with the bodybuilder, protein supplements should not be normally used.

In addition to various protein supplements, amino acid supplements can also be found on the shelves of health food stores. One particular form of an amino acid supplement is called a free-form amino acid. Free-form amino acids are available in isolated form, that is, one specific amino acid is contained in the supplement. Free-form amino acids are also available in combination form, in which several amino acids are combined into a single supplement. The most popular combination form of an amino acid supplement contains all of the essential amino acids. Other free-form amino acid supplements contain all the amino acids, both essential and nonessential. The advantage of a free-form amino acid supplement is that it does not have to be digested in order to be absorbed. This makes them particularly valuable in treating certain conditions, such as rebuilding the lining of a compromised digestive tract. In another example, the body's nutritional requirement of the branched-chain amino acids leucine, isoleucine and valine are elevated in bodybuilders. Amino acid supplements are available in specifically formulated products to meet this increased demand in the bodybuilder. Amino acids are also the precursors to certain neurotransmitters. If a decreased level of a neurotransmitter is found, dietary supplementation of the appropriate free-form amino acid will, in many cases, restore the neurotransmitter level.

A term called Biological Value measures how well the body can absorb and utilize the amino acids from a particular protein source. The higher the Biological Value, the greater the value of that particular protein source is to the body. Eggs are traditionally assigned the highest Biological Value score, and have been rated at an arbitrary 100. Eggs were initially assigned an arbitrary score of 100, since it was the most complete protein known when the scale was originally developed. Recently, isolated whey protein has been rated at a Biological Value of 104, suggesting that isolated whey protein is of greater Biological Value than the protein found in eggs. Table 4.3 identifies the Biological Value of some common protein sources.

The ideal protein source would have all the required amino acids needed by the body in the exact proportions. Such a food cannot possibly exist since the nutritional needs of the body for specific amino acids, although well documented, can vary from day to day, based upon activities and lifestyle. As previously mentioned, the branched-chain amino acids are required in higher levels by athletes in training and bodybuilders, and this increased requirement occurs because of activities involving increasing muscular development. By obtaining protein from various sources, the probability of any specific amino acid deficiency significantly decreases.

Amino acids obtained through the digestion of protein are reassembled by the body to form specific proteins. Every protein has a unique sequence of amino acids associated with it. Proteins are found in every cell of the body, and serve many purposes. Proteins are very specific in nature, performing a specific function vital to life. Actin and Myosin are two proteins involved in muscular contraction. Antibodies, also known as immunoglobulins, are yet other proteins that are specific to protecting the body against infection. Hemoglobin is a protein involved in transport of oxygen to tissues. Considering these few examples, understanding why any specific amino acid deficiencies can have widespread consequences to health is not hard. If the body lacks the required amino acids to make these proteins, the protein simply cannot be made.

Protein Source	Biological Value
Isolated Whey	104
Eggs (whole)	100
Eggs (whites)	88
Poultry	79
Fish	70
Lean Beef	69
Cow's Milk	60
Brown Rice	57
Whole Wheat	49
Corn	36
Beans	34
White Potato	34

Table 4.3   Biological Value of Selected Foods

Amino acids are also precursors to certain neurotransmitters. In other words, specific amino acids are converted in the brain through various biochemical mechanisms to these neurotransmitters. Deficiency of these amino acids in the diet can lead to decreased production of the associated neurotransmitter. In many cases, supplementation of the diet with the appropriate precursor amino acids will help to restore the levels of the neurotransmitters dependent on that amino acid. This is especially true if neurotransmitter availability is limited due to a nutritional cause. Table 4.4 identifies the precursor amino acids to certain neurotransmitters.   Other amino acids act as neurotransmitters themselves. Glycine, taurine, glutamate, and aspartate are examples of amino acids that also act as neurotransmitters.

Antacids and acid suppressing medications inhibit the digestion of protein. The antacid raises the pH of the stomach, neutralizing the very environment required for protein digestion. Certain medications, broadly referred to as proton pump inhibitors, cause long term suppression of stomach acid. As a result of inhibited protein digestion, specific amino acid deficiencies can easily occur. This can subsequently lead to the decrease in certain neurotransmitter levels, easily resulting disorders such as depression, anxiety, and other mental disorders.

Neurotransmitter	Amino Acid Precursor
Dopamine	Tyrosine
Serotonin	Tryptophan
Norepinephrine	Tyrosine
Phenylethylamine	Phenylalanine
Epinephrine	Tyrosine
GABA	Glutamine

Table 4.4   Neurotransmitter Precursory Amino Acids

To properly correct balance or correct neurotransmitter levels, the current levels of neurotransmitters must be determined. Specialized tests can be performed by a natural health practitioner to determine the levels of the various of neurotransmitters in the brain. While these tests do not measure the level of the neurotransmitter directly, what they do measure, in fact, are the by-products of metabolic processes associated with the neurotransmitter. These tests, therefore, give an excellent indication of both neurotransmitter levels and the balance of the neurotransmitters. When the current state of the neurotransmitters has been determined, appropriate supplements, vitamins, or dietary changes can be prescribed to correct any imbalances. In addition to correction of nutritional issues, making certain changes in lifestyle activities, such as reduction of stress and increasing physical activity, are also imperative in restoration of neurotransmitter levels.

Carbohydrates

Carbohydrates provide the primary energy source for the body. In the body, carbohydrates are converted to glycogen. Glycogen is stored in the muscle tissue, liver, and, to some degree in other organs, until it is needed. Any excess carbohydrate, no matter the source, is converted to fat and is stored in adipose, or fat, tissue. Carbohydrates are the most efficient source of energy for the body. One gram of carbohydrate contains four calories.

The body can store approximately 350 grams of glycogen, a third of which is found in the liver, and two-thirds of which is stored in the muscles. Strenuous physical activity depletes the body's reserves of glycogen. It takes the body about 24 to 48 hours to fully replace these reserves following severe depletion. When the reserve of glycogen runs low, the body turns to the utilization of fat for energy. The lower the carbohydrate reserve becomes, the greater the percentage of fat is used for energy. If the percentage of fat used for energy gets too high, however, ketosis, a dangerous condition where toxic ketones accumulate in the body, can result.

Glucose	Turbinado sugar
Fructose	High fructose corn syrup
Table sugar	Raw sugar
Confectioner's sugar	Corn syrup
Dextrose	White sugar
Brown sugar	Honey
Molasses	Sucrose
Cane sugar	... and just plain Sugar

Figure 4.5   Refined Sugar

Unrefined carbohydrates, also called complex carbohydrates, are the most desirable form of carbohydrate for the body. Unrefined carbohydrates are carbohydrates found in their natural state. These are normally found in vegetables, fruits, and natural whole grains. Digestion of complex carbohydrates takes a long time as compared with digestion of simple sugars. Consequently, the digestive system does not get quickly overloaded with an enormous amount of sugar at once. Consumption of unrefined carbohydrates therefore helps to keep blood sugar levels relatively constant.

Refined carbohydrates, also called simple carbohydrates or simple sugars, can be found under many different names. These refined sugar products are often disguised under names as *natural* or *organic*. While these terms may be accurate, they are still refined carbohydrates nevertheless. Figure 4.5 lists just a few of the common names associated with refined carbohydrates.

Ingestion of refined carbohydrates causes blood sugar levels to rise and fall rapidly. When the blood sugar level rises, an energetic period, lasting for an hour or two, results. As the age-old proverb states, whatever goes up must come down. The pancreas, as a result of the ingestion of all that refined sugar, floods the bloodstream with insulin, which facilitates the transport of glucose across the cell membranes. Blood sugar levels then drop and the person feels tired. Cravings for more carbohydrates result from the drop in blood sugar, and when more refined carbohydrates are ingested, the cycle simply repeats itself. This results in blood sugar levels that look like a roller coaster. This constant overloading of the body's biochemical mechanisms by ingesting refined carbohydrates has the undesirable side effect of causing the excess carbohydrate to be converted to fat.

The nervous system, specifically the nerves themselves, cannot store glycogen. As a result, when blood sugar levels drop, the nervous system is particularly affected. Nerves get very irritated when the blood sugar level begins to fall. If blood sugar levels fall low enough, delirium may result. Even further drops can result in a coma. Certain disorders can be aggravated by wide swings in blood sugar. Depression, bipolar disorders, and any number of psychological disorders can be aggravated by, and, in some cases caused by, unstable blood sugar levels. By selecting foods containing unrefined natural carbohydrates, dramatic swings in blood sugar can be avoided.

Sugar substitutes are commonly used by individuals who are trying to lose weight, who have a fear of gaining weight, or are diabetic. Sugar substitutes simply should not be used, and no room for negotiation can be found regarding this issue. Sugars are broken down by the digestive system to form glycogen, the body's primary source of fuel. Digestion of sugar substitutes, if they can be digested at all, does not yield any source of fuel. If a sugar substitute can be broken down by the digestive system at all, the breakdown usually results in chemicals that are toxic to the body. No one would add liquid fertilizer to the fuel tank of their automobile and expect the automobile to run. Ingestion of sugar substitutes, similarly, is of no benefit to the body. In ingesting these artificial chemicals, the body is fooled into believing that some nutritional requirement has been satisfied. A short time later, when the expected nutrients are not found, hunger returns, and the person eats more food. This explains why sugar substitutes actually lead to weight gain, not weight loss.

If the patient is diabetic, the use of sugar substitutes seems to be a way of life. The sugar substitutes, as stated earlier, are of no nutritional value to the body, and ingestion of such products should be simply avoided. Eating high fat cakes and cookies manufactured with chemicals to make it taste sweet is not sound nutrition, and this practice will contribute to other problems commonly associated with diabetes, such as increased risk of heart disease and circulatory problems. Diabetics are typically instructed to select foods with a low glycemic index. This is good advice not only for the diabetic, but for everyone else as well. Natural foods with a low glycemic index are superior in every way to artificial chemical sweeteners manufactured in a chemical laboratory.

The glycemic index is a numerical rating associated with carbohydrate food sources. The rating system takes into account how fast the carbohydrate is digested and absorbed. A food with a low glycemic index will digest slowly and result in a small rise in blood sugar levels. Conversely, a food with a high glycemic index will digest rapidly or need no digestion at all, and will result in a dramatic spike in blood sugar levels. A glycemic index of 70 or more is considered high. A glycemic index of 56 to 69 is considered intermediate or moderate. A glycemic index of 55 or less is considered low, this category comprising the most desirable types of carbohydrate foods. Rather than ranking foods by numerical value, foods are often ranked by which category into which they fall. This makes much more sense, since the difference in effect of a food with a glycemic index of 30 and another with a glycemic index of 31 is negligible.

Foods with a moderate or high glycemic index not only cause dramatic spikes in blood sugar, but also facilitate an overgrowth of yeast in the intestines. Overall, foods with a low glycemic index do not cause the same disruption of the microbial flora of the intestines.

Any properly formulated diet should contain carbohydrates that are primarily of a low glycemic index. This applies to everyone who is interested in maintaining good health, not only those who have a chronic disease or diabetes. The following three figures identify the glycemic category of some common foods. If a food is listed in two categories, the glycemic index of that food is known to increase with ripeness. Bananas, for example, have a high glycemic index when the fruit is very soft and ripe, but a moderate glycemic index when the fruit is firm and less ripe.

Foods assigned a low glycemic index may be consumed without a great concern of inducing large variations of blood sugar levels. Foods with a low glycemic index, listed in Figure 4.6, are assumed to have no added sugar. Adding sugar to any food raises the glycemic index of that food. Dried fruit of the types listed have the same glycemic index as the undried fruit, providing no sugar was added during processing. The following three figures identify those foods with a low, moderate, and high glycemic index. Foods with a moderate glycemic index can be consumed in small quantities from time to time, and should not constitute a significant part of the diet. Foods with a high glycemic index should be avoided completely.

Fruits	Vegetables	Grains	Beverages
Apples	Artichokes	Barley	Carrot Juice
Berries	Apsaragus	Bran Cereals	Grapefruit Juice
Cherries	Azuki Beans	Parboiled Rice	Milk
Grapefruit	Black Eyed Peas	Rye	Soy Milk
Oranges	Broccoli	Wheat kernels	Tea
Peaches	Butter Beans	Whole Grain	
Plums	Bulgur	Pasta	
Pears	Cauliflower	Breads	
	Celery		
	Chickpeas		**Dairy**
	Cucumber		
Nuts and Seeds	Eggplant		Cottage Cheese
	Green Beans		Plain Yogurt
Almonds	Kidney beans		
Flax Seeds	Lentils		
Peanuts	Lettuce		
Pumpkin Seeds	Navy Beans		
Sunflower Seeds	Onions		
Walnuts	Peppers		
	Soybeans		
	Spinach		
	Tomatoes		
	Zucchini		

Figure 4.6   Foods With a Low Glycemic Index

Fruits	Vegetables	Grains	Beverages
Apricots	Beets	Basmati Rice	Apple Juice
Banana	Carrots	Brown Rice	Blueberry Juice
Figs	Corn	Buckwheat	Cherry Juice
Grapes	Lima Beans	Most Pasta	Orange Juice
Mango	Peas	Pita Bread	
Pineapple	Potatoes	Popcorn	
Raisins	Yams	Wild Rice	**Dairy**
Watermelon			
			Custard

Figure 4.7   Foods With a Moderate Glycemic Index

Fruits	Sweeteners	Grains	Beverages
Banana	Brown Sugar	Bagels	Soft Drinks
Papaya	Cane Sugar	Baguette	Sports Drinks
Sweetened Fruit	Corn Syrup	Most Cereals	Sweet Tea
Watermelon	Dextrose	Corn Chips	
	Fructose	Doughnuts	
	Glucose	Millet	
Vegetables	Honey	Muffins	
	Maltodextrin	Pancakes	**Dairy**
Carrots	Molasses	Pretzels	
Parsnips	Sucrose	Shredded Wheat	Ice Cream
Sweet Corn		Waffles	
Yam		White Bread	
		White Rice	

Figure 4.8   Foods With a High Glycemic Index

Fat

Fats, or lipids, are the secondary source of energy for the body. During digestion, fats are broken into smaller molecules. These smaller molecules are termed *fatty acids*. Once absorbed, the majority of these fatty acids are transported to adipose, or fat, tissue where it is stored. Fatty acids are also incorporated into cell membranes, and many other biochemical compounds. Although not as efficient of an energy source as carbohydrate, fats are the most efficient long term storage source of energy for the body. One gram of fat contains nine calories.

Two polyunsaturated fatty acids that cannot be synthesized by the body are linoleic acid (Omega-6) and alpha-linolenic acid (Omega-3). Because they cannot be synthesized by the body, they are termed essential fatty acids. The body, however, can convert these two fatty acids to other fatty acids. Alpha-linoleic acid can be converted by the body to eicosapentaenoic acid and docosahexaenoic acid, which are other members of the Omega-3 group. Linoleic acid can be converted by the body to gamma-linolenic acid and dihomo-gamma-linolenic acid. These essential fatty acids are often sold in supplement form, such as Evening Primrose oil, purified fish oil supplements, and Flax seed oil to name just a few. Alpha-linolenic acid (Omega-3) is an essential fatty acid that is very commonly found to be deficient in the Western diet. Omega-6 and Omega-3 essential acids should be consumed in a 1:1 ratio, in other words, if one gram of Omega-6 is consumed, one gram of Omega-3 should also be consumed. Unfortunately, the ratio of Omega-6 to Omega-3 in the typical Western diet is approximately 20:1. An Omega-3 supplement is therefore generally indicated for most people consuming the typical Western diet. Table 4.9 summarizes the Omega-3 and Omega-6 essential fatty acids.

Class	Fatty Acids	Natural Sources
Omega-3	Alpha linoleic acid, Eicosapentaenoic acid, Docosahexaenoic acid	Flax seeds, Walnuts, Butternuts, Cold water fish, Free-range meats, Cruciferous vegetables
Omega-6	Linoleic acid, Gamma-linolenic acid, Dihomo-gamma-linolenic acid	Nuts, Whole grains, Vegetable oils, Eggs, Meats, Fish

Table 4.9   Essential Fatty Acids

Linoleic acid, an Omega-6 fatty acid, can also be converted in the body to arachidonic acid, a semi essential fatty acid. In this case, *semi essential* means that the body can perform the conversion of linoleic acid to arachidonic acid, but only in limited quantities. Arachidonic acid is the precursor to the biochemical compounds involved in inflammation. On a technical level, arachidonic acid is converted in the body to the cyclooxygenase enzymes COX-1 and COX-2, and subsequent conversion to various prostaglandins then takes place. Drugs marketed as COX-1 or COX-2 inhibitors, commonly known as anti-inflammatory medications, attempts to control inflammation by preventing this conversion from taking place. The actual mechanism of inhibiting the conversion varies from drug to drug. By decreasing the dietary intake of arachidonic acid, a natural limiting effect of inflammation will occur. Arachidonic acid, therefore, should be limited in the diet of anyone who has any chronic inflammatory condition, including autoimmune diseases and heart disease. Foods found to have high levels of arachidonic acid are primarily from animal sources, and include fatty red meats, egg yolks, and organ meats.

Fat substitutes, as with sugar substitutes, are commonly used by individuals who are trying lo lose weight, or who have a fear of gaining weight. Fat substitutes simply should not be used, and again, no room for negotiation can be afforded on this issue. Worse yet are drugs that prevent the body's absorption of fat, which are commonly used for weight loss. If the absorption of fat is inhibited, essential fatty acids are not being absorbed. This can lead to a myriad of disorders that are difficult to detect. In cases where the patient is morbidly obese, use of these fat absorption blocking medications should be used only under the supervision of a competent health practitioner. The health practitioner will monitor the patient and make sure the patient is not deprived of essential fatty acids or other vital nutrients. If a fat blocking drug must be used, essential fatty acid supplementation to the diet will be required. The essential fatty acid supplement, in this case, should be taken at a time as far away as possible from the time the fat blocking drug is taken.

Vitamins

A vitamin is an organic compound required in relatively small amounts by the body, and is used in various biochemical reactions that occur in each cell. A vitamin is defined in the context of an exclusionary nutrient, meaning that it is required by the body, and does not fall into the classification of an amino acid, carbohydrate, fat, mineral, or water. Vitamins are classified as either water soluble or fat soluble. Fat soluble vitamins include A, D, E, H, and K. Water soluble vitamins include the B complex and Vitamin C.

Vitamins are essential for normal growth and development, and play a part in many biochemical reactions of the body. Vitamins can act as catalysts or substrates in biochemical reactions, and are found in every cell of the body. A deficiency in one of these nutrients is certain to result in disease. For example, a Vitamin B1 deficiency causes Beriberi, a Vitamin D deficiency causes Rickets, and Vitamin C deficiency causes Scurvy.

Some vitamins can be stored by the body. These include Vitamins A and D, which are stored in fat cells and the liver, and Vitamin B-12, which is stored in the liver. Significant quantities of other vitamins cannot be stored by the body, and therefore must be obtained through the diet on a daily basis.

Vitamins are primarily obtained through food. Some vitamins can also be obtained through other sources. Vitamin K, which is synthesized by microorganisms in the intestinal tract, is one example of a vitamin that can be obtained from a source other than food. Vitamin D, which is synthesized in the skin in the presence of natural sunlight, is another example. A vague belief exists that, if someone eats a well-balanced diet, a vitamin or mineral supplement is not required. In an ideal world, where the food is naturally grown, and everyone has a perfect diet, this might be true. Much of the food available today, however, is grown is soil depleted of nutrients, hydroponically grown, or grown in foreign countries where the farming industry is unregulated, allowing dangerous chemicals to enter the food supply. Consequently, a vitamin supplement is a necessity for most people living in today's society. If a vitamin supplement is taken, it should generally be taken with the largest meal of the day. Some vitamin supplements are formulated so that two or three tablets are taken per day, in which case one tablet should be taken with breakfast, and the other with dinner. The divided dose of these supplements provides a more constant supply of nutrients to the body. Megavitamin supplements, which contain many times the Recommended Daily Allowance (RDA), should be avoided unless specifically prescribed for a particular condition.

Table 4.10 identifies the vitamins required by human nutrition. A vitamin, unlike other nutrients, is classically designated by a letter, either A, B, C, D, E, H, or K. This is because many forms of any given vitamin are found to exist naturally in plants and animals. For example, Vitamin D has five common forms found in food; Vitamin D1 (ergocalciferol bound with lumisterol), Vitamin D2 (either ergocalciferol or calciferol), Vitamin D3 (cholecalciferol), Vitamin D4 (22-dihydroergocalciferol), and Vitamin D5 (sitocalciferol). If those names are not confusing enough, the International Union of Pure and Applied Chemistry (IUPAC) name of cholecalciferol, the most common form of Vitamin D, is written as:

$$(3\beta,5Z,7E)\text{-}9,10\text{-secocholesta-}5,7,10(19)\text{-trien-3-ol}$$

Since the chemical names of each form of a vitamin can be complicated, letters have been designated to simplify reference to the vitamin. As with Vitamin D, other vitamins can be found in nature in various forms. The name of the vitamin shown in the table is the most common form. The amounts suggested in the table are guidelines for a normal, healthy adult. The actual vitamin requirements of the body depend on many factors, including current health status, physical activities, stress levels, sex, age, and many other factors that vary from person to person. For example, the Vitamin D requirement of the body increases with age. This increased requirement is because the biochemical mechanisms associated with Vitamin D metabolism decrease in efficiency as a person gets older. The same increased requirement with age is true regarding Vitamin E. The amounts in the table are not the amounts that should be obtained through a vitamin supplement. Taking a vitamin supplement adds to the total daily vitamin intake, much of which has already been obtained through the diet.

All vitamins have a U.S. Recommended Daily Allowance (RDA) associated with them. The Recommended Daily Allowance is published by the National Institute of Health (NIH). Many countries have similar organizations and researchers who publish their own recommendations based upon their own findings. All of this in-depth research concludes that the recommended intake level of a particular vitamin varies from country to country. Since the biochemistry of the human organism is relatively constant from country to country, the variation in recommendations is due to differing conclusions from expert researchers. Many factors determine the required level of a particular nutrient, and vitamins are no exception. Factors such as diet, stress levels, and overall health all contribute to the nutritional requirements of the body, and adjustments to the daily allowance must subsequently be made based upon these factors. This could explain, in part, why the body's requirement of certain vitamins varies from one civilization to another.

Vitamin	Name	Water / Fat Soluble	Recommended Amount *
A	Retinol	Fat	1000-5000 IU
B1	Thiamine	Water	10 - 50 mg.
B2	Riboflavin	Water	10 - 50 mg.
B3	Niacin	Water	15 mg.
B5	Pantothenic Acid	Water	10 - 150 mg.
B6	Pyridoxine	Water	10 - 100 mg.
B9	Folic Acid	Water	400 - 800 mcg.
B12	Cyanocobalamin	Water	10 - 100 mcg.
C	Ascorbate	Water	500 - 3000 mg.
D	Cholecalciferol	Fat	200 - 600 IU
E	alpha-tocopherol	Fat	200 - 1000 IU
H	Biotin	Water	30 - 300 mcg.
K	Phylloquinone	Fat	10 - 60 mcg.

Table 4.10   Vitamins

* The recommended amount is NOT the RDA

Any well-versed biochemist would agree that the Recommended Daily Allowance of certain vitamins is inaccurate. Vitamin C is a perfect example of this. At one time, the RDA of Vitamin C was 60 mg. The Recommended Daily Allowance of Vitamin C was recently revised upward to 90 mg. for the average adult. The biochemistry of the body suggests that even the revised figure be still inadequate. It appears, in some cases, that the RDA is an amount that is set to prevent the onset of illness or disease. Since illness is often determined to exist when some symptom has appeared, this is a poor way to determine the body's requirements for any nutrient. Nearly all nutritional requirements of the body are raised, for example, during physical activity. Bodybuilders, who are very meticulous about exercise and nutrition, have a much higher vitamin requirement than the person who leads a sedentary lifestyle. Limiting the diet of the bodybuilder to the recommended daily intake of nutrients is sure to result in a nutritionally deficient state, decreased performance, and possibly disease. The recommended amounts depicted in the table, therefore, represent a consensus of various reputable international organizations.

Vitamin supplements are used to ensure that adequate amounts of these nutrients are present for the biochemical reactions that they support. If the appropriate vitamins are not present, the associated biochemical reactions in the body cannot go to completion. A biochemical reaction that cannot go to completion is essentially "hung" in that state, awaiting some nutrient to become available. An accumulation of these hung reactions is not good for the body, and is direct evidence of malnutrition. When the vitamin becomes available, the hung reaction then can proceed toward completion.

Minerals

Minerals, in reference to nutrition, are the ionized form of the chemical elements that are required by the body. A mineral is an inorganic compound, as opposed to proteins, carbohydrates, fats, and vitamins, which are all organic compounds. Minerals are sometimes sub-classified, and sometimes referred to as electrolytes, macrominerals, or trace minerals. Minerals, however they are classified, are still minerals. Any subclassification is done merely for convenience sake.

The group of macrominerals consists of Calcium, Phosphorus, and Magnesium. They are termed *macrominerals* because the daily requirement of these minerals is quite significant when compared with trace minerals. Sodium, Potassium, and Chloride are commonly known as the electrolytes. Some authorities also consider Calcium and Magnesium to be electrolytes. Table 4.11 identifies the minerals that are required in human metabolism.

Minerals play a vital part in just about every metabolic process of the body. Minerals, particularly trace minerals, act as catalysts for many biochemical reactions that occur in the body. Minerals also play an important role in the transmission of nerve impulses. Muscular contractions are largely dependent on proper mineral balance. The crystalline structure of bone is made up of minerals, primarily Calcium and Phosphorus. Other minerals are also found in bone tissue. Minerals play an important role in the water balance of the body. The importance of minerals in metabolism cannot be understated. With minerals involved in every facet of metabolism, the dietary importance of obtaining adequate amounts of these nutrients is vital to good health.

When it comes to minerals, obtaining the appropriate quantities of each mineral through the diet or through a mineral supplement is the key. Taking more minerals than that which is required by the body is not necessarily better. For every nutrient of the body, a certain dietary requirement exists, and this particularly applies to trace minerals. Trace minerals are required in only small amounts by the body; this is why they are called trace minerals. Excess consumption of trace minerals usually results in toxicity. Excessive consumption of Manganese, for example, can cause Parkinson like symptoms.

An overdose of Iron or fluoride has been known to cause death. This does not mean that minerals should be avoided, but emphasizes the fact that there is an appropriate amount required by the body.

Some authorities consider certain minerals, such Strontium, to be required by the body, but the nutritional need for this mineral is reported to be not fully understood. The reason that the need for Strontium is not fully understood is because no biochemical reaction can be found in the body supporting the necessity of Strontium. Strontium is radioactive, and the belief that there is a need for this mineral in human metabolism is absurd. Strontium, however, has been detected in human bone tissue. Lead has also been found in human bone tissue, and is nothing more that an indicator that the person has been exposed to Lead, and perhaps suffers from Lead poisoning. The presence of a mineral in the body does not necessarily suggest a need for that mineral, but is an indicator of the toxicity of the environment in which we live.

A commonly available mineral supplement is available that is reported to contain more than 50 naturally occurring minerals. This dietary supplement states, on the label, that the minerals are in their natural concentrations as found in natural seawater in varying trace amounts. Among the minerals reported to be in these supplements are Rubidium, Nickel, Strontium, Lanthanum, Cerium, Yttrium, Gallium, Cesium, Beryllium, and Holmium. The label on this type of supplement often states something to the effect of "plus other minerals naturally found in seawater." These *other minerals* are left unmentioned by name for obvious reasons, and include Lead, Aluminum and Uranium. No biochemical basis exists whatever for the presence of any these minerals in the human body. Nickel, in fact, can cause an immune system reaction, and the dangers of Lead and Aluminum are well documented. Manufacturing a supplement that contains an element such as radioactive Strontium is absurd. Any mineral supplement of this character is, based on the label alone, to be considered toxic, and therefore should be avoided. If such a supplement is already owned, it should be discarded. Do not crush the tablets and use them for plant fertilizer. The content of the supplement may actually harm the plant.

Blood tests are generally a poor method of determining the need for a particular mineral. Tissue levels of minerals are more important in determining the need for a specific mineral nutrient, but are difficult to measure analytically. Deficiency of some minerals can be determined by symptoms and the patient history. For example, whenever a patient complains of muscle spasms, the levels of Calcium and Magnesium in the muscle tissue are generally found low. Blood levels of Calcium and Magnesium, however, will most likely be found within normal limits. This is because the physiology of the body maintains a serum Calcium level of 8.5 to 10.2 mg/dl and a serum Magnesium level at 1.5 to 2.6 mg/dl. To maintain constant serum levels of these minerals, the body will transfer Calcium from the bones and Magnesium from the muscles to the blood. Another example of a mineral imbalance involves muscle cramps in the calves, feet, hands, forearms, or in any combination. Cramps of this nature are usually due to a deficiency of the mineral Potassium. Increasing the dietary intake of Potassium either through a supplement or foods high in

Potassium should relieve the muscle cramps. In short, blood tests cannot always be relied upon in determining the need for a specific mineral.

Most minerals have a U.S. Recommended Daily Allowance (RDA) associated with them. The Recommended Daily Allowance of these minerals is published by the National Institute of Health (NIH). As with all nutrients, various other countries have similar organizations that publish their own recommendations, based upon their research findings and understanding of nutrition. Again, as with other nutrients, the published recommended amounts vary from government to government. Significant research efforts are always underway to determine the requirements of specific nutrients by the body. The conclusion of this research is significantly skewed based upon many dietary and other factors. One such dietary factor involves the metabolism of Calcium. Ingestion of carbonated beverages, which contain phosphoric acid, have been linked to osteoporosis. Phosphoric acid is known to disrupt the Calcium / Phosphorous ratio of the blood. This subsequently leads to a decreased serum level of Calcium. In response to this decreased Calcium level, Calcium is transferred from the bones to the blood. As a result of this effect of carbonated beverages, the Calcium requirement can significantly increase in persons who consume such beverages. Many dietary factors may account for the variation in recommendations from expert researchers.

The daily requirement of certain minerals also varies with activity level. The body's requirements of certain other minerals are less affected by activity levels. Calcium and Magnesium requirements are significantly increased with prolonged heavy physical exertion. Bodybuilders, weight lifters, athletes, and anyone with a job that entails physical exertion require more Calcium and Magnesium than the RDA would normally suggest. Calcium and Magnesium should be ingested in a 2:1 ratio; that is, two parts Calcium to one part Magnesium. If 1000 mg. of Calcium is ingested, 500 mg. of Magnesium should also be ingested. Electrolyte levels decrease with physical exertion, particularly in hot weather. For this reason, Calcium, Magnesium, Sodium and Potassium must be replenished during physical activity in hot climates. Not a year goes by that a high school football player dies of a cardiac arrhythmia or dehydration caused by electrolyte imbalances during Summer training. The sad part is that this loss of life could have been completely avoided by a few dollars of supplements and adequate water intake. What we should learn from this tragedy is that the nutritional requirements of the body, particularly when it comes to certain minerals, depend greatly on physical activity level and environmental conditions.

Mineral	Recommended Amount *	Comments
Calcium	800 – 3000 mg.	Requirement is proportional to physical activity level.
Chloride	1000 – 2500 mg.	Supplementation usually is not needed.
Chromium	35 – 200 mcg.	A common dietary deficiency.
Copper	0.5 – 2 mg.	Overdose leads to toxicity.
Fluoride	≤ 1 mg.	Adequate amounts are obtained through the diet.
Iodine	150 mcg.	Deficiencies rare due to iodized salt.
Iron	5 – 20 mg.	Overdose leads to toxicity.
Magnesium	400 – 1500 mg.	Requirement is proportional to physical activity level.
Manganese	2 – 4 mg.	Overdose leads to toxicity.
Molybdenum	25 – 200 mcg.	Overdose leads to toxicity.
Phosphorus	800 – 3000 mg.	Supplementation usually not needed. Should be equal to Calcium intake.
Potassium	3000 – 6000 mg.	
Selenium	50 – 250 mcg.	Overdose leads to toxicity.
Sodium	1000 – 3000 mg.	Supplementation is usually not necessary.
Zinc	10 – 20 mg.	

Table 4.11   Minerals Required for Human Nutrition

* The recommended amount is NOT the RDA

Water

Water is a vital nutrient to the body. Water is also the most abundant nutrient in the body. Cells are made up of mostly water, and every biochemical reaction that occur in these cells takes place in the presence of water. On a larger scale, the wastes and by-products of metabolism are eliminated in a medium of water.

Most people do not drink enough water and are in a chronic state of dehydration. The question always arises "how much water should I drink?" The answer is quite simple. A good general rule is to drink 1 ounce of water for every 2 pounds of body weight. In other words, if a person weighs 150 pounds, they should drink a minimum of 75 ounces of water a day. The intake of water should be increased above that level during hot weather and days of heavy physical activity, such as exercise. A decrease in sodium intake causes the body to eliminate more water, and may require an increased water intake, particularly in hot weather. Limiting the intake of sodium, therefore, can disrupt the water and mineral balance of the body.

Large quantities of water should not be consumed with meals. Excessive water ingested during a meal dilutes the digestive enzymes, resulting in the incomplete digestion of food. Drinking a small amount of water, however, with a meal helps with digestion. Drinking a large glass of water, for example eight to sixteen ounces, an hour or two following a meal will help transport the digested food through the intestinal tract.

Consumption of enormous quantities of water is dangerous. Large quantities of water must be flushed out of the body, taking with it vital electrolytes and other minerals. The continued intake of water far beyond the recommended amounts can cause significant damage to the Hypothalamus gland.

A popular belief is that drinking tea and coffee do not contribute to the daily total of water consumption. This belief is based upon the thought that coffee and tea contain caffeine, and that, since caffeine is a diuretic, it will eliminate water from the body. While caffeine does have mild diuretic properties, the diuretic effect from the amount of caffeine present in either coffee or tea is insufficient to eliminate anywhere near the water contained in the drink from the body.

Fiber

Fiber is an important part of the diet. Specifically, the role of fiber in human nutrition is to promote and maintain the health of the digestive tract. Although fiber cannot be digested, is not a nutrient required for human nutrition at the biochemical level, and technically has no nutritional value, fiber is very important in the digestive process. Fiber is inherently found in many foods of the diet. A diet with appropriate fiber has been shown to decrease the likelihood of certain diseases, such as elevated cholesterol, diverticulosis, and constipation. Increased fiber intake has been shown to decrease the risk of some cancers. A diet rich in fiber is also associated with improved glucose tolerance.

Two types of dietary fiber, soluble and insoluble fiber, exist. Both soluble and insoluble fiber play different roles in digestion. Soluble fibers are those that dissolve in water, insoluble fibers are those that do not dissolve in water.

Soluble fiber, which dissolves in water, absorbs excess liquid in the colon, forming a thick gel and adding bulk as it passes intact through the intestines.

This gel keeps the intestinal muscles stretched slightly, aiding in the peristaltic contractions of the muscular wall of the intestines that move the digested food through easily. Soluble fiber is valuable in preventing both diarrhea and constipation. Excess cholesterol found in the intestines is absorbed by soluble fiber. Soluble fiber has also been found to help in the normalization of blood sugar levels.

Insoluble fiber plays a vital role in maintaining the health of the digestive tract. Insoluble fiber increases bulk, softens the stools, cleanses the small and large intestine, and shortens the transit time of the digested food through the intestinal tract. By decreasing the transit time of the digested food, regularity is promoted. Many colon cleansing products are found to have high amounts of insoluble fiber.

Foods that contain fiber generally contain both insoluble and soluble fiber. The diet should contain approximately 30 grams of fiber daily. Approximately one-half the daily fiber intake should be insoluble fiber, and one-half should be soluble fiber. Consuming excessive amounts of fiber, as with the excessive consummation of any nutrient, is not recommended. When the diet contains an appropriate balance of fiber, regularity of elimination of waste is promoted.

The best sources of fiber are natural foods. Fruits, vegetables, grains, and seeds are all excellent sources. Highly processed foods are generally devoid of fiber. If a dietary supplement of fiber is used, the supplement should be properly formulated to contain appropriate amounts of soluble and insoluble fiber. Avoid supplements which only contain exclusively soluble or insoluble fiber unless otherwise directed by your health practitioner.

When it comes time to purchase a supplement of any type, how, then do we choose a quality vitamin, mineral, fiber, or other supplement? The question always arises as to what is a quality supplement and what supplements are a waste of money. With many brands of supplements lining the shelves of grocery stores, pharmacies, discount houses, and health food stores, it becomes increasingly complicated and confusing to decide which supplements are high quality and which supplements are of poor quality. Calcium supplements, for example, can be found in the form of Calcium oxide, Calcium carbonate, Calcium citrate, and a few other forms as well. While the lower cost of the Calcium oxide supplement may look like a good deal when compared with the Calcium citrate supplement, Calcium citrate has a far superior absorption rate in the intestinal tract than does Calcium oxide. When the absorption rate is factored into the equation, the supplement containing Calcium citrate actually is less expensive than the poorly absorbed Calcium oxide product. Calcium citrate, in this example, is clearly the better product. In addition, any advice in determining which supplements are appropriate for any particular condition will simply not be found in a grocery store or pharmacy. When purchasing a supplement, clearly the best place to purchase quality products is through a store that specializes in vitamins and health foods. Independent health food or vitamin stores stock a variety of high quality products. The owners of these independent stores are usually well known by their customers, and are often willing to order special products for them upon request. In addition, the employees of the independent store are generally very knowledgeable about the products they sell. These stores often work with natural health care providers, stocking products recommended by the health care providers in the area.

The components that make up the cells of the body are replaced on a continual basis. The chemical nutrients resulting from the digestion of food are assimilated into the body, and incorporated into the cells of the body. When a chemical is not needed, it is eliminated by the body. In this sense, the body attempts to maintain a balance of nutrients, retaining what is expected to be needed in the future, and eliminating what is of no immediate value. In an ideal situation, an individual would only consume exactly what is needed to fulfil the body's short term needs. This, however, is an unreasonable and unattainable goal. What is attainable, however, is developing a diet that will come close to meeting the nutritional needs of the body, taking into consideration certain issues of biochemical individuality.

Any deficiencies, excesses or imbalances of nutrients in the diet will eventually lead to undesirable effects on health. These undesirable effects can lead to specific diseases, such as obesity, Beriberi, or osteoporosis. Nonspecific diseases, including many syndromes, are often a result of an improper diet. Improper nutrition will also have some effect on any disease of psychological origin.

Malnutrition typically occurs when a nutrient or nutrients are missing from the diet. Malnutrition will ultimately result in disease; the type of disease that develops is largely determined by which nutrient or nutrients are missing from the diet. When we think of malnutrition, we usually think of third world countries where people are starving with little or no food to eat. This is not always the case. Malnutrition, by definition, simply means bad nutrition. Bad nutrition can mean the deficiency of one nutrient, multiple nutrients, or the excessive consumption of any nutrient. When we see someone who is morbidly obese, we do not think that they are suffering from malnutrition, but, in fact, this is the case. The nutrition of the morbidly obese person is hardly within the realm of proper and adequate nutrition. In some cases, the obese person is lacking some specific nutrients, and the over consumption of foods occurs as a result of the body making a desperate attempt to obtain that nutrient. Many cases involving the overweight patient reveal a specific amino acid that is found deficient in the diet, easily revealed by an amino acid profile laboratory test. Food cravings typically involve the desire for fatty foods or carbohydrates. Rarely, however, does a person crave protein, the source of amino acids. If proper nutrition is restored along with other dietary and lifestyle changes, the cravings for foods will most likely subside.

With any nutrient, a proper amount exists that is needed by the body. This amount depends on many factors, such as age, sex, activity level, and the environment to name a few. These amounts can vary from time to time, and change based upon certain factors, such as stress level, muscle strains, or any illness such as the common cold or influenza.

If a nutrient is found in deficient quantities for any reason, the biochemical reactions that involve that nutrient cannot occur, or occur at a level that is insufficient to meet the body's metabolic requirements. In our three causes leading to disease of the body, this falls into the category of:

Something that should be in the body is not in the body

If excess nutrients are ingested, the body becomes overloaded, and is unable to utilize the excess. When this happens, the nutrient must either be stored or eliminated from the body. In many cases, the body is unable to eliminate the excess efficiently, saturating the body not only with nutrients it cannot use, but the by-products of its breakdown as well. Of the three causes leading to disease of the body, this falls into the category of:

Something enters into the body, but, for some reason, the body can no longer process it correctly

In this case, *for some reason* refers to the saturation of the body's biochemical mechanisms designed to handle the particular nutrient. When the biochemical mechanisms designed to process any nutrient become overloaded, the excess nutrients accumulate and ultimately interfere with any number of other biochemical processes that are occurring. This invariably causes a problem at the biochemical level. Problems at the biochemical level are often the origin of disease.

When dietary excess or dietary deficiency of any nutrient is found to exist, disease can result. This is the root cause, or the beginning, of the disease process, and is almost never accompanied by symptoms. In fact, improper nutrition can occur for several years before the first symptom is even apparent.

With all the simultaneous biochemical reactions occurring in the body, many nutrients are required for these reactions to complete. A particular biochemical reaction may require several key components to complete properly. These may include amino acids, various enzymes, vitamins, and minerals to name just a few. If one or more of the vital components of these reactions are not present, the biochemical reaction started cannot go to completion. When this is the case, the biochemical reaction is suspended in a "hung" state, waiting on some nutrient to be provided to enable its completion. When the missing component finally becomes available, the biochemical reaction then may proceed to the next step, and barring any other unavailable components, going to completion and accomplish the purpose for which it was originally started. Obtaining adequate nutrition will virtually eliminate these hung reactions, therefore, eliminating one potential factor in the development of disease.

Competition among biochemical reactions for the available nutrients is frequently found. When adequate nutrients are present, all reactions requiring that particular nutrient occur unhindered and go to completion. Whenever a deficiency of a particular nutrient exists, the body must decide which biochemical reaction is more important. Whenever the body is presented with this dilemma, survival always wins over comfort. The conversion of tryptophan to either niacin or serotonin exemplifies this quite well. While both are ultimately important, niacin is more important for survival than is serotonin. If the body has a deficiency of niacin, any tryptophan ingested will be promptly converted to niacin. If an adequate level of niacin is present, the conversion of tryptophan to serotonin is then facilitated. Low serotonin levels have been implicated in depression. If low niacin levels exist due to improper nutrition, seeing why depression can result is not hard. In this example, restoration of niacin and tryptophan levels through the temporary use of dietary supplements would logically cause the depression to resolve.

An accumulation of hung biochemical reactions is the first step in the development of certain diseases or disorders. This is evident with specific vitamin deficiencies, where a specific deficiency subsequently leads to a very specific and well-defined disease. Hung biochemical reactions, however, are not limited to vitamin deficiencies. Other nutrients, such as amino acids, essential fatty acids, and minerals are all vital components in biochemical reactions. If these nutrients are not present in adequate quantities, especially over the long term, many disorders can subsequently result. Some of these disorders are vague, and some are very specific in nature. Copper, for example, is a mineral involved in electron transfer reactions in certain critical metabolic pathways. These pathways involve cellular respiration, pigment formation, connective tissue formation, neurotransmitter synthesis, and protein formation, among others. The result of Copper deprivation produces very vague symptoms, all of which can easily be explained by any number of disorders. Essential fatty acids are yet another example. Essential fatty acids play a part in many metabolic processes, and any deficiency of these required nutrients have widespread consequences in the body. A deficiency of the essential fatty acids often produces no discernable symptoms, but tissue damage proceeds to occur nevertheless.

Lack of nutrients can also occur on a larger scale as well. Protein deficiency is common among persons taking antacids and medications designed to suppress hydrochloric acid secretion in the stomach. These medications are commonly prescribed for ulcers and acid reflux disease. Unfortunately, these medications also inhibit protein digestion by either neutralizing the acid medium of the stomach or suppressing the secretion of the acid required by the enzymes that perform protein digestion. As a result, amino acids, which are the products of protein digestion, become scarce. Amino acids are vital nutrients in rebuilding damaged tissue of the intestinal lining. The result is that the body does not have adequate nutrients to rebuild the lining of the digestive tract. This lack of nutrients is precisely why persons taking these acid neutralizing and inhibiting medications never really get well, but instead get worse as time goes on. The very nutrients needed to rebuild the intestinal lining become scarce and unavailable as a result of the medications used to alleviate the symptoms. The lack of amino acids, however, is not confined to the intestinal tract. Every cell in the body requires amino acids, as does the synthesis of neurotransmitters, digestive enzymes, and immunoglobulins. As a result, long term deficiency of these nutrients can lead to serious consequences, including depression, decreased immune system function, and muscular weakness to name a few.

Over saturation of nutrients in the body presents a similar problem. Excessive nutrients must either be stored or broken down and eliminated from the body. In the case where the nutrient must be broken down, a burden is placed on various organs to carry out the steps required for its elimination from the body. This breakdown process usually involves the liver and kidneys. In the liver, enzymes break down the nutrient into smaller components that can readily be eliminated from the body. Following the enzymatic breakdown of these nutrients in the liver, they are dumped back into the bloodstream and eventually make their way to the kidneys. The kidneys then eliminate the toxic waste through the urine. What may not be obvious is the fact that the toxic waste from the breakdown of the excessive nutrients is circulating in the bloodstream for days before being completely eliminated. Since the blood travels through all bodily tissues, an accumulation of these toxins in the tissues occurs. This accumulation of waste in the tissues is often seen in persons with chronic disorders, such as fibromyalgia, chronic fatigue syndrome, or chronic stress.

The effect of excessive ingestion of a nutrient can be examined, again using tryptophan as an example. Someone may have heard or read that tryptophan helps with depression, and subsequently purchases a tryptophan dietary supplement, and then proceeds to take many times the recommended dose, against all reasonable recommendations. Excessive tryptophan consumption upregulates the kynurenine pathway, the body's tryptophan elimination mechanism, allowing more efficient degradation and elimination of the excess tryptophan. This excess tryptophan will activate a liver enzyme *tryptophan pyrrolase*, which breaks down the surplus tryptophan. To cope with the increasing levels of tryptophan, the liver compensates by synthesizing more of the enzyme *tryptophan pyrrolase*. In addition, when ingested tryptophan levels return to normal, usually when the supplement bottle is empty, the up-regulated elimination mechanism is still present, and will require time to down-regulate back to a normal level. With the ingestion of tryptophan returning to a normal level, and excess levels of *tryptophan pyrrolase* now found in the liver, any ingested tryptophan is efficiently eliminated rather than being utilized. The practice of ingesting excess nutrients always comes at cost. Excess nutrients require energy to break down, and the toxic by-products as a result of this breakdown circulate in the blood and accumulate in the bodily tissues. Ingesting excessive nutrients, therefore, is of no benefit to the body.

The use of megavitamin supplements is another instance in which the body becomes over saturated with nutrients. With some vitamins, such as Vitamin C and most of the B complex, the body readily excretes any excess. This is not true with several other vitamins, such as Vitamins A and D, where any excess is stored in the liver and adipose, or fat, tissue. Excessive ingestion of Vitamin A, for example, is very toxic to the liver. Just a few of the symptoms associated with Vitamin A toxicity include fatigue, vague gastrointestinal complaints, headaches, muscle pain, joint pain, changes in bone structure, alopecia (hair loss), and, to the unborn fetus, birth defects. Remember that symptoms are always the last thing to appear in any disease process. In the case of Vitamin A toxicity, the symptoms are as a result of tissue damage that has been occurring for quite some time. Whereas appropriate vitamin levels in the body are beneficial to health, excessive consumption of vitamins can be just as detrimental to health as a vitamin deficiency.

As a general rule, no nutrient should be consumed in quantities significantly greater than is found naturally in foods. Any exceptions to this rule would be in treating specific nutritionally related conditions that have arisen as a result of some disease process. When treating specific conditions, the appropriate use of supplements would generally dictate short term use rather than long term use. Long term use of supplements may be required under certain circumstances, and are generally indicated when certain genetic factors, biochemical individuality, specific disease processes, or any combination of these are present. Prolonged use of certain vitamin supplements can result in dependancy states requiring the elevated levels of the particular vitamin be always present. Vitamin dependancy states are most often observed with the B-complex. Overloading the body with excess nutrients is of no benefit to the body, and is actually counterproductive.

Nutrients are normally obtained through the food we eat. With all these considerations of the various nutrients to take into account, what, then, constitutes a normal meal? To answer this question, we must remove ourselves from the modern day technologically-based society, and examine how the average person would eat given a more primitive society without a grocery store or restaurant on every corner. Before modern technology, many chronic diseases of today's society were rare or nonexistent. Examining the dietary practices of civilization before modern technology came on the scene will reveal significant differences in the way the population ate. Mass transportation, refrigeration, and technology to preserve foods have all contributed significantly to the ease of obtaining just about any food product desired. On one hand this is a major advancement of society, on the other hand it leads to dietary practices that are unnatural and subsequently lead to the decline of health. Societal advancements, in this regard, have virtually eliminated diseases such as Scurvy, but, in their place, have opened the door to the development of food allergies and food hypersensitivities. In essence, what has happened is that one problem was traded for another.

Until the early twentieth century, people were forced to eat what foods were readily available and are in season. Refrigeration was nonexistent, transportation of food was limited, short term preservation was done with salt, and any long term preservation was done by canning. Consequently, most foods had to be consumed shortly after being harvested. This food was organically grown, not genetically modified, grown without the use of pesticides, and arrived at the dinner table fresh. Crops were rotated on the land on which they were grown, and at the end of the season the dead plant material was recycled and used as fertilizer for next year's crop. Food was not highly processed, most often sold fresh, and artificial chemicals, such as dyes and preservatives, were never used. In addition to the fresh produce available in the local market, many people grew their own fruits and vegetables, providing a constant supply of fresh food for the duration of the growing season.

Foods naturally grown contain many types of beneficial bacteria on the surface. These beneficial bacteria are found in or on most foods obtained from a natural source, including fruits and vegetables. The beneficial bacteria are passed on to products manufactured by these foods providing nothing is done to destroy them. One hundred years ago, a piece of fruit would have been picked from a tree, possibly rinsed off, and then eaten. Modern methods of processing food, such as Pasteurization or irradiation, are intended to destroy any harmful bacteria that may be present on the food. Unfortunately, the processes of Pasteurization and irradiation also destroy the beneficial bacteria required for normal digestive system health. Today, fruit available from modern retail outlets has most likely been washed, irradiated, washed again, gassed, sprayed with fungicide, and shined up for display Saturday morning in the produce section of the grocery store. Before it is eaten, it is washed again, ensuring that it is sterilized to the highest degree before entering the digestive tract. Lacking any beneficial bacteria, much of the health benefits of the food have been lost. Oddly, the act of picking a piece of fruit off a tree and eating it is commonly thought of as poor hygiene. Anyone who has ever picked an ugly piece fruit off a tree and eaten it realizes that the naturally grown fruit tastes better than the fruit from the grocery store.

Today, many more types of foods are available than decades ago. The corner grocery store carries thousands of products, many of which are imported from foreign countries. As a result, anyone can walk into a grocery store and select any of the products they want. By having a choice, many people fall into the same repetitive dietary habits, selecting only those foods that they really like to eat. Limiting the selection of foods in the diet causes several problems. The first problem is, due to the lack of variety, certain nutrients may be lacking in the diet. The second problem, again due to lack of variety, an excess of certain nutrients may be present in the diet. The third problem is repeated exposure to the same foods can cause an immune system reaction, such as either a food hypersensitivity or a food allergy. Finally, over exposure to certain foods can cause gastric complaints, such as indigestion or irritation to the intestinal lining.

Most gastric complaints are as of a result of improper food combining. These problems can be eliminated if food were eaten in appropriate quantities and combined correctly. Following a few simple rules should prevent any digestive problems, and ensure that the food consumed is fully digested and assimilated properly. To understand how to combine foods correctly, the process of digestion must be understood, at least on a basic level. In addition, some knowledge of the six classes of nutrients is desirable to make informed decisions and choices regarding the diet.

Digestion of food is performed by enzymes. Each enzyme is very specific in its action. Certain enzymes act upon proteins, other enzymes act upon carbohydrates, and yet other enzymes act upon fats. Enzymes are very specific, the enzymes that act upon one class of food do not and cannot act upon another class of food. Different enzymes are also required at the various stages of digestion. The proper action of an enzyme at any given stage is dependent on the previous stage of digestion being completed by the appropriate enzymes. If the digestive system is overloaded in any single meal by either too many types of foods or too much food, the enzymes cannot properly do their job. Meals, then, should be kept as simple as possible.

Any meal should only contain a few different types of foods. By limiting the number of types of foods at each meal, it ensures that the enzymes participating in digestion can do their job, and each stage of digestion can be properly completed. On the other hand, eating a large variety of foods during any meal decreases the likelihood that the food is digested properly. By making appropriate choices, digestion can be properly completed, and assimilation of the nutrients can properly occur.

Soups, salads, breads, and other appetizers are customarily served with or before the modern day meal. If soup is to be served with the meal, it should be served before the meal, and the portion size should be limited to a cup, not a large bowl. Any salad should be served with the meal or eaten afterwards, not before. The practice of serving bread with meals is of little nutritional benefit, and simply should not be done. Breads made from refined grains, typically served with butter or dipped in high fat oil and spice combinations, are empty calories and will be added immediately to the body's fat reserves. Eating something that will eventually have to be worked off later during exercise is of no benefit. It is simpler, and healthier, not to eat these foods in the first place.

Appetizers are also a part of the modern day dining experience. Appetizers present an entirely different problem. An appetizer, as typically served in a restaurant, is a meal in itself. The typical appetizer is a high fat, low nutrition food, and, as with breads, should simply be avoided. Occasionally, raw vegetables are served before a meal, and are generally not a problem providing the high calorie dipping sauce often served with the vegetable tray is avoided. Oddly, after eating an appetizer, most people are no longer hungry, yet they continue with the dining extravaganza with the main course, and continue all the way through dessert.

When it comes to eating bread, only whole grain bread made without processed sugar or flour are of any nutritional benefit. If butter needs to be spread over the bread to make it taste good, the bread, and the butter for that matter, is best left uneaten and thrown away. Bread manufactured from highly refined and processed flour should not be consumed. This includes most of the breads found in the grocery store. If having bread is desirable, homemade whole grain bread is simple to make and will provide much greater nutrition to the body than the grocery store brands. Local farmers' markets often make their own bread made with natural, unprocessed ingredients. These also make a much better choice.

The main course of any meal, traditionally meat, should be kept as simple as possible. Meat, whether it is fish, chicken, beef, pork, lamb, or other meat, should be kept to a portion size that is readily and completely digestible by the body. For an adult over the age of 25 or 30, this size is about three to eight ounces. Anything more than this amount is unnecessary to consume since it will not be completely digested. Not mixing different types of animal protein sources in any given meal is desirable, and is easier for the body to digest. If the meal is chicken, keep it to chicken, if the meal is pork, keep it to just pork.

Vegetables are also traditionally part of the main course. While having a variety of vegetables in the diet is important, during any single meal it is preferable to only eat two or three different types. Choosing fresh vegetables that are organically grown and are in season is the best choice. Vegetables are an excellent source of carbohydrates, and, since the carbohydrates found in vegetables are not highly concentrated, it does not overload the digestive system and does not cause drastic blood sugar swings. While many different types of vegetables are typically available, most people limit their choices to only a few that they happen to like. Limiting the diet in this manner paves the way to immune system reactions, food hypersensitivities, and food allergies. By eating a variety of vegetables, the likelihood of an immune system reaction is significantly reduced. A good practice to avoid overexposure to any particular vegetable is to try a new vegetable every week. Vegetables can generally be a part of any meal, however, vegetables that are very acidic should be avoided in a meal where protein is served.

Most vegetables are preferably eaten in the raw or minimally cooked state. Excessive cooking destroys much of the nutritional content of the vegetable, including many vitamins. Raw food often contains certain enzymes that aid in the digestion of the food. Enzymes have a very specific three-dimensional shape and are structurally unstable at high temperatures. Cooking, especially at high temperatures, destroys these enzymes by distorting their structure, rendering them inactive. The technical term of this distorted enzyme is a *denatured enzyme* or a *denatured protein*. Vegetables also contain various strains of natural beneficial bacteria on the surface. Cooking at excessively high temperatures destroys these bacteria, decreasing the overall nutritional value of the food. Organically grown raw vegetables from a home garden should be part of any healthy diet.

Starches, such as potatoes and rice, can be added to the meal provided the portions are kept small. The combination of starches and protein together in the same meal inhibits digestion. Therefore, eating protein foods and starches at different times is best. Since starches do not combine well with proteins, this is evidence that the classical steak and potato dinner is not exactly the best meal choice. The quantity of starch foods typically consumed supply more calories than the body's immediate requirement. Since starches are very dense forms of carbohydrate, any extra calories consumed are quickly converted to fat. It makes no sense to consume more calories in the form of carbohydrate foods than meets the short term needs of the body. The excess fat resulting from eating excess carbohydrates will only result in extra exercise later to burn it off.

Water is the best drink to consume during meals, and should be kept to a small amount. Excessive liquid consumption during a meal will dilute digestive enzymes, inhibiting the digestion of the food consumed. Unsweetened tea is also a good beverage choice at mealtime. Carbonated beverages contain acids, specifically carbonic and phosphoric acid, which interfere with the digestion process. Sweetened drinks contain refined sugar and should be avoided. The refined sugar in soft drinks and sweetened tea also causes tremendous blood sugar swings, which contributes to the sleepiness that often follows an hour or so later. Diet drinks containing chemical artificial sweeteners should be avoided. Milk is another beverage to be avoided during meals. In Western society, milk seems to the standard issue drink for children at mealtime. This constant exposure to milk over a period of years explains why milk is among the leading food allergens in adulthood.

Occasionally, eating between meals is necessary. A piece of fruit makes an excellent choice. Dried fruit is another alternative, providing it is not loaded with preservatives. Since dried fruit is dehydrated, some water must be drunk with the fruit so that it will be rehydrated in the stomach. Other good choices for snacks are nuts, however, since nuts can take several hours to digest fully, they are best eaten as a snack between meals, and not right before a meal. Nuts are also rich in essential fatty acids, a vital nutrient that is often found deficient in the Western diet.

Certain foods should never be combined with other foods. Nuts and melons fall into this category. Digestion of these foods is not compatible with the digestion of other foods. Either make a meal out of that holiday melon spread stuffed into the watermelon shell, or avoid it.

A digestive enzyme supplement may be indicated for persons who feel uncomfortable after eating a normal sized meal. Digestive enzymes are normally produced by the pancreas. The production of certain digestive enzymes decreases with age, therefore, at times, supplementation may be indicated. Three classes of enzymes are produced by the pancreas, protease, lipase and amylase. Protease enzymes break down protein, lipase breaks down fat, and amylase breaks down carbohydrates. Within each classification, many different specialized enzymes exist, each performing a specific phase of digestion. Lack of these enzymes will result in poor digestion of proteins, fats and carbohydrates, potentially allowing incompletely digested food to pass through the intestines. Absorption of incompletely digested food molecules, particularly undigested proteins, can lead to food allergies and food hypersensitivities. Using a digestive enzyme supplement will help to ensure that food is more completely digested. The appropriate time to take a digestive enzyme is halfway through the meal. Both full spectrum and specialized digestive enzyme supplements can be purchased in any good health food store.

Properly combining foods during a meal may be difficult or impossible at times. This is especially true during the holiday season, while on the road for business, or away on vacation. During these times, the diet changes quite abruptly, with indigestion being a frequent complaint. Consequently, a broad-spectrum digestive enzyme supplement may be beneficial to ensure any food consumed is more fully digested, therefore averting some potential digestive problems. Digestive enzymes, however, are not a license to overindulge and eat everything in sight.

As a final topic in this chapter on nutrition, visiting some older, forgotten knowledge of the nutritional value of certain foods is in order. Examining the knowledge and wisdom of older civilizations, and looking at this knowledge through the eyes of modern research, we find that modern research validates what has been discovered hundreds of years ago.

Regarding nutrition, it has been said that "you are what you eat." This statement is more true than the average person may realize. The wisdom of ancient civilizations can be easily seen in the *Doctrine of Signatures*, a philosophical treatise originated by Paracelsus, the father of modern chemistry. This philosophy has subsequently been developed and expanded upon by herbalists over the ages. The Doctrine of Signatures contends that every naturally occurring food has a pattern that resembles a body organ or physiological function, and this pattern is representative of the benefits provided by that particular food. The Doctrine of Signatures is not, however, limited to food, but extends to herbs as well. This philosophy, popularized by the writings of Jakob Bööhme of Göörlitz, Germany, became part of medical thinking in the middle of the seventeenth century.

Modern research has concluded that certain foods have both healing and protective effects on the body's organs and systems. Interestingly, this modern research has validated the knowledge and wisdom known by natural health practitioners for hundreds of years. Examining a few foods and their signature pattern reveals an astonishing correlation of this older wisdom and the discoveries of modern research. Just what are these patterns, or signatures, found in foods and herbs that have a relation to the vital processes of the body? In examining a few common foods, the signatures described by the older philosophers become readily apparent. The examples cited below are but a small representation of this topic.

Cross-sectional views of a sliced carrot reveal that it closely resembles the human eye. The pupil and radiating lines of the iris of the eye look astonishingly similar to the cross-section of a sliced carrot. Carrots contain Beta Carotene, a precursor to Vitamin A, which is necessary for good eye sight.

A tomato has four chambers, is red, and contains a red liquid inside. The heart is red, and has four chambers, and is filled with blood. Research shows that tomatoes have beneficial effects on the circulatory system. Tomatoes contain lycopene, a very powerful antioxidant. In recent times, the label on certain tomato-based foods boasts that it is good for the heart.

Grapes hang in a cluster that has the shape that resembles the heart. Each grape looks like a blood cell, and the small branches resemble the branching of arteries. Extensive research today shows that grapes, rich with antioxidants provide protective benefits to the heart and blood vessels. Wine, made from grapes, has been shown to decrease the risk of cardiovascular related disease. The health related benefits of wine have been popularized in recent news articles, not a month goes by that another benefit of wine is found.

Inside a walnut, the actual nut looks like a miniature brain, with a left and right cerebral hemisphere, a cerebellum, and membranes resembling the meninges. The folds appear on the nut just as is seen in the cerebral cortex. Walnuts are rich in linoleic and alpha-linolenic acid, essential for myelin formation.

Walnuts also are a good source of tryptophan, the amino acid precursor to the neurotransmitter serotonin and the hormone melatonin, both of which are found in the brain.

Kidney beans look very similar to a kidney, as the name suggests. Kidney beans are reported to help maintain kidney function. The dried pod of certain kidney beans has been demonstrated to have a strong diuretic effect.

Modern research may dismiss the Doctrine of Signatures as unscientific. Not even aware of the Doctrine of Signatures, researchers are inadvertently uncovering proof that the philosophy, in many regards, is correct. Not a week goes by that new health benefits are discovered regarding specific, naturally occurring foods. Little, if any, protective health benefits are discovered by research regarding highly processed foods.

Perhaps the most memorable Thanksgiving day dinner I can remember was a gathering of more than 20 people. As the food was being passed around, I took a little turkey, few vegetables, and made a small salad. This is about what I would normally eat at any other meal. One of the guests was sitting across the table from me. He asked whether I was sick or something. Not understanding why he would ask this question, I simply answered "no." He then asked "What's the matter, you can't eat?" I assured him I was fine. As he persisted in this line of questioning, he continued to pile huge amounts of food on his plate, perhaps enough for five meals. Not surprisingly, he had gone back for seconds and thirds. Also not surprising is it looked as if he had a basketball under his shirt. I finally had to tell him I was in training, just to quiet him down. Sadly, he died young.

Chapter 5
The Immune System

An illusion exists that the world around us is largely hostile. Bacteria, viruses, fungi, or parasites, all of which are commonly termed *germs*, are found in every nook and cranny, and we are taught from a very early age that they are to be avoided like the plague. When any of these germs enter the body, it is then termed an infection. We are forever conquering nature, creating antibiotics to destroy every strain of bacteria, antiviral drugs to stop viruses from replicating, insecticides to eliminate insects, and herbicides to kill plants, and fungicides to kill mold and fungi, instead of learning to cooperate with nature in a harmonious order. The vague rule to destroy completely and eliminate any organism that presents even a minor inconvenience can only end in a negative outcome. The hostile attitude of conquering nature completely ignores the basic interdependence and cooperation of all organisms that were designed to occupy the same environment. As a result, we end up destroying the very environment from which our whole life depends.

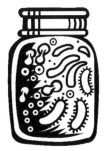

Bacteria live everywhere in the environment. They are found, on plants, on food, in the ground, and in water. Many bacteria produce toxins that can damage the body. These harmful bacteria can enter the body in any number of ways. Some enter along with our food, others may enter through the respiratory system, and others can break through the skin. If any of these harmful bacteria should somehow get into the body, they must be eliminated. The body is perfectly equipped to handle most of these harmful germs that can gain entry. The elimination of these germs is accomplished by our immune system.

Not all bacteria are harmful, some are termed beneficial as they have a desirable purpose and benefit the host in some way. Some bacteria live in other organisms, including humans. Others, such as *Staphylococcal aureus*, live harmoniously on our skin, but can cause havoc if the bacteria enter the inside of the physical body. The intestinal tract contains dozens of strains of bacteria proven beneficial in many ways. One of the most commonly known beneficial bacteria found to reside in the human digestive tract is *Acidophilous sp*. The body develops a symbiotic relationship with these beneficial bacteria, in other words, a relationship in which both the bacteria and host benefit.

Viruses, also, can be found most anywhere in the environment. A virus can attack a plant, a human, an animal, or any other type organism. Unlike most bacteria, a specific virus typically can only attack a specific type or organism. A virus able to attack a plant is harmless to a human, and a virus able to attack a human is harmless to a plant. No one has ever heard of a houseplant catching the flu. If a particular virus can attack a human, even then, the virus is limited in the tissue type in which it can gain entry and replicate. The influenza virus, for example, specifically attacks the respiratory system, the hepatitis virus attacks the liver, and the Human Immunodeficiency Virus (HIV) attacks specific cells of the immune system. In addition, a virus is generally specific to the organism that it attacks. The virus that causes the common cold in a human does not cause the same cold in other animals. When a virus remains in check without any outward signs of disease, the person or animal hosting that virus is called a *carrier*. Human transmission of viruses generally occurs through the respiratory system or through the secretions of a mucous membrane. Viral infections can also occur by the virus directly entering the bloodstream.

Very few pathogens cannot be handled by a normal and healthy immune system. The question arises about whether the immune system can successfully destroy the pathogen faster than the pathogen can kill the infected person. The Ebola virus is a perfect example of a pathogen in which the immune system is in a critical race of time. The immune system is perfectly capable of destroying the Ebola virus. The Ebola virus is a rapidly multiplying and highly destructive pathogen, resulting in approximately 85 percent mortality rate. The immune system, however, requires time to develop the specific defenses necessary to destroy the virus. If the immune system can work fast enough, the virus will be successfully eradicated, and, as a result of the formed immunological memory, immunity to the virus will be gained. When time is of the essence, a healthy immune system can mean the difference between life and death. While most pathogens are not nearly as destructive as the Ebola virus, nearly any pathogen can cause death in the presence of an unresponsive immune system.

Two primary defensive strategies are in place for the immune system to handle any of these pathogenic foreign invaders. The first type of defense is nonspecific defense, which does not discriminate based upon the type of invader. The second type of defense is a more specific type of defense in which the invader is identified and marked as a pathogen, and is subsequently eliminated by any number of subsequent immune system mechanisms.

Nonspecific defenses include the integumentary system, consisting of the skin, hair and nails. This is the body's first line of nonspecific defense against a pathogen. The secretions of the stomach, particularly hydrochloric acid, are other examples of nonspecific defenses. Most pathogens do not survive the highly acidic environment of the stomach. *Helicobacter pylori*, a gram negative bacteria, is one exception to this rule. *Helicobacter pylori* is well able to survive in the acidic environment of the stomach, and an infection involving this bacterium can lead to ulceration of the stomach lining. Other nonspecific defenses include an elevated body temperature as a result of an infection. In the case of elevated body temperature, the details of a specific pathogen are unknown, but a cascade of events causes this nonspecific immune response to occur.

Natural specific immunity can be of two types. The first type is innate immunity, also known as natural immunity, and refers to the specific immune system components that are in place at birth. Innate immunity also includes the natural activity of passing of immunoglobulins from mothers' milk to the newborn. Innate immunity is genetically based. The second type is acquired immunity, also known as active immunity, is the immunity that occurs resulting from exposure to pathogens. Another type of immunity, called passive immunity or artificial immunity, can be obtained through administration of a vaccine. Technically, artificial immunity is a type of acquired immunity.

Acquired immunity has two major mechanisms of action. The first mechanism is known as either humoral immunity or antibody mediated immunity. In humoral immunity or antibody mediated immunity, certain proteins, called either immunoglobulins or antibodies, initiate the defense against an invading pathogen. The second mechanism is known as cell-mediated immunity, in which immune system cells, known as either leukocytes or white blood cells, destroy the invading pathogen. Many immune responses involve a combination of humoral and cell-mediated responses.

The first mechanism of acquired immunity is called humoral immunity, and is also known as antibody mediated immunity. Humoral immunity involves the use of various proteins, called either immunoglobulins or antibodies. These antibodies initiate the initial defense against an invading pathogen. Antibodies are found in the blood, lymph, intestinal tract, and other bodily fluids. Antibodies identify foreign invaders such as viruses and bacteria, and attach to them, marking them for elimination. Five different types of antibodies exist in the human immune system, each performing different functions. Antibodies are commonly designated by a letter, and are called IgA, IgD, IgE, IgG, and IgM, where Ig stands for immunoglobulin and the letter A, D, E, G, or M designates the type of antibody. Within each type of antibody, several different subclassifications exist. Differences in the structure and biological properties of these types of antibodies facilitate differing abilities to counteract specific antigens in specific ways. Table 5.1 identifies these five types of antibodies and a brief description of their function. An elevated level of a specific class of immunoglobulin is often an indicator of what type of infection may be present in the body.

A foreign invader, such as a virus, bacteria, venom, or allergen, is commonly termed an antigen. Specific receptor sites on the immunoglobulin or antibody have the ability to recognize the antigen and subsequently bind to the antigen in several different ways. When an antibody is bound to an antigen, it is termed an antibody-antigen complex. The antibody-antigen complex is destroyed by specific leukocytes (white blood cells) known as macrophages and by other immune system cells.

In addition, the antibody-antigen complex sets other immune responses into action, such as activation of the complement system. The complement system is another method by which the immune system eliminates foreign invaders. Three variations of the complement system are documented, and are termed the classical pathway, alternative pathway, and the Lectin pathway. The complement system consists of proteins, which are found in the blood, which target the specific cells by disrupting the membrane structure of that cell. More than 20 proteins have been identified as part of the complement system.

Immunoglobulin	Function
IgA	Prevents colonization of pathogens along mucosal membranes. Found in the digestive tract, tears, saliva, and breast milk.
IgD	Functions as an antigen receptor on B-Cells.
IgE	Involved in allergic responses, primarily in identifying the pathogen. Triggers histamine release from mast cells. Protects against parasitic worms.
IgG	Protection against invading pathogens
IgM	Involved in elimination of pathogens in B-Cell mediated immunity

Table 5.1   Immunoglobulins

The second mechanism of acquired immunity, called the cell-mediated immune response, involves leukocytes. Leukocytes are commonly called white blood cells. Many different types of leukocytes exist, each type having a specific function associated with it. All leukocytes originate from a specific type of cell found in the bone marrow known as a hematopoietic stem cell. Leukocytes often carry the label T-Cell or B-Cell. This designation is assigned based upon where the leukocyte matures. T-Cells mature in the thymus gland, and B-Cells mature in the bone marrow. The number of leukocytes in the blood is often used as an indicator of whether an infection is present or not. This analysis

Why Am I Sick? And What To Do About It

commonly called a blood count. The type of leukocyte appearing with an elevated count is often an indicator of what type of infection is present. For example, if neutrophil counts are found elevated, a bacterial infection would be suspected. Table 5.2 identifies the types of leukocytes involved in cell-mediated immune responses.

The primary type of leukocyte involved in cell-mediated immune response are the class of lymphocytes called T-Cells. T-Cells come in many varieties, each of which plays a highly specific role. Cytotoxic T-Cells (also called killer T-cells), Suppressor T-Cells, and Helper T-Cells are all different types of T-Cells. Helper T cells direct the activities of other immune system components, such as initiating and directing the activity of Cytotoxic T cells. Helper T cells are also involved in activating B-Cells to produce antibodies. CD4 and CD8 cells are very publicized types of T-Cells, primarily due their involvement in many common diseases of society. CD stands for Cluster of Differentiation, and the nomenclature identifies which molecules are present on the surface of the cell. A CD4 cell is a specific type of Helper T-Cell. A CD8 cell is a specific type of Cytotoxic T-Cell.

It should be no secret by now that the inner workings of the immune system are very complicated. We have only touched the surface of the intricacies of the immune system in the discussion. Fortunately, only a basic understanding of the immune system is required to avert or correct some of the health problems facing today's society. For the remainder of the discussion, the emphasis will be primarily placed on the areas of the immune system specifically involved in the particular diseases and disorders discussed elsewhere in this book.

Leukocyte	Percent	Function
Neutrophils	40 – 60	Bacterial and fungal defense
Lymphocyte	20 – 40	Cell-mediated immunity, active in viral infections
Monocyte	2 – 8	Phagocytosis, defense against blood-borne pathogens
Eosinophil	1 – 4	Parasitic infections
Basophil	0.5 – 1	Allergic responses, production of histamine.
Macrophage	Varies	Phagocytosis. A macrophage is a highly differentiated form of a Monocyte

Table 5.2   Leukocyte Types

The immune system is a collection of processes using specialized proteins and cells by which pathogens are identified and systematically destroyed and eliminated from the body. Pathogens may be either bacteria, viruses, parasites, pollen, or any form of foreign matter. To carry out the process of destruction and elimination of these pathogens, the immune system utilizes these various types of proteins and cells, and, in addition, specific tissues and organs. These components of the immune system interact in a sophisticated way to identify precisely and eliminate the pathogen. Pathogens continually adapt and evolve in many ways to evade detection in order to continue infecting the host organism. The immune system must be able to identify these changes, and reprogram itself to detect, destroy and eliminate the modified pathogen. This adaptation process forms immunological memories and allows a faster, more effective response during a future encounter of these, or similar, pathogens. Immunity is like playing a game in which the rules are constantly changing without ever being made clear. Such a game can never be won, unless, of course, the pathogen kills the host or the host eradicates the pathogen. Oddly, should the pathogen kill the host, the pathogen will most likely die as well.

Simply put, then, the immune system recognizes the foreign invader as not part of the body, and, depending on the type of invader, initiates the appropriate immune response to eliminate it. During this process, the immune system creates a memory of the foreign invader, enabling more efficient destruction of the pathogen in the future should the pathogen be encountered again. If all goes well, the unwelcome invader is destroyed and eliminated, and, should the invader ever appear again, it will be eliminated even quicker during subsequent encounters. If all does not go well, however, we have a problem. Immunodeficiency, hypersensitivity, allergic responses, and autoimmunity are a few of the problems that can occur with the immune system. When a problem occurs, which involves the immune system, it will eventually affect any of the systems of the body.

A compromised immune system, or immunodeficiency, occurs when the immune system is less active than normal. This results in opportunistic infections, recurring infections, and prolonged infections. In some cases, life threatening infections could occur, which would normally be of no consequence. Immunodeficiency can be a result of genetic factors, caused by certain drugs, or caused by an infection, such as Human Immunodeficiency Virus (HIV). Immunodeficiency can also be simply a result of fatigue or malnutrition. The immune system has many different facets to it. The possibility exists for certain facets of the immune system to be in an immunodeficient or suppressed state, while other parts are functioning at a normal level.

In modern day Western civilization, certain acute diseases are a clear indication of a compromised immune system. Meningitis and *Staphylococcal aureus* are prime examples of infections that normally would not occur in a person with a healthy immune system. Meningitis outbreaks are usually confined to a particular school, whether it is an elementary school, high school, college or university. Students often have a poor diet, are under stress from deadlines for papers and final exams, and have a schedule that is more rigid than steel reinforced concrete. It is no surprise at all that the immune system becomes compromised, resulting in any number of opportunistic infections. Whenever such an outbreak occurs, the infection itself is reported by the news media as the problem. Parents want to remove their son or daughter from the school as fast as possible, and understandably so. In all likelihood, their son or daughter's immune system is most likely in the same immunodeficient state as the unfortunate few who caught the disease. In reality, a pandemic of compromised immune systems is the real problem in this situation, not the pathogen. No one should be overly concerned about *Staphylococcal aureus* or Meningitis, what should be of greater concern, however, is the compromised state of the immune system. If the immune system was not in a compromised state, an opportunistic infection is unlikely to occur.

Hyperactivity and hypersensitivity of certain facets of the immune system often result in exaggerated immune responses. Allergies and autoimmune diseases fall into this category. Each type of exaggerated immune response involves a different cascade of events. One event in the cascade of events of an allergy is the release of histamine by mast cells. An antihistamine inhibits the release of histamine, thus relieving the symptoms of the allergy. In the case of autoimmune disease, one event in the cascade of events is the release of proinflammatory cytokines by T-Cells. Drugs used to combat rheumatoid conditions target these T-Cells, specifically inhibiting the release of these cytokines by various mechanisms. In the case of either allergy and autoimmune disease, suppression of histamine or proinflammatory cytokines respectively, do not cure the disease. Suppression of these immune components merely suppresses the symptoms. The cure can only be found in restoring the proper function of the immune system. When the different facets of the immune system are brought back into balance, exaggerated immune responses do not generally occur.

Allergies are a relatively new phenomenon affecting modern day society. In examining the society that lived in the beginning of the twentieth century, the concept of an allergy was foreign to the people living then. At the beginning of the twenty first century, the number of people suffering with allergies is estimated to be approximately 20 to 30 percent of the population living in modern industrialized areas. Interestingly, persons living in third world countries, where they must grow their own food and raise their own livestock, do not have a high prevalence rate of allergies. The dramatic increase in allergies found in industrialized society lead us to believe that something in industrialized society has changed in the last one hundred years. What has changed is the diet, stress levels, and the widespread use of certain medications that can lead to certain imbalances in the body.

Allergies occur when an exaggerated immune response occurs in reaction to a pathogen. Allergic responses come in many different varieties. Environmental allergies, food allergies, and allergies to medications are among the most commonly seen. Allergies involve both genetic and environmental factors. Research into the genetic basis of allergies, however, has not been accomplished to the extent that it has with autoimmune diseases. T-Cells, specifically Th2 cells (Thymus Helper Type 2 Cell), play a significant role in the allergic response. Various interleukins and immunoglobulins are also involved in the cascade of events of the allergic response. The types of immunoglobulins, and the type of immune system cells involved determine the type of allergy.

Allergens, whatever the method of entry into the body, provoke an initial immune response by B-Cells or macrophages. The allergen, also termed an antigen, is engulfed by the immune cell by a process called phagocytosis. The immune system cell then destroys the antigen by essentially dismantling it. These dismantled sub-components are ejected from the immune system cell, and come in contact with allergen specific Th2 cells. In response, the Th2 cells secrete chemicals known as cytokines, such as interleukin-4, interleukin-5, interleukin-6, and interleukin-10. The presence of these interleukins subsequently stimulates and recruits other immune system cells. This cascade of events normally occurs in response to a pathogen in individuals both with and without allergies. In the individual with allergies, however, the Th2 response of secreting cytokines is greatly exaggerated. This exaggeration is commonly recognized as the excessive release of histamine, with the individual often taking an antihistamine to relieve the symptoms.

Autoimmune diseases result when a different portion of the immune system has become hyperactive, attacking the body's tissues as if the tissue itself was a foreign invader. As often seen with allergies, autoimmune diseases require both a genetic and environmental factor in order to be expressed. Autoimmune disorders are often referred to as the family of inflammatory disorders because inflammation of a particular tissue occurs as part of the disorder. The possibility exists for certain facets of the immune system to exhibit exacerbated responses while other facets are functioning at a normal level. In the individual with autoimmune disorders, the Th1 (Thymus Helper Type 1 Cell) response of secreting cytokines is greatly exaggerated. These cytokines, released during the cascade of events associated with autoimmune disorders, play a major role in the inflammatory response found with autoimmune disease.

The presence of immune system hyperactivity often results in other quirks that are not readily obvious. Hyperactivity of the Th1 associated immunological response has been linked to autoimmune disease. In persons with an active autoimmune issue, Th1 activity is exaggerated. Since Th1 activity is also linked to fighting the common cold, persons with an active autoimmune condition rarely catch a cold. Much less obvious is that Th1 cells also are involved in the body's defenses against cancer. Hyperactivity of the Th1 immunological response would increase the body's defense against cancer.

It should be clear by now that if something goes wrong with the immune system, by whichever mechanism, disease of the body results. What else is clear is that when certain diseases are present, the immune system, in many cases, is either hyperactive or hypoactive, i.e., out of balance in some respect. One might wonder if there really can be that many separate and distinct diseases that can occur, or could they perhaps be different expressions of the same immune system failure. If the specific facet of the immune system determined to be out of balance can be identified and corrected, it would logically follow that the disease process that was set into motion as a result of that imbalance would be cured.

Th1 and Th2 immune cells have a natural balance to them. Autoimmune diseases occur as a result of an exaggerated Th1 associated immune system response. Allergies, on the other hand, occur as a result of an exaggerated Th2 associated immune system response. If the Th1 / Th2 balance was restored, autoimmune diseases and allergies would cease, or at least alleviated to great extent. Restoration of Th1 / Th2 balance, in fact, has been shown to benefit both the allergy and autoimmune patient. The question arises of what actually caused the imbalance in the first place. While multiple factors are known to influence immune system function, the specific factors involved in Th1 / Th2 balance are well documented.

In today's society, technology and science have given us the ability to eradicate disease causing pathogens. In modern times, we attempt to sterilize everything that we may potentially contact, eat, or breathe. Antibacterial soap, antibacterial wipes, germ killing bathroom cleaners, ammonia, bleach, high tech cleaning solutions, chlorination of water, and ultraviolet sterilization are but a few ways to kill potentially harmful germs. Lack of exposure to pathogens is seemingly beneficial to health. When the immune system is not exposed to pathogens, however, the future disease fighting ability of the immune system is subsequently compromised. This reduced disease fighting ability of the immune system is technically a form of environmentally acquired immunodeficiency. Specifically, in this type of immunodeficiency, the immune system has the ability to fight disease adequately, but environmental factors did not allow the immune system to develop to the level required to handle certain pathogens adequately. Factors leading to environmentally acquired immunodeficiency include antibiotic usage, over sterilization of the environment, and living a life primarily indoors.

In an article originally published in 1989 in the British Medical Journal, epidemiologist David P. Strachan developed and documented what is known as the Hygiene Hypothesis. The observation was made that both eczema and hay fever was far less common in children from larger families. In larger families, greater exposure of any child to infectious agents, such as bacteria and viruses, through their siblings is evident. Specifically, the greater number of older siblings a child had, the less likely they are to contract certain diseases. In families with only one child, exposure to infectious agents would be considerably diminished. The increased exposure to infectious agents in larger families subsequently resulted in a better developed immune system, ultimately resulting in a healthier individual. The Hygiene Hypothesis suggests that a decreased exposure to pathogens subsequently increase susceptibility to various diseases. The Hygiene Hypothesis also suggests that the maturation of the immune system requires exposure to infectious agents.

Since the original hypothesis in 1989, many additional observations regarding pathogen exposure and the immune system have been documented. The following are just a few observations made.

> *Higher infant sibling exposure in the first six years of life is associated with decreased risk of Multiple Sclerosis.*

Persons living in tropical regions having the most infections and parasitic diseases are the least affected by Type-1 Diabetes.

A disproportionate high incidence of childhood Leukemia is observed to occur in industrialized countries, as opposed to developing countries.

A decreased risk of heart disease has been observed in individuals exposed to a greater number of childhood infections.

A significant decreased incidence of inflammatory bowel disease has been observed in nations in which an overall low level of hygiene and greater environmental microbial exposure.

Exposure to environmental pathogens is not necessarily bad. Constant exposure to these pathogens is, in fact, necessary to develop the immunity required to live in modern day society. When a person living in one country travels to a different area of the world, they are often afflicted by pathogens to which the local population has gained immunity. Never being exposed to the pathogens found in the distant society, the traveler is at a much higher risk to develop disease as a result of an immune system unfamiliar with the pathogens of another land. The same principle applies to any local community. The immune system of anyone living in a sterilized environment is weak and underdeveloped as compared with the person who has been exposed to a variety of pathogens present in the environment.

Exposure to a pathogen does not infer that disease is inevitable. The average person is exposed to many pathogens every hour of every day. The immune system, in the great majority of these exposures, is very successful in fighting off the pathogen. Many of these pathogens are able to cause disease, but, in most cases, the immune system is successful in quickly eradicating the pathogen. If the immune system has been compromised for one reason or another, such as stress, poor diet, or lack of sleep, the pathogen that should have been successfully fought off is now able to gain a stronghold and cause disease. The immune system in a compromised state, while still able to eliminate the pathogen, has a more difficult time in doing so.

In the case of the common cold, we are taught to believe that a virus is the root cause, and that "nothing can be done to cure the common cold." However, twenty people can all be exposed to the same virus at the same level, and two may catch a cold, and the other eighteen may not. Careful examination reveals that it is not the virus, but it is either a suppressed immune system or an out of balance immune system that allowed the pathogen to become established. In the eighteen who did not catch the cold, the immune system was successful in fighting off the pathogen. Frequent colds, therefore, is a symptom of a weakened immune system. While the cold is typically treated with decongestants, inappropriately by antibiotics, and other over-the-counter remedies, little, if anything, is ever done to restore the weakened immune system. What is of concern, however, in the patient with frequent colds is that the immune system is suppressed. Either the entire immune system is suppressed, or the Th1 and Th2 segments of the immune system are out of

Why Am I Sick? And What To Do About It

balance. Specifically, in this case, over activity of the Th2 segment, and under activity of the Th1 segment would be suspected. In the case of the Th1 / Th2 imbalance, the patient is who catches frequent colds is also more susceptible to cancer. Frequent colds, then is a wake-up call to get the immune system healthy and back in balance before something worse happens. The age-old saying that there is no cure for the common cold is completely false, purely in the realm of *ad falsum*. The body's immune system is perfectly capable of curing the common cold, but it just needs to be kept in a strong and healthy condition to do so.

The person who is 50 years old, playing tennis, hiking in the mountains, waterskiing, and enjoying the outdoor life most likely has an optimally functioning and balanced immune system. This adequately developed immune system comes as a result of a lifetime of healthy activities. This is not to say that they will never get sick, but if they do, their immune system has an appropriate response and they are quickly restored to health.

In an exaggerated immune response, such as anaphylactic shock, the immune system attacks the foreign invader with such voracity, that death of the body is apparently an acceptable outcome.

Why Am I Sick? And What To Do About It

Chapter 6
Digestive System Restoration

Restoration of the digestive system is the first step in the restoration of health. Regardless of the health issues facing any individual, a properly working digestive system is an imperative part of restoring and maintaining good health. Restoring the normal functioning digestive system, however, is only the first step in this process. Adopting new dietary habits to prevent any problems that may have developed in the past is also required for anyone to remain healthy.

Serious health problems that have arisen in recent years have made headlines in the news. Food poisoning caused by E-coli, Salmonella, Campylobacter, Shigella, Listeria, botulism and other pathogenic bacteria have become more common in recent years. The range of symptoms caused by these pathogens, or any pathogen for that matter, can range anywhere from mild to severe. What, then, decides the severity of any particular occurrence of food

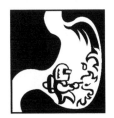

poisoning? When the beneficial bacterial flora of the intestine is properly in balance, the symptoms associated with food poisoning are drastically less severe than when either the normal bacterial flora has been all killed by antibiotics, a yeast overgrowth is found in the intestines, or both. This explains why, when ten people consume the same contaminated food, four have serious symptoms, four have only mild discomfort, and two may be hospitalized due to life-threatening dehydration or other serious issue. It is not the quantity of the pathogen consumed that is responsible for the difference in the severity of the symptoms. Any of the bacteria listed can easily multiply to pathogenic levels in the small intestine if no beneficial bacteria are present to keep them in check. What is responsible for the differing levels of symptoms from one person to the next is the overall health of the digestive tract, including the proper balance of the microbial flora, and a properly balanced immune system. If a person is hospitalized due to food poisoning, both a suppressed immune system and disrupted beneficial bacterial flora of the intestines should immediately be suspected. While treatment of the acute symptoms of food poisoning is very important, what is more important is to evaluate carefully and correct any immune system and digestive system issues that are obviously evident.

Health of the digestive system requires that the organs associated with digestion are functioning correctly and the natural balance of beneficial bacteria and yeast exists in the intestinal tract. When this is the case, the digestive system can properly digest and assimilate food presented to it, followed by a quick and effective elimination of the waste. If the integrity of the stomach or intestinal wall is compromised to any degree, such as is found in leaky gut syndrome, food will not be digested or assimilated correctly. Compromised integrity of the intestinal lining lays the foundation for many chronic diseases. If the organs of digestion, for example the liver or pancreas, are not functioning normally, digestion can become impaired. As we have discovered in the chapter discussing nutrition, improper eating habits can also lead to improper digestion, resulting in poor absorption of nutrients and absorption of toxic compounds.

The disruption of the normal bacterial flora in the intestinal tract has been identified with many chronic disease states. These include autoimmune diseases, fibromyalgia, chronic fatigue syndrome, immune hypersensitivity, environmental allergies, and food allergies. The presence of these chronic disease states subsequently leads to yet other more advanced diseased states of the body. Current research into probiotics has led to a deeper understanding of their role in health. Dozens of species of bacterial flora normally inhabit the human intestinal tract. Many strains have been extensively studied and their beneficial effects on overall health have been well documented. This research has recently gone to such depth that specific probiotic bacterial strains have been identified to facilitate correction of Th1 / Th2 immune system imbalances that are largely responsible for allergies and autoimmune diseases. The intestinal flora interfaces with the immune system, nervous system and endocrine system through various means. The presence of this interface makes it easy to understand how disruption of the intestinal flora can lead to serious chronic disease.

Disruption of the digestive system usually does not occur overnight. Any problems associated with the digestive system most likely have been going on for several months before any symptoms are realized. As with most chronic disorders, the symptoms begin to appear slowly over time, often so slowly that the symptoms are not even recognized until they begin to interfere with daily life. In the case of digestive system related chronic disease, the disruption of the digestive system most likely began many years before the chronic disease was diagnosed. Likewise, digestive system problems do not resolve very quickly, even under optimal conditions. This is due, in part, to the fact that tissue repair, such as the healing of ulcerations, takes a significant time to occur. In addition to damaged intestinal tissue resulting from ulcerations, yeast overgrowths become firmly imbedded in the intestinal lining. This yeast overgrowth not only has to be eliminated, but any damage to the intestinal lining caused by the yeast must be also repaired. Once any tissue damage has been repaired, probiotic supplements are used to restore the natural flora of the intestines. This process, again, takes time. Complete restoration of the digestive tract can therefore take many months to complete. The exact duration of each phase of the restoration process depends on many factors, all of which vary from person to person. Optimal results are generally obtained when supervised by a qualified health care professional who specializes in not only the digestive tract, but any associated chronic conditions as well. The skilled natural health care provider has extensive knowledge regarding restoration of the digestive tract, and does not rely upon a trial and error approach. The approach that he or she takes is largely dependent on the presenting condition and patient history.

Antibiotics are one reason the normal bacterial flora in the intestines has been disrupted in many people. Complicating the issue further is the fact that many antibiotics prescribed today are the broad-spectrum type, which are often prescribed without any clinical rationale. Antibiotics are prescribed for patients with viral infections, such as the common cold, even though a virus is completely unaffected by the antibiotic. Antibiotics are "tried" for sinus infections, and after failing to eliminate the infection, it is found that the sinus infection was a fungal origin after all. Broad-spectrum antibiotic usage poses yet another problem. Specifically, by killing off most of the beneficial bacteria present in the intestines, only the antibiotic resistant strains of bacteria remain. If the antibiotic resistant bacteria are pathogenic, meaning that they have the potential to cause disease, they now have free rein of the intestinal tract to multiply. The beneficial bacteria that were not antibiotic resistant are now, for the most part, gone, therefore unable to keep the pathogenic bacteria in check. As a result, any number of gastrointestinal problems can occur, many of which are not evident until several months after the course of antibiotics. These problems are usually initially recognized by the patient as digestive problems, intestinal discomfort, indigestion, or colitis, all of which are the precursors to more serious gastrointestinal disease. If the disrupted intestinal flora is not corrected following antibiotic use, the immune system will also eventually be affected, paving the way for even more disorders in the future.

Prescription antibiotics, however, are not the sole cause of a disrupted digestive system. Antibiotics, found in beef, pork and poultry raised in modern industrial farms, are also significant contributors to the destruction of intestinal flora in those persons who consume these products. Antibiotic laden foods cause antibiotics to trickle through the intestines meal after meal, day after day, killing the beneficial bacteria that normally reside there. For this reason, only free range, antibiotic free meats and poultry should be consumed. While these products often carry a higher cost, the extra expense is well justified.

Another reason of disrupted bacterial flora is the consumption of refined sugar. Products manufactured with refined sugar are found everywhere in Western society. Cake, soft drinks and other sweetened beverages, cookies, pastries, and ice cream consumption is frankly enormous. Examining the labels of prepared food products often reveals refined sugar in one form or another. The presence of refined sugar in the intestines provides an ideal environment for a yeast infection to proliferate. Yeast primarily live on sugar, and thrive on refined sugar. The yeast ferments the sugar, and excretes their metabolic waste directly into the host's intestinal tract. Much of this metabolic waste is subsequently absorbed into the bloodstream, where the liver and kidneys must then detoxify and eliminate it. Any left over nutrients not consumed by the yeast are available for digestion and utilization by the body. Restoration of the digestive system requires that these issues surrounding sugar and yeast infections be addressed.

When someone contracts diabetes, they are told to avoid refined sugar to regulate blood sugar better. If someone must take an antibiotic for some reason, refined sugar, similarly, must be avoided to decrease the likelihood of an intestinal yeast overgrowth. The recommendation to avoid refined sugar is, however, rarely made by the prescribing physician. Since autoimmune disease is associated with disrupted intestinal flora, persons with autoimmune disease should also avoid consuming refined sugar. Avoiding refined sugar is good advice for any chronic disease sufferer, but, since the effects cannot readily be demonstrated on a blood test, as with diabetes, it is therefore assumed that the sugar presents no harm. If a biopsy were routinely performed of the intestinal lining of the chronic disease sufferer, they would no doubt be instructed to avoid refined sugar just as the diabetic. For the healthy person who is not suffering from any chronic diseases, avoiding refined sugar will drastically reduce the likelihood of certain disease processes in the future.

One of the most important considerations to improve digestive system function is to drink more pure water. Lack of water leads to chronic dehydration, resulting in decreased intestinal motility. The dehydrated bowel content also results in inflammation of the intestinal lining. Drinking chlorinated water should be avoided completely. Chlorine is added to water to kill bacteria and other water borne pathogens that may be present in the public water supply. Chlorine will also kill the beneficial bacteria in the gastrointestinal tract, particularly in the upper gastrointestinal tract. Chlorinated water is particularly detrimental to the Lactobacillus strains that live in the small intestine. The Bifidobacteria that inhabits the large intestine will generally be spared from the full effects of chlorine because most of the chlorine has been absorbed into the body by the small intestine.

The first step in correcting any digestive system problem is to eliminate leaky gut syndrome should it be proven to exist. Leaky gut syndrome is a condition of increased permeability of the intestinal wall. Increased permeability of the intestinal wall allows bacteria, toxins and partially digested food to leak through the intestinal lining and enter the bloodstream. Leaky gut syndrome occurs when the intestinal lining becomes inflamed and subsequently damaged. An inflamed intestinal lining is not able to absorb nutrients correctly. Both undigested or partially digested proteins can also be absorbed, laying the foundation for IgG mediated food allergies. Inflammation of the intestinal lining also affects secretory IgA, an immunoglobulin that provides a first line of defense against antigens such as bacteria, yeast, protozoa, and viruses. In cases where the digestive system function is compromised, the levels of IgA are often demonstrated to be low. A decrease in IgA and increased intestinal permeability allow these pathogens to enter the bloodstream where they can travel through the body and set up an infection just about anywhere.

In advanced cases of leaky gut syndrome, IgG antibodies bind to undigested proteins that have been allowed to pass through the intestinal wall and have entered the body. Food allergies associated with IgG are the delayed onset type, in which symptoms generally appear from eight hours to several days following exposure to the antigen. The IgG antibody binds to the protein, and this antibody and antigen pair is called an antibody-antigen complex. Since IgG levels increase with exposure, levels of these antibodies can reach highly elevated levels over time. IgG ELISA (Enzyme-Linked Immunosorbent Assay) food allergy testing is used to identify elevated IgG antibody levels specific to food antigens. Four different types of IgG antibodies are known to exist, and are called IgG1, IgG2, IgG3, and IgG4. IgG antibodies account for approximately 75% of serum antibodies. IgG antibodies, specifically IgG1, IgG3, and IgG4 are unique in the sense that they can cross the placenta, potentially imparting food allergies to the unborn fetus. IgG1 and IgG4 are commonly implicated in food allergies. Anyone with leaky gut syndrome should have an IgG food allergy panel performed. Any reactive foods revealed by the test must be avoided until the foods are proven unreactive.

It must be noted that IgG ELISA testing is sometimes termed *experimental* by modern medicine and other various organizations. The most common reason cited for this classification is lack of supporting research. Significant research supporting the effects of IgG mediated hypersensitivity reactions, however, can easily be found. The real reason for this classification of *experimental* is that no medical treatment for an IgG mediated food hypersensitivity is known. The treatment of an IgG mediated food allergy or hypersensitivity solely consists of either the temporary or permanent removal of the offending food from the diet. Pharmaceutical companies, which fund much of medical research, have no incentive to undertake expensive research studies for any disease or disorder for which no pill can be manufactured to address. IgG ELISA testing will be quickly removed from the experimental category if a drug is ever developed to treat the hypersensitivity. It is quite odd that the one test that can actually identify the source of many forms of serious chronic diseases is termed *experimental*. Because this test is classified as experimental, most insurance companies will not pay for the test, therefore most medical doctors will not consider ordering the test. As a result, many patients continue suffering with illnesses unnecessarily.

Leaky gut syndrome, in conjunction with disruption of the normal bacterial flora found in the intestines, has been implicated in autoimmune diseases and allergies. A high correlation of leaky gut syndrome with other chronic disorders is found as well. Reversal of the autoimmune disease, allergy, or other chronic disorder depends on healing the lining of the gastrointestinal tract, restoration of the normal bacterial flora, and, most of all, obtaining proper nutrition through a proper diet.

Leaky gut syndrome is also responsible for malnutrition. Because of the disrupted integrity of the intestinal lining, damaged carrier mechanisms can no longer effectively transport certain nutrients across the intestinal lining to the bloodstream. For example, hypomagnesemia, a serum deficiency of Magnesium, is quite common in conditions like fibromyalgia. Despite a high Magnesium intake through both the diet and supplementation, transportation across the intestinal lining is impaired, resulting in a deficiency state. Over time, tissue levels of Magnesium decrease, resulting in muscle spasms. Muscle spasms result in the accumulation of toxins, such as lactic acid, causing pain. This again exemplifies why restoration of the digestive system is an imperative step in the reversal of all chronic diseases.

Leaky Gut Syndrome is, in reality, a state of auto toxicity of the body. Several factors of auto toxicity are present. First, the increased permeability of the intestinal lining allows toxic undigested food to enter the bloodstream. Detoxification must then be carried out by the liver. Secondly, parasitic organisms, specifically *Candida albicans* and *Candida krusei*, have made their way into the intestinal tract where they digest and consume food intended for the host. These organisms then excrete toxic waste into the intestines of the host, which subsequently gets absorbed into the bloodstream. This waste must also be detoxified by the liver. Thirdly, the disruption of the beneficial bacterial flora is disrupted, interfering with a variety of immune and biochemical processes of the body, leading to autoimmune and other disorders. A state of auto toxicity is not conducive to health, in fact, it leads to even more disease. The first step in restoring health, therefore, is elimination of leaky gut syndrome.

When leaky gut syndrome is present, one cannot just go to the local health food store, purchase some probiotic supplements, take them, and expect any digestive problems to go away. Taking probiotics in the presence of leaky gut syndrome can create even more problems, and, in fact, is quite dangerous under certain circumstances. Specifically, the increased permeability of the intestinal lining may allow the beneficial bacteria contained in the probiotic supplement to be absorbed into the bloodstream. The beneficial bacteria found in probiotic supplements are only beneficial in the intestines, not in the bloodstream or other bodily tissues where they can cause infection. This is why finding a natural health practitioner to serve as a guide in restoration of health is desirable in all circumstances.

In severe cases of a compromised intestinal lining often found in leaky gut syndrome, the intestinal lining must be rebuilt and healed to a certain extent before addressing the issue of balancing the intestinal flora and eliminating any yeast overgrowth that may be present. This is because the compromised intestinal lining seen in leaky gut syndrome is too permeable. This increased permeability will not only allow the absorption of probiotic bacteria, but the absorption of undigested or partially digested food, and components of the enzymatic breakdown of the yeast overgrowth. A natural health care provider will prescribe a course of action to restore the health of the digestive tract in several phases. The course of action is largely based upon the condition of the patient. The duration of each specific phase is dependent on the progress of the patient, and is carefully evaluated by the health care provider. Adherence to the suggested care plan is, therefore, very important.

The intestinal barrier consists of chemical, physical, and immunological components. Most often, the clinical presentation of leaky gut syndrome reveals compromises of all three components. The first step in the correction of leaky gut syndrome is repair of the intestinal lining. Rebuilding this lining takes protein. Often, however, the digestive system is not working at a sufficient level to facilitate proper digestion of protein. This is particularly the situation when the patient is taking antacids and acid suppressing medications prescribed by a medical doctor. When this is the case, supplementation of the diet with essential amino acids is necessary, giving the body the building blocks needed to repair the damaged intestinal lining. A properly formulated essential amino acid supplement to restore the intestinal lining should contain all of the essential amino acids. It is important that these amino acids be in *free-form* because they can be absorbed directly into the bloodstream and do not have to be digested. The last thing a person with leaky gut syndrome needs is even more work for the digestive system to perform, therefore the free-form amino acid supplement is ideal in this situation. Three to six weeks of amino acid supplementation should be sufficient to rebuild the intestinal lining. Longer periods may be required if extensive damage has occurred.

Amino acids are also needed to repair any ulcerations in the intestinal lining. When the word ulcer is used, we often think of a gastric, also known as a stomach ulcer, but an ulceration may occur anywhere in the intestinal lining. This includes the large intestine, where an ulceration is termed ulcerative colitis. Ulcerations of the gastrointestinal lining are a serious matter and must be corrected. A severely ulcerated gastrointestinal tract could potentially lead to a perforation of the lining, which can subsequently lead to peritonitis, a condition of bacterial contamination of the abdominal cavity. Peritonitis is a medical emergency that requires immediate attention.

The rate at which a tissue heals decreases predictably with age, and is more noticeable each decade. This applies to all tissues of the body, including the intestinal tract. Several methods to speed the process of healing and recovery are, however, well known. One factor that determines the rate of tissue healing is growth hormone levels. Growth hormone levels decrease with age, and this decrease is largely responsible for the aging process. At 60 years old, the Pituitary typically secretes about 25 percent of the growth hormone secreted by a person in their twenties. Growth hormone levels are also often decreased in persons who have several health issues. Restoring growth hormone levels is an effective way to restoring the healing and recuperative powers of the body.

One difference between growth hormone and other hormones, such as estrogen and testosterone, is that the body continues to produce significant quantities of growth hormone during a person's entire life span. This growth hormone is stored in the Pituitary gland. The problem is that, although the hormone is present at significantly high levels, it is not being released at the same levels it was during youth. The challenge, therefore, is to release the stored growth hormone from the Pituitary so that it can be put to use in maintaining a youthful and a healthy state. This can be accomplished using a specialized class of product called a secretagogue, which causes secretion of this stored growth hormone from the Pituitary gland. One such product is Meditropin®, a growth hormone secretagogue manufactured by Nutraceutics Corporation. Meditropin® is available through many natural health practitioners.

When leaky gut syndrome is present, it is likely that an overgrowth of undesirable yeast can be found in the small intestine. This yeast is called *Candida albicans* and *Candida krusei*. An overgrowth of this yeast is called candidiasis. Other types of yeast may be involved as well. Elimination of the yeast overgrowth is imperative in the restoration of the digestive system. This is accomplished quite easily, and involves a simple dietary change accompanied by the short term use of a particular dietary supplement containing various enzymes that are specifically designed to break down and destroy the yeast.

Yeasts contain a cell wall, as do plants. The cell wall is what differentiates a plant, yeast, or fungus from an animal. The cellular material comprising the cell wall of the yeast cannot be digested or otherwise broken down by the human digestive system. Consequently, yeasts are particularly difficult to eliminate from the digestive tract. An enzyme supplement can be taken to break down the cell wall of the yeast, effectively killing the yeast organism. Enzymes used to break down the yeast cell wall primarily include cellulase and hemicellulase. Certain enzymes, such as amylase, glucoamylase, invertase, and malt diastase also play an important role in the elimination of intestinal yeast infections. Particularly effective products to eliminate a yeast overgrowth can be found in Appendix I. Products of this sort often contain other enzymes and proprietary blends to aid in the elimination of an intestinal yeast infection. Yeast infections can take several months to eliminate, with three months being a good period for the initial treatment.

Treating a *Candida albicans* and a *Candida krusei* infection can be a big challenge if the consumption of refined sugar is allowed to continue. Survival of *Candida albicans* and *Candida krusei* depend on the presence of sufficient quantities of sugar in the intestinal tract. Eliminating refined sugar from the diet decreases the likelihood the yeast will thrive, and will hasten the elimination of the yeast infection.

Concurrently performed with the elimination of a yeast infection is restoration of the normal bacterial flora of the intestines. This is easily accomplished with a probiotic supplement. A yeast overgrowth in the intestine suppresses colonization of the probiotic bacteria, since they are both competing for the same space in the intestine. When the yeast is systematically removed by the specialized enzymes, space along the intestinal wall becomes available for colonization of the beneficial probiotic bacteria. Effective probiotic products are listed in Appendix I. A natural health care provider will, in certain circumstances, recommend that the probiotic formula be taken at a level above the recommendation on the supplement bottle. Always follow the recommendation of the health care provider.

In the small intestine, the most commonly found types of beneficial bacteria are strains of the species of *Lactobacillus sp*. In the large intestine, most of the

Why Am I Sick? And What To Do About It

beneficial bacteria are mainly of the species *Bifidobacteria sp.* A properly formulated probiotic product will contain many strains of each of these species, all of which are beneficial in different ways. When taking a probiotic, using a brand that will survive the acidic environment of the stomach is important. Taking the probiotic formulation with a large glass of water on an empty stomach is imperative. This insures that the bacteria make their way into the small intestine, and are not digested with food or killed by the acid environment of the stomach.

Once the bacterial flora of the intestines is properly restored, and any yeast infection is eliminated, consideration must be given to the presence of specific chronic diseases. Specifically, the presence of autoimmune diseases and allergies must be considered. Most autoimmune diseases involve a Type-1 Thymus Helper cell (Th1) response. Allergies, on the other hand, involve a Type-2 Thymus Helper cell (Th2) response. Over activity of either the Th1 or Th2 cell type can cause down regulation of the other. In the patient with autoimmune diseases, Th1 cell activity is found hyperactive, and Th2 activity is suppressed. In the patient with allergies, Th2 cell activity is found hyperactive, and Th1 activity is suppressed.

Specific strains of probiotics have been shown to suppress Th1 activity, and other specific strains of probiotics have been shown to suppress Th2 activity. If the proper probiotic strains are applied under the appropriate circumstances, balance between Th1 and Th2 cell activity can be therefore restored. *Lactobacillus plantarum*, *Lactobacillus acidophilus*, and *Lactobacillus paracasei* have been shown to suppress Th2 activity, and therefore would prove beneficial for patients with chronic allergies. *Lactobacillus salivarius* and *Bifidobacterium lactis* have been shown to suppress Th1 activity, therefore beneficial to patients with autoimmune diseases. The company Original Medicine® has developed products containing these specific strains. Th2S™ is specifically formulated to suppress Th2 activity. Th1S™ is specifically formulated to suppress Th1 activity.

Since specific hypersensitivity responses, allergies, and autoimmune responses are often indistinguishable from each other, care must be given in selecting the correct probiotic strains to suppress the Th1 or Th2 response. Selecting the wrong product can cause manifestation or exacerbation of a disease process. For example, administration of the Th2S product in a patient with an exaggerated Th1 response will lead to the aggravation of any autoimmune disorders present. This is why consulting a natural health care provider who can properly identify and appropriately treat any condition that may exist is valuable.

Adverse reactions to foods are very common in today's society. Many terms are used to describe these adverse reactions to foods. Food allergy, food intolerance, and food hypersensitivity are a few terms commonly used when referring to an adverse reaction to food. Any food associated with an adverse reaction must be eliminated from the diet. In many cases, certain steps can be taken to reintroduce these foods to the diet after a period of abstinence from the offending food. In other cases, the food may have to be eliminated from the diet permanently.

Food intolerance refers to an abnormal physiologic response to an ingested food component. A food allergy is a specific type of food intolerance, but a food intolerance is not necessarily a food allergy. Food intolerance can refer to an abnormal physiologic response to a food additive, a toxic response to the ingested food, or to an idiosyncratic response. A genetically missing, a deficient, or a defective enzyme, which is required to digest a particular food, is one type of food intolerance. Celiac disease, a common gastrointestinal disorder, is an example of this type of food intolerance. In Celiac disease, the enzyme *tissue transglutaminase* modifies gliadin, a gluten protein, and the immune system subsequently attack this modified protein, causing an inflammatory reaction in the intestinal lining. This inflammatory reaction causes destruction of the villi, consequently resulting in the malabsorption of nutrients, which is termed a malabsorption syndrome. Lactose intolerance is yet another example of food intolerance. Levels of the enzyme *lactase*, which is responsible for the breakdown of lactose, decreases in certain individuals with age. As a result of the decreased levels of the enzyme, lactose does not get properly digested, leading to various gastrointestinal complaints.

The term food allergy refers to an abnormal immunological response to an ingested food component. In the allergic response, a target organ is the site of the immune reaction. Two primary types of food allergies are documented. These are the IgE mediated allergic response and IgG mediated allergic response. IgE allergic responses are typically evaluated by a skin prick test or blood test. IgG mediated responses are evaluated with a blood test.

IgE mediated food allergies are an acute reaction to an ingested food. IgE reactions are often termed an immediate allergic response, generally occurring within four hours following ingestion of the offending food. Hives and the feared anaphylactic reaction are examples of IgE mediated food allergies. The target organs of an IgE mediated food allergy are typically either the skin, the respiratory system, or both. In recent times, severe reactions to peanuts have become common IgE food allergies. Since an anaphylactic reaction can easily cause death, any food known to cause an anaphylactic reaction must be avoided completely.

IgG mediated food allergies are also termed a delayed hypersensitivity reaction. This is because the immune system reaction is, as a result of a cascade of events, delayed. The delayed reaction occurs anywhere between eight hours and several days following the ingestion of the offending food. Consequently, identifying problematic foods is particularly difficult. Some type of IgG mediated allergic response is implicated in many chronic diseases. Gastrointestinal disorders, asthma, and autoimmune disorders can all be caused or exacerbated by an IgG food allergy. Multiple IgG allergies are highly suggestive of Leaky Gut Syndrome.

Food allergies are often caused by over exposure to specific foods. By consuming the same foods repeatedly, the risk of developing an immune mediated response to the food increases greatly. The probability of developing a food allergy is greatly increased during times when the immune system is stressed. This includes emotional stress, the stress incurred by the body fighting off either a cold, the flu, or mononucleosis, or any type of physical stress. Certain foods appear to be more allergenic than others, a characteristic that is primarily due to the widespread use of these foods in modern day society. The most common food allergens are egg, milk, peanut, wheat, soy, seafood, and shellfish. Chicken, beef, corn and potatoes are not too far behind on the list. The casual observer might recognize these foods as a significant part of the great American diet.

Food allergies can be easily avoided though proper dietary practices. Maintaining the health of the digestive tract is imperative in the prevention of immune mediated responses to food. This includes maintaining the integrity of the intestinal membrane, presence of the normal bacterial flora in the intestinal tract, and proper diet and nutrition. Any foods demonstrated to cause an allergic response should also be avoided until such time the allergy has been proven to have resolved. Consuming a variety of foods is suggested to avoid developing any IgG food allergies.

If Leaky Gut Syndrome is known to exist, or a food allergy is suspected for one reason or another, an IgG ELISA (Enzyme-Linked Immunosorbent Assay) food allergy testing is warranted. This test is used to identify elevated IgG antibody levels specific to food antigens. This test is a specialized test, and is not typically performed by walk-in laboratories. Any reactive foods identified by the test must be eliminated from the diet. The time and quantity of which reactive foods can be reintroduced vary from patient to patient, and is best determined by a qualified practitioner. Typical waiting times are minimally three months, with four to six months generally appropriate. In some cases involving a severe immune system reaction, the abstinence period may be even longer.

When the abstinence period of reactive foods is completed, the period of which may be substantially different for different foods, reintroduction of any food previously causing a problem into the diet can usually begin. If multiple sensitivities were present on the initial IgG allergy test, retesting may be deemed appropriate at this time. When foods are reintroduced into the diet, only very small quantities should be initially consumed. In addition, any food reintroduced should initially be limited to one or two small servings a week. If large quantities of the food are suddenly reintroduced into the diet, the hypersensitivity may quickly return. Therefore, great care must be given to the process of reintroduction of any food that has been previously known to cause a problem.

The subject of colon cleansing always arises when digestive system restoration is discussed. Many colon cleansing products exist, and primarily contain fiber, and possibly other herbal additives to accomplish a specific purpose, such as elimination of certain types of parasites. Colon cleansing is often recommended for people suffering from constipation, have irritable bowel syndrome, or when a toxic state of the body is suspected.

The colon does not normally need to be cleansed. The question arises as to why the person suffering from constipation, a toxic state of the body, or other chronic ailment, has a problem with the colon in the first place. Any problems with the colon generally result from an improper diet, food allergies, or disrupted flora of the intestinal tract. A diet that contains 30 grams of fiber a day will keep the colon in a healthy condition. Approximately 50 percent of this fiber should be soluble fiber, and approximately 50 percent should be insoluble fiber, unless otherwise directed by your natural health care provider. Ingesting excessive amounts of processed fiber can actually be harmful, and result in acute mineral imbalances. Acute mineral imbalances can result in various types of cardiac arrhythmias, and possibly lead to other problems. Anyone who feels better following a colon cleansing regimen most likely has other unaddressed intestinal issues.

Another subject that arises quite often is that of a gallbladder flush. The gallbladder is a hollow organ that is found adjacent to the liver. The gallbladder supplies bile, used to emulsify fats and oils, to the digestive tract. Bile is manufactured in the liver, stored in the gallbladder, and released into the intestinal tract following a meal to emulsify fat. When sediment forms in the gallbladder, gall stones can form. If gall stones get large enough, the cystic duct or the common bile duct can become blocked, often requiring emergency surgery. A vague belief exists in the medical profession that gall stones that do not cause any symptoms subsequently do not require any treatment. Belief in this position also requires the belief that symptoms are the sole indicators in determining when medical intervention is required. When symptoms involving gall stones appear, the disease process has obviously become quite advanced. The medical solution to any gallbladder problem is to remove the gallbladder. Since the gallbladder is not an extra or unnecessary organ, steps should be taken to keep it healthy.

The purpose of a gallbladder flush is to eliminate any gall stones that may be present. In eliminating the gall stones, the overall health of the gallbladder is maintained. All gallbladder flush protocols follow roughly the same principle. Fat is eliminated from the diet for a short period, usually a few days, followed by the introduction of a large quantity of fat to the digestive system. When the fat is consumed, the gallbladder forcefully contracts, emptying its contents into the intestinal tract, gall stones and any sediment that are found in the gallbladder. Because of the possibility that a gall stone can get lodged in the cystic duct or common bile duct, any gallbladder flush should be done only under the supervision of a qualified and experienced health practitioner.

The gallbladder can be flushed abruptly in one day or over a period of several days. A gallbladder flush involves an abrupt change in diet, which may not be appropriate for some people, such as people with diabetes, hypoglycemia, or certain other health conditions. This is yet another reason that a gallbladder flush should be done only under the supervision of a qualified health practitioner. The following two methods of flushing gallbladder work quite well for most people. Hundreds of variations of these flushes can be found, but the basic principles remain the same.

The one-day gallbladder flush is a quick and effective method to eliminate any small gall stones and sediment that may have accumulated in the gallbladder. For two weeks prior to the flush, eat a low fat diet and drink two glasses of apple juice each day. The apple juice helps to soften any gall stones, thus allowing them to pass more easily through the ducts. On the day of the flush, eat only green organic apples. Green apples are generally preferred to red apples for flushing the gallbladder. At least five apples should be consumed, during various times throughout the day. Drink only pure water, herbal teas, or unsweetened apple juice. Refrain from eating anything for approximately two hours before bedtime. Right before bedtime, mix 2/3 cup of olive oil and 1/3 cup of freshly squeezed lemon juice. Warm the mixture to body temperature. Drink the mixture, which will not taste too good, and then immediately go to bed. Lie on your right side with your right leg drawn up and left leg straight. This position should be maintained for at least one-half hour, and typically no longer than one hour. In the morning, all gall stones should pass in the stool, and will typically appear as a greenish tint in the feces. Some gall stones may be clearly visible.

For persons who cannot tolerate a one-day drastic gallbladder flush, a variation of the one-day flush may prove sufficient in eliminating a good portion of any gall stones that may exist. In this alternative method, apples are consumed for a period of four to five consecutive days, in addition to a low fat diet. Drink only pure water and herbal teas. On each of the four or five days, right before bedtime, mix three tablespoons of olive oil and two tablespoons of lemon juice, and warm the mixture to body temperature. Drink the mixture and then immediately go to bed. Lie on your right side with your right leg drawn up and left leg straight. This position should be maintained for at least one-half hour, and, again, typically no longer than one hour. This flush can be repeated a month or two later.

Once the integrity of the intestinal lining has been restored, any yeast overgrowths eliminated, the normal bacterial flora restored, and food allergies eliminated, keeping the digestive tract in good working condition would be most beneficial to future health. This is best accomplished by changing the diet to one that is more conducive to good intestinal health. The chapter on nutrition gives several suggestions on how to develop good dietary habits. One thing is for sure, and that is going back to the same eating habits will ultimately result in the same problems resurfacing.

A twenty-three-year-old was diagnosed with Crohn's disease by a gastroenterologist. With no other suggestion than extensive reconstructive surgery offered by the gastroenterologist, the patient sought alternative treatment. The patient entered the office, and presented with classical signs and symptoms of delayed onset food allergies. Clearly a case of leaky gut syndrome, an IgG1 and IgG4 ELISA combination panel was ordered. The test results indicated hypersensitivity to wheat, barley, rye, malt, green peppers, egg, milk, navy beans, pinto beans, cashews, lemon, pineapple, and almonds. All of the hypersensitivities were in the moderate to severe range. The patient had recently graduated from college. A close examination of the allergens reveals a typical college diet - beer, pizza, chili, and assorted snacks found at most any college. Removal of these foods from the diet for several months, combined with supplements to restore the integrity of the digestive tract brought the condition into "complete remission," as verified by a follow-up colonoscopy. The patient, to this date, has been in excellent health.

Chapter 7
Autoimmune Disorders

Autoimmune disease is a result of the failure of the immune system to recognize a part of the body as itself. In a response against its own cells and tissues, the immune system destroys these parts of the body as if they were a foreign invader or some sort of pathogen. Autoimmune diseases can affect connective tissue, nerves, joints, muscles, glands, digestive system, and just about any other tissue or organ in the body. Statistically, most autoimmune diseases occur in women, primarily during childbearing years. Genetic factors have a strong influence on who will and will not potentially develop an autoimmune disease.

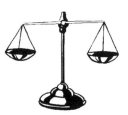

Autoimmune diseases generally occur as a result of an immune system imbalance. When portions of the immune system become out of balance, one part of the immune system becomes dominant as compared with another part. In autoimmune disorders, the Th1 / Th2 balance has been disrupted, with the Th1 response becoming very dominant, and, in comparison, the Th2 response becoming relatively depressed. The Th1 dominance, in conjunction with other factors, leads to the immune system components attacking the body's tissues as if they were a foreign invader. Autoimmune diseases generally require both a genetic and environmental factor to be expressed. Often referred to as the family of inflammatory disorders, the list of diseases that have an autoimmune basis is constantly expanding. Figure 7.1 identifies a partial list of diseases that have an autoimmune component, and the structure or tissue affected by the inflammatory response.

Autoimmune Condition	Antibody Target
Addison's disease	Adrenal cortex cells
Alopecia Areata	Skin
Ankylosing Spondylitis	Spine
Autoimmune Hemolytic Anemia	Erythrocytes
Antiphospholipid syndrome	Blood clotting mechanism
Aplastic Anemia	Bone Marrow
Bursitis	Bursae
Chronic active hepatitis	Hepatocytes
Celiac disease	Small intestine
Crohn's disease	Large Intestine
Diabetes Mellitus Type 1	Pancreas (islet cells)
Eczema	Skin
Goodpasture's syndrome	Kidneys, Lungs
Graves's disease	TSH receptor of Thyroid
Guillain-Barré syndrome	Brain and Nerves
Hashimoto's Thyroiditis	Thyroid
Hypoparathyroidism	Parathyroid cells
Iritis	Iris of the eye
Kawasaki's disease	Arteries around the heart
Multiple Sclerosis	Myelin sheath of nerves
Myasthenia Gravis	Acetylcholine receptors
Pemphigus	Intercellular substance of skin
Pernicious Anemia	Gastric parietal cells
Polymyalgia Rheumatica	Muscle cells
Psoriatic arthritis	Skin
Rheumatoid arthritis	Joints
Rheumatoid fever	Heart
Sjögren's syndrome	Nuclei
Systemic Lupus Erythematosus	Nuclei, DNA, RNA, connective tissue
Ulcerative Colitis	Large Intestine
Wegener's granulomatosis	Primarily Kidneys and Lungs

Figure 7.1   Diseases With an Autoimmune Component

Autoimmunity cannot be contained. When an autoimmune disease is diagnosed, other autoimmune diseases are often found present in varying degrees. The autoimmune diagnosis most commonly is assigned the title of the disease that has the most readily obvious signs and symptoms. Grave's disease and Multiple Sclerosis are autoimmune disorders that appear to share the same mechanism of pathogenesis. A significant co-occurrence of Hashimoto's disease, an autoimmune thyroid condition, can be found in patients with either Multiple Sclerosis or Grave's disease. Other concurrent autoimmune processes that may be present, such as eczema or hypothyroidism, often take a back seat and are usually dismissed as unrelated conditions by the medical doctor and referred out to the appropriate specialist.

The patient with rheumatoid arthritis, eczema, and hypothyroidism ends up seeing a rheumatologist, dermatologist, and endocrinologist. These practitioners are all treating different symptoms of the same autoimmune process, but none are addressing the root cause of the disease. Medical treatment of the inflammatory aspect of autoimmune disease typically consists of anti-inflammatory medications, pain medication, steroids, hormones, and many other medications targeted toward symptomatic relief. Hypothyroidism would be treated with a synthetic thyroid hormone, and the eczema would typically be treated by topical steroid creams. If the root cause was addressed, all autoimmunity would cease, and the related conditions, which were seemingly unrelated, would all subsequently disappear. The need for these medications prescribed for treatment of the symptoms would also disappear.

While autoimmune disease has traditionally been viewed as a disease of the immune system, there is increasing evidence that specific genetic factors are involved. Each year, scientists and researchers are finding more specific genetic links associated with autoimmune diseases. As advancements in technology allow, specific genes are identified with various autoimmune diseases. Research into these specific genes has been occurring for decades, but until the entire sequence of the human genome is precisely mapped and accurately examined, the genetic mechanism of autoimmunity will remain incomplete. When the genome is mapped completely, and research into the science of genetics moves into its final stages, the result will reveal the specific genes associated with and responsible for all autoimmune diseases. Modern genetic research is currently revealing variants of genes affecting a specific part of the immune system. The specific immune system component involved in autoimmunity are the receptors on T-Cells associated with other immune system components called interleukins. Interleukins are proteins, which instruct other specific immune cells called natural killer cells (NK cells), to attack the pathogen.

In many diseases that have a partial genetic basis, an environmental factor must also be present in order for expression of the disease to occur. Autoimmune disease is no exception. This can be seen in families where everyone has inherited the genes linked to the disease, but not everyone contracts the disease. While genetics cannot be controlled, environmental factors leading to the expression of the disease can be controlled to a great degree. If the environmental factors can be identified and controlled, the disease process can be avoided.

Four types of immune hypersensitivity are known to exist. These are termed Type I, Type II, Type III, and Type IV hypersensitivity. The basis of the classification is determined by the different mechanisms involved. Hypersensitivities are often incorrectly called allergies. Hypersensitivity reactions result in responses that causes damage the body's tissues. Autoimmune diseases generally fall into the category of either the Type II or the Type III hypersensitivity mechanism.

A Type I hypersensitivity is an immediate immune response. Symptoms can range from mild discomfort to death. Type I hypersensitivity is mediated by the immunoglobulin IgE. Atopic dermatitis is one example of a Type I hypersensitivity. Others include allergic rhinitis, conjunctivitis, asthma and hay fever. IgE mediated food allergies are also a Type I hypersensitivity reaction. Anaphylactic shock is an extreme case of a Type I hypersensitivity, causing a reaction that is so severe it can possibly lead to death. Exposure to pathogens associated with a Type I hypersensitivity reaction generally occurs at the mucous membranes in the respiratory and digestive tracts. A Type I hypersensitivity immune reaction involves the subsequent activation of a Th2 response.

Type II hypersensitivity, sometimes called a cytotoxic reaction, occurs when an antibody binds to an antigen on the host's own cells, marking them for destruction. This has all the inner workings of autoimmunity. Type B insulin resistant diabetes, Raynaud's syndrome, Grave's disease, Myasthenia Gravis, and some forms of asthma are all classified as a Type II hypersensitivity, although other mechanisms may be involved as well. Type II immune reactions are mediated by IgG and IgM antibodies. Autoimmune Type II hypersensitivities are very difficult to treat. This difficulty in treatment arises because the antigen must be specifically identified and its presence removed. ELISA (Enzyme-Linked Immunosorbent Assay) and EIA (Enzyme Immunoassays) panels are used to test the presence of IgG antibodies in patients suspected of food hypersensitivities.

Type III hypersensitivity reactions are a bit more complex. Immune complexes of IgG, IgM and complement proteins are deposited in various tissues, resulting in the tissue being subsequently attacked by other immune components. This invariably leads to tissue damage. The release of cytoplasmic enzymes from these damaged tissues and influx of pro-inflammatory cells prolong the hypersensitivity. Systemic Lupus Erythematosus, Rheumatoid arthritis, Goodpasture's syndrome, Pemphigus, and Hashimoto's Thyroiditis are all believed to be, at least in part, a Type III Hypersensitivity.

Type IV, or cell-mediated hypersensitivity, are mediated by T-Cells, monocytes, and macrophages. Contact dermatitis is an example of a Type IV hypersensitivity. Poison Ivy is one common Type IV hypersensitivity that everyone is familiar. Latex allergies also fall into the category of a Type IV hypersensitivity, and have become more common in recent years. Celiac disease is a Type IV hypersensitivity to gliadin, a glycoprotein (a carbohydrate and protein combination) found within gluten, a protein found in wheat, barley and oats. Hypersensitivity to gliadin causes destruction of the intestinal villi, subsequently resulting in the malabsorption of nutrients.

Consider for a moment that all autoimmune responses have similar biochemical responses initiated by the immune system. This is not unreasonable, since the same drugs used to treat the symptoms of one autoimmune disease also are effective for treating the symptoms of another autoimmune disease. Also, consider that all allergic responses also have similar biochemical responses initiated by the immune system. This is also reasonable, since a drug used to treat one allergic response is generally shown to be effective for any number of different allergic responses. The drugs used to treat an autoimmune disease act specifically to suppress one type of immune activity, and the drugs used to treat an allergy act to suppress a completely different type of immune activity.

Furthermore, persons who have autoimmune disorders rarely have allergies, and persons who have allergies rarely have autoimmune diseases. That being the case, it leads us to suspect that the two facets of the immune system that are responsible for autoimmune diseases and allergies must have some relation, or some state of balance, with each other. If this delicate balance is disrupted, disease develops. If we can specifically identify the imbalance and somehow restore the balance, the disease process would be theoretically reversed.

Thymus helper cells (Th cells) play a central role in the immune responses associated with allergies and autoimmune diseases. Thymus helper cells can be divided into two major subtypes, Th1 and Th2 cells. Th1 cells are responsible for cell-mediated immune responses, or immunity gained from inside the immune system cell. Th2 cells, on the other hand, are associated with antibody mediated immunity, which is primarily accomplished by the secretion of antibodies, such as IgE and IgG. Th1 and Th2 cells are both necessary, and must be in balance with each other for an appropriate immune response to any pathogen. Thymus helper cells produce chemicals called cytokines. The cytokines produced by Th1 cells are generally different than the cytokines produced by Th2 cells. The cytokines produced by Th1 cells have an inhibitory effect on Th2 cells, and vice versa. Th1 and Th2 cells should have a natural balance to them. Hyperactivity of Th1 cells inhibits Th2 function and hyperactivity of Th2 cells inhibit Th1 function, therefore creating an imbalance in the immune system. This specific type of imbalance is particularly problematic because the Th1 and Th2 components of the immune system have a delicately balanced relationship, or a seesaw effect, to them. The hyperactivity of one component virtually guarantees the suppression of the other component.

In persons with autoimmune diseases, the Th1 immunological response is exaggerated, thus suppressing the activity of Th2 cells. Likewise, in persons with chronic allergic responses, the Th2 immunological response is exaggerated, thus suppressing Th1 cell activity.

Th1 dominant conditions are the family of autoimmune disorders, which are discussed in the beginning of the chapter. Any chronic inflammatory condition is suspect of Th1 dominance. The Th1 immune system pathway primarily acts against intracellular pathogens. These pathogens include viruses and bacteria, therefore, any disease or condition caused by these pathogens activates a Th1 response. Suppressed Th1 activity during pregnancy may explain the higher incidence of infections in pregnant women. The postpartum restoration of Th1 function may also explain why the increased incidence of autoimmune disease often occurs at this time. It is also well known that any person with Multiple Sclerosis, an autoimmune disorder, rarely gets colds, especially during any exacerbation of the disease. Since a cold is caused by a virus, the intracellular pathogen is quickly extinguished by an exaggerated response by Th1 component of the immune system.

Th2 dominant conditions also include a variety of chronic illnesses. These include candidiasis, frequent colds, multiple allergies of various types, multiple chemical sensitivity disorder, asthma, viral hepatitis, and cancer, among many others. Any chronic allergic reaction is suspect of Th2 dominance. Hyperactivity of Th2 cells suppresses the activity of Th1 cells. The Th1 immune response acts against disease causing intracellular pathogens. If the Th2 immunological response becomes dominant, the Th1 response subsequently becomes suppressed. As a result of Th1 suppression due to Th2 dominance, conditions involving intracellular pathogens are more easily able to cause an infection. Interleukin-10, a cytokine produced by Th2 cells, is known to inhibit Th1 cytokine production. Interleukin-10 is just one example of how one facet of the immune system, if overactive, can suppress another facet of the immune system,

The cytokines produced by Th1 and Th2 cells have specific functions associated with them. Great benefit can be found in examining one mechanism of action of a particular cytokine to gain a better understanding of the Th1 / Th2 relationship. Interferon is a well-known cytokine produced by Th1 cells. One very well documented function of Interferon is to inhibit viral growth and tumor growth. In the case of Interferon, three variations of the cytokine are known to exist. These variations are named *Interferon-alpha*, *Interferon-beta*, and *Interferon-gamma*. Each variation has a specific effect on other types of immune cells. All variations of Interferon stimulate the activity of Natural Killer (NK) cells, which are a vital part of the immune system cascade in fighting cancer. *Interferon-gamma* specifically plays a part in the stimulation of B-Cell growth and differentiation. If Th1 cell activity is diminished due to Th2 hyperactivity, it would logically follow that Interferon levels would subsequently decrease since Interferon is produced by Th1 cells. This decrease in Interferon levels is just one example of why the patient with Th2 hyperactivity is more susceptible to diseases of both viral origin and cancer. What is also evident is that the decreased levels of Interferon have a marked effect on other immune system components as well. The subsequent effects on other immune systems components, such as in B-Cell growth and differentiation, have extensive effects on many facets of the immune system.

Despite the significant amount of research focused on the Th1 and Th2 responses in autoimmune diseases and allergies, it must be pointed out that external factors often skew evidence collected in human tests and observations. One such factor is long term use of pharmacologic agents to suppress certain immune responses. Specifically, any pharmacological agent in which the mechanism of action modifies any of the immune components involved is suspect in immune system modification. Antibiotics, antihistamines, anti-RA drugs, corticosteroids, the administration of Interferon, and certain medications that are prescribed off-label, are but a few examples of medications that can be involved in immune system modification. Finding test patients who have not been subjected to such medications is difficult, if not impossible. Finding a control group for research purposes who have never been subjected to these medications is even more impossible. The scientific methods utilized in research require, by definition, that a control group exist. As a result of no legitimate control group, the conclusion of any research, at best, represents opinion based on speculation.

In the case of any autoimmune disorder, at sometime during the patient's life the hypersensitivity was clearly allowed to manifest for any number of reasons.

In the discussion of health, three reasons were identified that lead to an unhealthy state. The hypersensitivity initially was allowed to manifest for the reason:

> *Something enters into the body, but, for some reason, the body can no longer process it correctly.*

Specifically, something that should have normally caused no harm to the body, as a result of some cascade of events, is now able to cause harm to the body. Backtracking may be difficult to find out specifically what caused the imbalance of the immune system leading to the unhealthy state. The usual suspects are the use of antibiotics, consumption of refined sugar, over exposure to certain foods, or poor diet. In most cases, however, multiple factors were involved for an extended time leading to the disease. Whatever the cause, any known biological or chemical disruptors linked to the development of an immune system imbalance should be avoided. Chlorinated water, causing biological disruption of the normal intestinal bacterial flora, is one example of a biological and chemical disruptor.

If we can restore Th1 and Th2 balance, any autoimmune disease, allergy, Th1 dominant condition, or Th2 dominant condition should then be resolved. Th1 and Th2 balance can be restored by eliminating any environmental factors that are responsible for the disruption. Identification and modification of environmental factors found contributing to the disruption of the Th1 / Th2 balance are then of the utmost importance.

In persons with autoimmune disease, the digestive system is invariably found to have a disruption of the normal bacterial flora. The integrity of the digestive system and balance of the beneficial bacterial flora must be corrected if the autoimmune condition is expected to resolve. An entire chapter has been devoted to discussing restoration of the digestive system. For the autoimmune sufferer, this is the first place to begin.

Once the digestive system has been restored, if an imbalance involving Th1 or Th2 activity is suspected, steps must be taken to adjust the Th1 and Th2 components of the immune system. This can be accomplished by specially formulated probiotic supplements designed to suppress the Th1 component of the immune system. Suppression of the Th1 component will result in enhanced activity of the Th2 component, thus bringing the immune system back into balance.

Specific strains of probiotics have been shown to suppress Th1 activity. If the probiotic strains with this characteristic were isolated and introduced to the digestive tract, the balance between Th1 and Th2 cell activity can be successfully restored. *Lactobacillus salivarius* and *Bifidobacterium lactis* have been specifically shown to suppress Th1 activity, therefore would be of great benefit to patients with autoimmune diseases. The company Original Medicine® has developed products containing these isolated strains. The Original Medicine® product, Th1S™ is specifically formulated to suppress Th1 activity.

Since the normal bacterial flora of the autoimmune patient was found in a disrupted state, steps must be taken to avoid future disruption of this delicate balance. Any factor involved in the disruption of the intestinal flora must be eliminated. These factors include the use of prescription antibiotics, consumption of antibiotic laden meats and dairy products, consumption of chlorinated water, and ingesting refined sugar, to name just a few. Adoption of a proper diet free of highly processed foods, therefore, is of utmost importance. The suggestion of adopting a healthy diet was made in the chapter on nutrition. In that chapter, it was also discussed that people living one hundred years ago were not afflicted with the diseases of people today. Autoimmune disease clearly is one of those diseases. With many factors contributing to disruption of the intestinal flora, understanding why this is so becomes very clear.

It must be taken into consideration that the immune system has a memory associated with it. This memory contains very specific details regarding antigens to which the immune system has been exposed. If the particular antigen is a food protein, the particular food containing that protein must be removed from the diet for a length of time. The period of abstinence will vary, depending on the severity of the associated immune system reaction. This time of abstinence is required for the immune system to lose memory, or forget about, the antigen. Specifically, the immune system does not continue to create more antibodies against antigens that do not pose a threat. By abstaining from the offending food, new antibodies against that food are therefore not created, and existing antibodies to that food will decrease over time.

Many external factors have been shown to affect the immune system in various ways. One such factor, stress, is well known to affect the immune system in a negative way. Anyone who has suffered with an autoimmune disease knows beyond any doubt that stress is a significant factor in exacerbation and remission of any autoimmune disease. When a person is under stress, they become more susceptible to contracting any number of illnesses. Considerable stress, in conjunction with poor diet and lack of sleep, is an open door for the disease process to begin. An entire chapter, therefore, has been dedicated to the subject of stress and the body's reaction to stress, known as the General Adaption Syndrome.

Herbs reported to strengthen the immune system should not be used by persons with autoimmune disease unless the herb has been specifically proven to correct any immune system imbalance associated with autoimmunity. Strengthening the immune system may very well strengthen the Th1 immunological response initially responsible for the autoimmune disease, therefore exacerbating the condition. The last thing a patient with autoimmune disease needs is to strengthen the Th1 immune response. The correct approach in addressing the immune system in persons with autoimmune disease would be to balance the immune system, suppressing the Th1 immune response and strengthening the Th2 immune response.

Autoimmune diseases have both a genetic basis and environmental factors involved. While little can be done to alter genetics, much can be done to adjust any environmental factors involved in autoimmune disease. Restoration of the digestive system, and proper balance of the normal intestinal bacterial flora is very important in keeping autoimmune disease in check. Proper handling of stress, as well, is important in keeping the immune system in balance. Several chapters, therefore, have been dedicated to these subjects.

A patient was distressed that she was recently diagnosed with Multiple Sclerosis by a neurologist. My response was "well, at least that is an easy one to fix." Her response, "easy, what do you mean easy?" quickly followed my statement. A 30 minute discussion of the immune system and how to balance the Th1 and Th2 components of the immune system gave the patient a better idea of what was going on. A change in diet, elimination of the yeast infection that was present, and administration of a probiotic supplement restored the digestive tract and immune system. The patient's neurological complaints disappeared, along with the eczema, which was overlooked by the neurologist.

Chapter 8
Chronic Stress

Stress is becoming more of an integral part of modern day society. With everyone working longer hours, almost no time can be found for leisure, vacation, or just a day off. The term "working vacation" has come into common use, and the term itself is a good indicator of not where society is headed, but already is. Substantial evidence can be found supporting the idea that the stressful modern human lifestyle is contributing to the decline in the overall health of society. If we, as a society, continue down the same path, the result will be increasing amounts of stress related disease. It seems then, that our need, as a society, is for some genius to come along and invent a new lifestyle that is free of stress. This better lifestyle would be a welcomed change to the modern way of life.

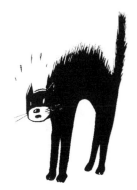

The environment of the modern day business world has been more competitive than a professional sports contest. Within business, fierce competition is not exclusive with the competitors in the marketplace, but internal competition within the ranks exists as well. Internal corporate politics have become a serious form of a one-upmanship competition because individual survival depends upon the salaries the corporations pay. To move up the corporate ladder, one must be able to "prove" themselves to the higher-ups in charge, which is traditionally accomplished by doing much more work than is normally expected. Since all employees have the desire to occupy the higher rungs of the corporate ladder, everyone can be found working longer and longer hours, thus setting the new standard of work performance. When the annual performance reviews come along, everyone is quite shocked when all those extra hours yield nothing more than "average" performance, and the suggestion that next year's performance should be better. Any salary increase is usually minimal, followed by the usual lecture regarding budgetary constraints and economic conditions. Suggestions by the management given to the employee are typically followed by the promise of a promotion and a raise next year if the goals are met. When someone is finally promoted within the group, it is usually the person who was the least expected to move up within the ranks, and it is later discovered that he is the nephew of the vice-president down the hall. This drives departmental morale to an all-time low, resulting in countless résumés and cover letters cranking out of printers after hours, emails being sent to every online employment website, and dedicated employees searching for better positions in new companies. When someone finally does leave the corporation, they find themselves again starting at the bottom, only to find themselves in a more fierce game climbing the corporate ladder, with a new and different set of rules, and in a worse mess than the job they left. The employee who left for that better situation quicky realizes that the grass is greener on the other side of the street because the dog has visited that yard more often. The person who decides to stay, after giving 110% and finally due that promotion that they have been looking forward to, finds out through the grapevine that their position, along with the rest of the department, has been contracted out to consultants in India who cannot speak English. At the same time, upper management pretends to know nothing about the situation, and the layoffs occur right before the holiday season, when no one is hiring. As it turned out, the color of that special credit card did not matter much in impressing upper-level management after all.

In most households, two wage earners are generally needed to make the monthly budget balance. With housing costs, utility costs, insurance premiums, college tuition, and other budget items outpacing any salary increases, other sources of income are required to maintain the same standard of living. Additional sources often include a second job, a spouse going to work, or joining some multi-level marketing group promising six-figure incomes while working only ten hours a week. Any of these usually result in even more stress, with any additional income earned ending up in the U.S. Treasury due to the new higher tax bracket and a daycare center to take care of the children during the longer working hours. If any additional money manages to make its way to the savings account, the water heater breaks or the car is suddenly in need of an overhaul. It is long forgotten that, in the 1960s, one wage earner is all that was required to support a family of five comfortably.

With the arrival of modern technology, everyone always seems to need the latest electronic toy. Cell phones, MP3 players, faster internet connections, and GPS navigation devices are all required to become an active member of the in-crowd. This is not limited to teenage social circles, but is evident among the adults as well. In teenage circles, however, the reasons for needing the newer, more modern technology goes far beyond reasons most parents can comprehend. These advanced reasons generally include indisputable facts such as their friends have one, or they will somehow feel left out. Having a cell

Why Am I Sick? And What To Do About It

phone is not only important, but it must be the right cell phone, with the right features, and the proper ring tone. The same applies to any other electronic gizmo, whether it is working properly or not, if it does not have the latest and greatest features, it is a social embarrassment and must simply be replaced. Modern day parents, in the eyes of a teenager, cannot simply comprehend these necessities of life. After all, in this complicated modern day society, it is next to impossible for a teenager to drive a half mile down the street to their friend's house without a GPS to tell them how to get there, a cell phone should they get lost, and an MP3 player to keep them entertained throughout the journey. While purchasing such items may cause financial stress upon the adults, not having the item often places social stress on the teenagers. With the teenager, whether this social stress is logical or not is, for the most part, immaterial. It is still stress, and carries the same burden of any other type of stress. The stress, in the case of either the teenager or the adult, is perceived as the same. As a result, the stress response in the body is the same.

The electronic generation has introduced another problem that is becoming more difficult to deal with, which affects almost every age group. The brain normally discards much of the sensory information it receives as irrelevant, or just simply background noise. At any given moment, much of this noise is present, such as a ticking clock, phones ringing, automobile traffic outside, conversations down the hall, radios playing, not to mention the background hum of flourescent lighting and air-conditioning equipment. This background noise is considered both irrelevant and unimportant, and therefore is ignored by the brain, thus preventing an overload of the senses. Modern society has brought a new type of background noise with which everyone must contend. In today's fast paced society, multitasking is becoming more common. Email piles up in the inbox, the newest hand-held gizmo demands immediate attention, cell phones are ringing, text messages are being sent back and forth, and instant messages come across the computer screen, all of which are top priority and must be addressed immediately. This puts us in a position where we must give constant careful attention to every form of stimuli around us, otherwise that important call or email might just be missed. This, in effect, is another form of a sensory overload. It is no different from listening to five radio stations simultaneously and expecting to make coherent sense out of every program. Simply put, the mind is not designed to function in continuous overload mode. Naturally, this type of continuous sensory and mental overload results in stress.

Modern electronics has brought us another highly technological group of inventions that promises to raise stress levels to even new heights. These new advances of technology are in the form of sophisticated snooping devices developed to watch a person's every action. Miniaturization techniques make it possible to place hidden cameras in just about any location. Telephone conversations may be listened to secretly, or recorded, so no one even feels comfortable placing a personal phone call from their corporate office. In attempts to avoid the corporate snoopers, personal calls are often placed from cell phones that appear to have much greater security. Most people, however, are unaware that anyone who has any knowledge of electronics can easily modify a radio scanner to listen in on these supposedly secure digital communications. Worse yet is knowing that someone can point a device at your home and listen to what has thought to have been said in private. Snooping is no longer limited to the video and audio level. Internet communications are monitored to the point that no personal business affairs dare be conducted at work in fear that one may lose their job. Spyware can be easily installed on most any computer, tracking every keystroke and website visited. If someone finds the spyware and removes it, they quickly are informed by a co-worker that a gateway-based employee monitoring tool tracks every website visited. The local intersection has even been fitted with a sophisticated camera connected to a computer that will send an automated traffic ticket to anyone caught running the red light. Newer technology, including biometric identification and radio frequency identification devices, (RFID) promise to end terrorism and make the world a safer place to live. However, once these tools get into the hands of corporations, they will be used at an absurd level to protect even the coffee machine from unauthorized users. The trend is clearly moving toward the end of any personal privacy at all. With no personal privacy, people often feel as if their life is put under a microscope, adding even more stress to any existing stress.

Another factor contributing to chronic stress is the time pressure exerted upon us because of social schedules. This is most commonly seen among parents of both preteens and teens who are involved in sports, after school activities, church groups, and other societal obligations. Planning a schedule in which every minute of every hour is accounted for has become the norm of today's society. Any free time is quicky filled with another activity, which is later found to conflict with that special event at school written on a notice that got lost on the school bus. Then comes the unplanned event, such as an unexpected trip to the doctor, which usually results in frantically trying to find someone to transport the remaining healthy kids to their scheduled events. With a schedule that demands such precise timing, we go from event to event without stopping, leaving no time to get a massage or read a book. Any means of escaping such a demanding lifestyle seems to be a glimpse into a fantasy world. This tremendous preoccupation with time and scheduling may as well be called an incapacity for pleasure. When rest and relaxation finally calls, it gets a busy signal.

Then, out of the blue, a symptom suddenly appears, and the patient attempts to make an appointment with the medical doctor. Not surprisingly, the doctor's office now has a computerized phone menu. So, after listening to "If you are a new patient, press one, if you are calling from a doctor's office, press two, if you are a telemarketer, press ten," the patient just presses zero and hopes for the best. Upon making their selection, the patient is now placed on hold for ten minutes, which seems like eternity. Everyone knows that no matter which number is chosen, the caller will still be connected with the same receptionist, but the new computerized phone system give the illusion that the medical office is bigger than it really is. When the patient finally gets to speak to a live person, they find out the doctor is no longer on the insurance plan, so they give the patient the name of another doctor down the street who takes the insurance plan. The patient calls, and the new doctor can surprisingly see them today. The trip to the doctor results in a complete physical, and a complete set of comprehensive laboratory tests. After the week of constant stress, the only problem the doctor can find is slightly elevated blood pressure, and suggests medication. The patient does not like this idea, so the decision is made to wait for the lab test results, and check the blood pressure again next week. During the follow-up visit, the patients blood pressure is normal, and the patient is also notified that all the laboratory tests were normal. But, since the patient's great-grandfather died of heart disease, the doctor suggests a cholesterol-lowering medication as a preventive measure. The doctor, while checking the patients blood pressure during the follow-up visit, suggests that an electrocardiogram should be done immediately, because he suspects a third degree heart block. Concerned, the patient then questions the doctor about this heart block. The doctor responds by telling her a heart rate of 40 beats per minute is not normal and is indicative of a third degree heart block, which is a potentially dangerous arrhythmia. At the end of this comprehensive examination and follow-up, it was somehow overlooked that the 26-year-old patient initially came in minor hip pain, which occurred while she was training for a triathlon, and only wanted a referral to her chiropractor. Casual examination of the patient should have revealed that the heart rate of 40 beats per minute is due to her exceptional physical condition, and not a third degree heart block. The doctor, picking up his cane, shakes it at the patient, sternly warning her how risky chiropractic can be, and leaves the room. Going to her chiropractor anyway, the patient pays out-of-pocket, and her hip gets completely better in two visits. Meanwhile, the bill from the medical doctor comes, and the insurance did not cover any of the $800.00 charges. Of course, in the mind of the medical doctor, no part of this fiasco should have caused the patient additional stress.

The word anxiety is really just another word for self-created mental stress. Anxiety comes about when a person is afraid some event will occur that will alter the future in a way thought to be undesirable. Everyone knows that whatever the problem is that is causing the anxiety is most likely not going to happen anyway, except, perhaps, for the person experiencing the anxiety. Opposing sound logic, the game of "what-if" never ceases, creating an enormous amount of self-inflicted mental stress, leading to physical diseases that would not have occurred otherwise. Even if the dreaded event did occur, often it turns out to be not nearly as disastrous as originally envisioned. The issue, however, is that it is the anxiety that leads to physical disease, and not the feared event.

All this seems seriously futile. The goal of moving up the corporate ladder, working endless hours, buying the latest technology, being controlled by plastic electronic boxes, schedules planned down to the minute, and dealing with a twisted and convoluted health care system all contribute to a stressful lifestyle. When one steps back and contemplates what is actually occurring, it appears to be, in a way, quite odd. What appears to be occurring is everyone is involved in a race in which the participants must keep running faster and faster. Once someone enters the race, they are told that continued participation is mandatory, and exiting the race is not an option. Unfortunately, the race never ends and the only winners are the ones who never chose to participate. The few who did not believe from the outset that participation in the race was mandatory subsequently are the happiest and healthiest people around. Not needing any electronic junk, they can be found laying aside some pool with their friends, on a beach, or climbing a mountain, seemingly out of touch with the rest of society. In reality, however, they are more in touch with themselves, other people, and their environment than the electronic driven society in which they refuse to participate. What is seen more in today's society is that people just choose to get out of the race altogether, move to the mountains or some other place they will be happy, and forget completely about the stressful society that caused all of their problems in the first place.

The difficulty in comprehending anything different other than the modern day stressful lifestyle has moved into a realm that conceptual thinking cannot easily grasp. The notion of not working continuously seems like a foreign concept to most individuals. Equally as foreign is the notion of not carrying a cell phone or having an email address. Every new generation creates a new form of reality, and thus redefines societal norms. The current generation could not easily survive in the society of one hundred years ago, just like the future generations will not be easily able to survive in today's world. With a pattern that keeps repeating itself, today's fast-paced society will appear slow and backward and archaic to future generations. As a consequence of increasing the pace, future generations must contend with even greater stresses, more stress related illness and disease, and subsequently more time and money maintaining what little health they have left.

Now that we have a basic understanding of where the various forms of stress come from, we must look at stress and examine what stress really is. When we think of stress, most commonly emotional stress comes to mind. Three types of stress, however, are known to exist. These are chemical stress, emotional stress, and physical stress. All three types of stress produce the same biochemical and physiological responses in the body. The body, contrary to what we may have been taught, does not differentiate between any of the three types of stress. No matter the type of stress, the end result is essentially the same. While stress seems bad, not all stress is detrimental. It is the unrelenting stress, for which there is no foreseen relief, that becomes problematic. This unrelenting chronic stress is what potentially leads to physical disease.

Chemical stress generally occurs when a chemical stressor is introduced directly into the body. Toxins, which are found in the air, water, and environment, are all sources of chemical stressors. The sources of chemical stressors, however, are not limited to only the environment. Medications, whether over the counter, recreational, or prescription, cause chemical stress to the body. Malnutrition is a different form of chemical stress, stressing the biochemical pathways of the body. In the case of malnutrition, chemical stress occurs due to the lack of, or excess of one or more nutrients. Chemical stress, then, is any stress that directly interferes with the biochemical pathways of the body.

When the term stress is used, most people immediately think of emotional stress. Commonly, emotional stress occurs as a result of certain thought patterns and emotions. Emotional stress is often linked to employment, day to day activities, and social situations. Emotional stress also occurs when a person watches a stressful movie in which horror, bloodshed, or otherwise

Why Am I Sick? And What To Do About It

stressful situations are depicted on the silver screen. Whether the source of the emotional stress is real or imagined, the stress is perceived in the same way by the mind. If one came across a Great White Shark while swimming in the ocean, emotional stress would instantaneously occur. In this respect, little difference is realized between watching a movie with a Great White Shark and actually encountering one. The only difference is the degree of the stress response. The physical response that occurs in the body from emotional stress is yet more evidence of the mind-body connection.

Physical stress occurs as a result of physical trauma to the body. Automobile accidents, slip and fall injuries, and athletic injuries are all types of physical stress. Repetitive trauma is also a type of physical stress, and is becoming more common in today's society. Repetitive trauma can occur as a result of any repeated activity. Carpal Tunnel Syndrome is one example of stress to the physical body, and is usually a result of repeated activities involving the hands, such as typing or writing. Bad posture is a chronic form of physical stress, causing unrelenting inordinate stress to be placed upon the muscles, tendons, and joints. Bad posture leads to muscle fatigue, toxin accumulation, and damage to the joints. In many cases, however, bad posture is a result of spinal subluxation, a condition best addressed by a chiropractor. Often, forms of physical stress are not readily apparent. Sleeping on an old and worn out mattress is an example of physical stress to the body that is often overlooked, and can result in physical stress to the joints and connective tissues, causing inflammation.

When someone is in a long, drawn out emotional argument, which lasts for days, they generally equate the overall feeling to being hit by a train or run over by a truck. In this regard, understanding how physical stress and emotional stress can have the same response in the body is not difficult. In all types of stress, muscles are found to be in spasm, the person does not sleep well, digestive issues may arise, along with a long list of seemingly unrelated complaints, which are, in fact, all due to the stress response. Stress in any form can quickly and easily take its toll on every system of the body.

Just what is this stress that is all too common in today's society? Does everybody react differently to stress? Are some fortunate few somehow been granted immunity to stress? Does this thing we call stress actually have a definition, or is it just another vague medical term? To understand stress, and understand what happens to the body during stress, we must look at stress from a biochemical and physiological viewpoint. In looking at stress at this level, we not only gain an understanding of stress, but the proper way to handle stress becomes evident as well.

In 1936, Hans Selye, a Canadian endocrinologist, described a model of stress called the General Adaption Syndrome. In this model, three stages of stress were identified. These three stages are the alarm phase, resistance phase, and the exhaustion phase. Dr. Selye showed that these three phases apply to all stress, no matter the origin or type of stress. Every year, more evidence from research accumulates supporting the principles of the General Adaption Syndrome model.

Initially, the inspiration for General Adaption Syndrome originated from an endocrine system experiment in which mice were injected with extracts of various organs. The result was that, for each substance injected into the mice, the same symptoms and physiologic responses were demonstrated to occur. These responses included many physiological responses, including atrophy of the thymus gland, liver, spleen, and lymph glands, loss of muscle tone, erosion (ulcers) of the intestinal lining, and multiple changes to the adrenal glands. These chemical irritants, termed "noxious agents" by Selye, were observed to produce similar physiological responses in people. Repeated injuries, excessive muscular exercise, and prolonged exposure to cold were also shown to cause the same physiologic response as did the noxious agents. Selye later used the term "stress" to describe the physiological response to these irritants, whether noxious agents (chemical stress), physical stress, or emotional stressors. Chemical stress, physical stress, or emotional stress, or any combination of the three, was found to initiate the General Adaption Syndrome.

If we were to research stress, we find a significant amount of work and literature suggesting that stress is very difficult to define. Organizations, purporting to be experts on the subject of stress, state that stress is a merely subjective sensation that is felt. If stress is subjective, the implication is made that stress cannot be measured. Stress, however, can be clearly measured in many ways. An elevated level of norepinephrine, for example, is a good indicator of acute stress. Biochemical markers can specifically identify oxidative stress. Elevated cortisol levels are an excellent indication of chronic stress. Various biochemical metabolites give an excellent indication of the biochemical health of an individual, many of which are affected in well known ways by stress. Many of these biochemical reactions, which result from stress, can be found in the cascade of events following engagement of the flight or fight mechanism. The engagement of the flight or fight mechanism is the beginning of stress. The cascade of events that follow varies from person to person, and is dependent upon many factors such as diet, overall health, activities, and genetic factors. If the fight or flight mechanism has not been engaged, the person will have no biochemical or physiological evidence indicting stress. Conversely, when the fight or flight mechanism is not engaged, the body is not under stress.

Stress, therefore, can be measured objectively, and can be defined quite easily. Stress can be defined, then, as:

> *Stress is the engagement of the flight or flight mechanism caused by a chemical, physical, or an emotional stressor.*

Selye also observed that the changes seen in the physiology of the body associated with stress is found to have two distinct components. The first component of stress is what he termed the General Adaptation Syndrome. The General Adaption Syndrome outlines the course that will be followed when an organism is presented with stress. The General Adaption Syndrome has three phases; progression through the phases is dependent on many factors. The second component of stress, left unnamed by Selye, is that, under the appropriate conditions, the stressors will ultimately cause disease. Any disease caused by stress is a result of chronically overloaded biochemical pathways and the associated cascade of effects on the tissues. In summary, the stress reaction follows a well-defined path. Figure 8.1 outlines the progression of stress, which is described in the following paragraphs.

The first stage of the General Adaption Syndrome is the alarm phase. The alarm phase is also known as acute stress. When the stressor is introduced, the initial response of the body is the state of alarm. Stressors may from either a chemical, physical, or an emotional origin, or any combination. During this stage, the body reacts by engaging the fight or flight response, causing adrenaline and norepinephrine to be released from the adrenal glands, and cortisol to be released from the adrenal cortex. The Hypothalamus and Pituitary Axis (HPA) is also involved, ultimately affecting the endocrine system. The fight or flight response also involves a strong sympathetic nervous system response. The primary neurotransmitter of the sympathetic nervous system is norepinephrine, which quickly sends the sympathetic nervous system into high gear. This results in an increased heart rate, the dilation of blood vessels supplying muscles, the constriction of blood vessels supplying the digestive and certain other organs, decreased digestive system activity, and other responses geared toward physical confrontation. Physiological changes associated with the first phase are apparent from six to forty-eight hours following the exposure to the stressor. Physiological changes, however, are only beginning to occur during the first phase.

The fight or flight mechanism is designed to be a response to acute stress. This is normally a short term response, lasting only a few minutes to a few hours. Biochemically and physiologically, the fight or flight response is not designed to be continually engaged for days. In addition, the fight or flight mechanism was not designed to be engaged multiple times a day, day after day. When such a degree of engagement is found to exist, steps must be taken to avoid the stressor.

Alarm Phase
↓
Resistance Phase → Physiological Changes
↓
Exhaustion Phase → Disease

Figure 8.1   The Progression of Stress

The second stage of the General Adaption Syndrome is called the resistance phase, and is entered approximately 48 hours following the initial exposure to the stressor. The resistance phase is inevitable when the source of the stress remains present, causing the body to develop some form of resistance to the stressor. The resistance phase is, therefore, the body attempting to find a method to cope with the continued stress. With the persistent fight or flight reaction, the thyroid becomes hypertrophied (increased in size), growth hormone levels decrease, the gonads become atrophied, and the adrenal glands remain enlarged. These biological changes are attempts of the body to increase the production of the hormones required to handle the stress response and ensure survival, and decrease other biological activities that are not associated with the stress response. During the second phase, the output of the glands associated with the stress response actually returns to normal for a short period. As the second phase continues, the patient, in response to the physiological changes in the body, may begin using caffeine, sugar, or other stimulant to maintain the energy levels required for daily life. The body, however, cannot maintain this state of increased stress indefinitely. Continued exposure to the stressors over a period of one to three months results in complete exhaustion of the body's resources. When these resources are depleted, the exhaustion phase is then entered.

The third and final stage of the General Adaption Syndrome is the exhaustion phase. In this final stage, all resources of the body have been significantly depleted, and, as the name of the phase suggests, the body is in a state of complete exhaustion. As a result, the systems of the body are unable to maintain normal function, and no longer is there any capacity for the systems of the body to adapt further. Impaired function of many of the body's systems is evident during this phase. In the exhaustion phase, insomnia, anxiety or both may be present, contributing to the already stressful state. Immune system function also begins to decrease, and other illnesses, such as frequent colds and infections, may occur. In the exhaustion phase, autoimmune disease may be found to be active in predisposed individuals. As a result of the fight or flight response being engaged for an extended period, nearly all of the body's systems have been compromised to some extent due to the unrelenting stress. This can cause damage to the organs involved, which will eventually manifest as some form of illness or disease. Ulcers, cardiovascular disease, depression, or chronic disease all can begin during the exhaustion phase, and, if the exhaustion phase is not exited, the disease process continues unabated. Perhaps the most overlooked and potentially most damaging manifestation of the exhaustion phase is a compromised immune system. A compromised immune system subsequently can lead to any number of chronic diseases. The digestive system, however, is usually the first to suffer in the cascade of events initiating the disease process. Long term examples of what can result from adrenal exhaustion are fibromyalgia and chronic fatigue syndrome. In these syndromes, cortisol levels often drop due to adrenal fatigue, resulting in loss of the protective benefits of cortisol.

Selye observed that the physiology associated with stress, under appropriate conditions, can cause disease. If stress, therefore, is not to result in disease, this pathway to disease must be circumvented. The pathway leading to disease can be best bypassed during the alarm phase before any physiological changes or diseases are allowed to occur. Once the resistance phase is entered, another pathway must be taken to reverse any physiological changes that may have occurred. Once the exhaustion phase has been entered, other factors must be taken into consideration in order to attempt to repair any damage to the body's systems that may have occurred. Reversal of the exhaustion phase is no simple matter. Fortunately, the good news is that each phase is reversible.

Phase one, the alarm phase, is primarily characterized as acute stress. If phase one has been entered, the fight or flight mechanism has been engaged by a chemical, physical, or an emotional stressor. During this phase, circumventing the natural progression of the General Adaption Syndrome is quite easily accomplished. By examining why the alarm phase is entered and what the purpose of the fight or flight reaction is, we will come to a clear understanding of how to circumvent the consequences of stress.

The response to any form of stress is termed the *fight or flight reaction*. This term did not come about for no reason at all, nor was it named the fight or flight reaction purely by accident. Before modern day society, the natural stress response of the body occurred to ensure survival by enabling the person to handle the natural stressors better, which presented themselves from time to time. Specifically, the intent of the fight or flight mechanism is to equip the person to confront an attacker, escape from an attacker, or handle any number of imminent physical threats with greater energy and strength. For example, a confrontation with a snake, tiger or angry dog would appropriately result in the fight or flight response. When such a confrontation occurs, adrenaline and norepinephrine levels rise suddenly, resulting in physical abilities that are far beyond what the body is normally capable. As a result of the increased adrenaline levels, the body fully expects some type of physical activity such as running, fighting, or both to follow. The fight or flight reaction is a short term physiological response, meaning the associated biochemical and physiological pathways cannot maintain functioning at an elevated level for an extended time.

In modern day society, unnatural stressors are more prevalent than natural stressors. Unnatural stressors, such as sitting in rush hour traffic, working extended hours, or a checkbook in the red should not qualify to engage the fight or flight response. For many people, however, these unnatural stressors engage the fight or flight response. When this is the case, the biochemistry and physiology of the body react in the same way as a result of these unnatural stressors as it did with the natural stressors. As a result, the fight or flight mechanism becomes engaged. A problem arises when the body has prepared itself at the biochemical and physiological level for a physical confrontation, yet no physical confrontation occurs. The sympathetic nervous system response, which occurs as a result of the fight or flight response, causes functional changes in many of the body's systems. When the alarm state is not carried through to completion, the expected release of energy is ultimately internalized in some manner that is inappropriate. This result of this internalization of the fight or flight response is highly dependent on the individual's personality. Since the associated mechanisms of stress in the situation of both natural and unnatural stress are the same, appropriate responses to unnatural stressors should be the same as with natural stressors. The appropriate response, whether the stressor is natural or unnatural, is physical activity. Physical activity, such as weightlifting, running, competitive sports, or any other activity in which significant physical energy is expended is the only viable method of carrying the fight or flight response through to completion. Counting to ten and smiling is an utterly useless method to release built-up stress. Stress, then, must be handled in a way that is compatible with the underlying biochemistry and physiology of the body. Physical activity is the only option.

Drugs, such as tranquilizers, are often prescribed for acute stress. While these medications may have their place, such as during severe acute stress, they do not eliminate the stressor or the stress response. No medication can cure stress. If one believes that stress can be cured by ingesting some man-made chemical, one must also believe that the stress was initially caused by the deficiency of that man-made chemical in the body. Medications used to combat stress are, themselves, yet another form of stress, specifically chemical stress. The additional burden on the body by this additional chemical stress hastens the progression to the next phase of the General Adaption Syndrome. When the body is already under stress, treatment should not consist of the burden of additional stress. The person using tranquilizers day after day to relieve stress, while they may feel better, is handling stress in a dangerous way.

The normal stress response, the fight or flight reaction, involves a sympathetic nervous system response. Decreased digestive system activity normally occurs as a result of this nervous system response. Often, an individual's response to stress is to eat. The type of food chosen varies from person to person, with sweets, particularly chocolate, being a common choice. No matter the food choice, eating during times of acute stress is not a normal biological activity. This abnormal activity of eating during times of stress is usually done to induce the release of serotonin in the brain, which is the body's "feel good" neurotransmitter, thus alleviating, to some degree, the feelings associated with stress. The normal and appropriate biological response to stress would be the opposite reaction, which is not to eat. Eating, then, during times of stress, causes a problem in that the food consumed is not adequately and fully digested. The behavior of eating when under acute stress, therefore, needs to be reversed. In reversing this behavior, the progression of the General Adaption Syndrome is slowed.

Circumventing the path to the second phase of the General Adaption Syndrome must obviously be done during the first phase. To circumvent this path, we need to look no further than the intended response of the body to the fight or flight reaction. Once adrenaline and norepinephrine have been released, the body expects physical activity to follow. Physical activity, therefore is the appropriate response to acute stress. Any form of elevated physical activity should suffice; the type selected depends only on the preferences of the individual. Some people prefer to go to the gym or engage in other athletic activities, others prefer to engage in a whirlwind session of cleaning the home, yet others prefer to engage in sexual activity. Those who prefer ranting and raving are actually releasing physical energy to some degree, although most likely at the expense of raising the stress of people around them. The point is, in each case, that physical energy is being released as a result of physical activity, which is what the physiology of the body expects.

The second phase, resistance, occurs when the body begins to develop resistance to the stressor. Most often, multiple stressors are present, all contributing to the net stress level. The natural physiological response to stress, the fight or flight reaction, continues unabated during the resistance phase. The body, however, begins to adapt, and it often appears to the patient that he or she is handling the stress quite well. This, however, is not the case. The body cannot maintain this state indefinitely, and unless this phase is interrupted, progression to the final phase, exhaustion, is inevitable.

While the resistance phase is underway, the digestive system is slowly being compromised. A compromised digestive system will ultimately lead to a compromised immune system, resulting in various disease processes. Restoration of the digestive system, therefore, is desirable to prevent any further decay of health. Temporary use of digestive enzyme supplements may be required, giving the digestive organs an opportunity to rest. Should the digestive system become compromised, malnutrition, food allergies, and compromise of the immune system are just around the corner, the effects of which may not be evident until months or years later. Consequently, adequate nutrition during times of stress is imperative. Since the mind is always involved in stress, particular attention must be paid to nutrients involved in the production of neurotransmitters.

Arresting all sources of stress is imperative during the resistance phase, whether the stress is from a chemical, physical, or an emotional source. This includes avoidance of any environmental toxins, which is a form of chemical stress. Any activities that are relaxing should be strongly considered. What is considered relaxing will vary from one person to another. Massage therapy, meditation, yoga, reading a book, and just laying on the beach are just a few activities that have relaxing qualities. Adequate restorative sleep is also mandatory, since lack of sleep is actually a form of stress.

During the resistance phase, exercise and physical activity are still options to address the physiological fight or flight response. The body's systems have not yet been compromised to a degree where exercise will prove detrimental. Excessive exercise, however, will quickly become counterproductive. This is because the addition of significant physical stress on the body's resources will deplete what little reserves are left. Exercise should therefore be initially kept to a minimal level, preferably to the level sufficient to reduce the effects of acute stress without causing significant additional physical stress to the body. Running a half marathon while in the resistance phase is of no benefit to the body. While running this distance may appear to reduce stress, any feeling of stress reduction is just an illusion. This feeling of stress reduction is coming from fatigue, the last thing anyone needs when in the resistance phase. What is actually happening is that the body is moving faster toward the exhaustion phase. As chronic stress is alleviated, exercise can be increased gradually.

The third phase, exhaustion, presents a unique situation in the sense that the person has entered a state of resource auto-depletion. In other words, the body's resources are being depleted and, at the same time, the very organs providing those resources are being damaged. This further decreases the ability of the body to handle any additional stress. During this phase, the chronic disease process is already in progress. This may be perceived by the patient as many seemingly unrelated illnesses, but, in fact, are all most likely simply a result of this final phase of stress. Chronic diseases that are often found in the patient who has entered the exhaustion phase are chronic fatigue syndrome, fibromyalgia, active and advanced autoimmune disease, allergies, leaky gut syndrome, and other ill-defined disorders such as metabolic syndrome. Since the chronic disorders found during the exhaustion phase are contributing to the stress already placed on the body, it is unlikely that the patient will ever recover from this phase without direct and specific intervention. In other words, if nothing is actively done to exit the exhaustion phase, it is highly unlikely that the condition will ever resolve on its own. This is often termed a *downward spiral*.

When a person has entered the exhaustion phase, seeking a natural or holistic health care provider to make specific recommendations to facilitate reversal of the condition is very wise. During this phase, the capacity of the endocrine system is markedly decreased. Temporary use of glandular supplements may be required, allowing the endocrine organs to rest, to facilitate healing. Glandular supplements, however, must be used with great care. Taking a glandular supplement for extended periods or using inappropriate dosages may cause additional damage to an already imbalanced endocrine system. The supervision of a qualified health care provider is strongly recommended when using glandular supplements. During the exhaustion phase, the digestive system is also compromised, invariably resulting in some form of malnutrition and multiple food allergies. Digestive enzyme supplements may be indicated, giving the severely stressed digestive organs an opportunity to rest. The immune system is often either suppressed, out of balance, or both, and must be addressed. With a plethora of simultaneous health issues that are occurring at the exhaustion phase, the need for professional guidance is very clear. The health care professional will most likely run several tests to determine the proper course of action to take. The tests prescribed and treatment indicated will vary from person to person.

Once a person has entered the exhaustion phase, exercise and physical activity become nearly impossible. Due to the compromised states of several of the body's systems, insufficient energy often exists to carry out day to day activities. Exercise, therefore, becomes counterproductive, adding the burden of physical stress on the body's resources that are already severely depleted. Exhaustion is not limited to the physical body. Primarily due to lack of sleep, depression, and other mental factors, the mind is exhausted as well. Neurotransmitters become severely depleted and out of balance, affecting thought patterns and mood. Since the endocrine system is also affected in the exhaustion phase, additional effects on the mood are expected, and, in fact, occur.

An important part in treating chronic stress is to identify what allowed the General Adaption Syndrome to progress to such an advanced stage. Various lifestyle changes must be considered to prevent the patient from entering the exhaustion phase again. Serious consideration must be given to making adjustments to specific circumstances contributing to the stress. These changes may involve relationships, employment, finances, social issues, physical activities, and daily schedules, to name just a few. Other changes often required are a change in cognitive thought processes, in other words, revised thinking patterns. Any necessary changes required will vary from person to person. Counseling may be beneficial to help identify these changes that need to be made, and should also include an implementation plan.

Only two possible choices are available when considering the course of action to be taken when dealing with a particular stressor. Either the person must completely change their response to the stressor, or the stressor must be eliminated. In some circumstances where the stressor cannot be eliminated, requiring the person to alter their response to the stressor is the only course of action. In other circumstances, expecting the person to alter their response to the stressor is unreasonable, therefore requiring the removal of the stressor. Regardless of any action taken, stress is what brought on the exhaustion phase, and cannot be allowed to continue.

Intervention beyond writing a prescription is water in which the medical profession is often unwilling to tread. Cases can be found in which the intervention that must be taken is significantly beyond the realm offered by modern medical care. The exhaustion phase of the General Adaption Syndrome is clearly one of these cases. The patient must often look beyond the health care system for emotional support to succeed at any adaptive changes to their lifestyle. Support from family, friends, and significant others are often needed regarding employment issues and certain financial considerations.

It is interesting that employment is a common source of stress for many people. When this is the case, it is often said that the person has a stressful job. In reality, however, there is no such thing as a stressful job. If the job is considered stressful, it is because the person holding that job is not properly matched with that the duties and responsibility of that position. When a job is considered less stressful, the person performing that job most likely well matched for the position, and is probably enjoying what he or she is doing on a daily basis. When chronic employment-related stress is found to exist, a change in career may be indicated.

Stress, then, has a clear definition. Stressors are well defined, and can be anything that initiates the fight or flight response. The fight or flight response involves very specific biochemical and physiological responses intended to be followed by a very specific response. This specific response is physical activity. Stress also has clear and defined consequences if it not handled in a way consistent with the expected biological response. The General Adaption Syndrome clearly defines how and why these consequences occur.

Noting that stress has been classified into the categories of *good stress* and *bad stress* is important. Stress is stress no matter the source, and these classifications of stress into either good or bad stress are really unnecessary. However, since the classification has already been made popular, examining exactly what factors are involved in determining the classification would be appropriate. The determining factor of whether stress is classified as either good or bad is whether or not the stress is followed by the appropriate biological response of elevated physical activity. If the stress is accompanied with or followed by physical activity, the stress would be classified as good stress. Rock climbing, bicycling, or a trip to the gym following a hard day at work would be categorized as good stress. Any physical activity would be considered good stress, because any norepinephrine or adrenaline release is quicky utilized by the sporting activity. If stress is not followed or accompanied by physical activity, the stress would be classified as bad stress. Fear, an unexpected flat tire, or lack of sleep due to anxiety would be categorized as bad stress. So-called bad stress can be turned into good stress if the normal biological response to stress is initiated. A good workout session following a bad day at the office is all that is needed to prevent the acute stress response from causing any adaptation to occur.

Stress cannot be eliminated from anyone's life. Stressful events will happen, and when they do, handling them in an appropriate manner is important. Any stressor that overwhelms the body's ability to handle the stress will result in the body adapting in a very specific and predictable way. Unrelenting chronic stress is the main ingredient in the recipe for any chronic disease.

Once stress is brought under control, it must be kept under control by appropriately responding to the stressor. This is most easily done by not entering the alarm phase, but this is not always possible. If the alarm phase is entered, the body expects physical activity, therefore physical activity is the best way to circumvent progression of the General Adaption Syndrome to any of the advanced stages.

To understand the extent of the consequences of stress better, gaining an understanding of one response to stress, that the medical community typically does not even consider a stress related response, would be desirable. The disorder is known as Multiple Personality Disorder, which has been recently renamed to Dissociative Identity Disorder. The former term, Multiple Personality Disorder, is a more accurate description of the condition, suggesting that multiple personalities do, in fact, exist. Both terms, however, lead us to believe that an actual disorder exists, and the presence of a disorder implies that the person is in need of treatment. The term *multiplicity*, as we will see, is a more accurate term, suggesting that the individual is capable of expressing separate and distinct personalities. Multiplicity does not require medical treatment. For purposes of discussion in this chapter, we will refer to the condition using both the medical term *Multiple Personality Disorder* and the more accurate term *multiplicity,* instead of inaccurate term *Dissociative Identity Disorder.*

Multiple Personality Disorder has become a controversial disorder in the sense that the mere existence of the disorder is now under question. Since no medication exists found effective in treating Multiple Personality Disorder, diagnosing this condition places the patient in a category for which there is no medical treatment. With no medical treatment, the physician has put forth a dead end diagnosis. The fact that no medication exists to treat the disorder sufficiently explains any controversy regarding the existence of the disorder. Should a medication be developed to suppress the symptoms of the disorder, the number of diagnosed cases of Multiple Personality Disorder will undoubtably skyrocket.

Multiple Personality Disorder was a relatively unknown condition until the late twentieth century, with only 200 cases reported between 1880 and 1979. The vast majority of cases reported have been reported after 1980, with 20,000 cases reported from 1980 to 1990, and 40,000 cases reported between 1985 and 1995. Documented cases are found proportionally high in the United States of America when compared with other countries. The question arises of what has changed during this period that would cause such a dramatic increase in the diagnosis of a disorder that was extremely rare and unheard of fifty years earlier. In addition, identifying any contributing factors found in the United States that are not typically found in the rest of the world might give further insight into the increased diagnosis rate of the disorder.

One does not have to look far to realize that societal stresses have dramatically increased since 1980. The fast paced society began with the arrival of the personal computer, paving the way to increased productivity in the workplace. Modern day employment carries no guarantees, the corporate pension plan is ancient history, employees are considered a disposable resource, and working hours are longer than ever. Technological advances occur at lightning speed, enabling even greater advances in productivity rates, further increasing job-related stress. The neighbor who had that secure corporate position has been laid off, and is now studying for a real estate license, only to find out that the real estate sector is saturated with agents who were laid off from their position last year. The real estate market, flooded with record numbers of foreclosures, is evidence of a fragile economy, despite what any economic indicators or the experts may say. The young person entering the working environment is more concerned about health insurance, the future of the economy, and debt than the people generations ago. Outside the workplace, the same technological advances provide a greater level of convenience and save time at the expense of dramatically increasing stress. As a result, many people are living in fear. More people are becoming fed up with the many forms of societal stress, and move to the mountains, beach, or other peaceful setting where the ways of life are at a much slower pace. All the wheels of modern day society appear to be turning, but what no one notices are that they are turning way too fast because the main spring is wound too tight. Stress levels clearly have markedly increased since 1980. The problem is that no one has noticed because the ways of life found in prior decades are unknown to the present generation. Sitting on the porch for two hours a day and talking to the neighbors who walk by is an unknown activity in modern day society.

Multiple Personality Disorder is one response of the mind to stress, and, in fact, is a natural stress response. This response to stress, should it occur, is not limited to only the mind, but manifests in body and spirit as well. Stress, in this case, refers to stress in which there is no method to escape, or no viable means available to deal with the stress. The stress can be of either chemical, physical, or emotional origin. When presented with this type of stress, the person with Multiple Personality Disorder has two options available to them, not only one option. The first option is to accept the stress, and therefore be forced to accept the physical, mental, and spiritual consequences of the stress. If the stress is allowed to manifest in the usual manner, the mechanisms associated with the General Adaption Syndrome go into motion, which will invariably lead to disease. The second option is to undergo a personality switch, thus escaping from the stress and therefore avoiding any physical, mental, and spiritual consequences of the stress. The act of personality switching circumvents progression of the General Adaption Syndrome, and in doing so, the consequences of stress in the body, mind, and spirit are successfully avoided.

The personality switch of Multiple Personality Disorder is actually a highly sophisticated response of the mind to stress. Personality switching is the preferred response by the individual as compared with the misery of entering the latent phases of the General Adaption Syndrome. It is almost certain that the person with Multiple Personality Disorder has, at one time, been subject to some form of stress in which no viable method of escape was found. Severe consequences were most likely were incurred as a result of this stress. It must be pointed out that the stress experienced by the person before the initial personality switch was perceived by that person to have no method of escape, whether a method of escape actually existed or not. Likewise, the stressor could have been easily identified or remain a mystery. When examined closely, the act of personality switching, then, is highly desirable in consideration of the consequences of not switching. The switch, therefore, is the best choice available to the person in consideration of the presenting situation.

It is not known whether every individual is capable of undergoing a personality switch. For those individuals who do have this capability, multiplicity, or the ability of undergoing a personality switch, can actually be a blessing. The person capable of multiplicity who is fully aware of their ability is able to undergo a personality switch at will, has a unique ability of avoiding stress and the consequences of stress. The ability to switch at will, or handle properly any personality switches that may occur has been termed a *non-disordered multiplicity* by those who have experienced this ability. In comparison to the consequences of the latent phases of the General Adaption Syndrome, the response to stress of a non-disordered multiple is quite a healthy neurological response.

The newly entered personality state is one that is very familiar to the person capable of multiplicity. Specifically, the new personality state is one that is unaffected by the stress presented to the prior personality state. In switching, either stress or an undesirable situation has thus been averted. The newly entered personality state is one that is more suited to handle whatever may be characteristic of the new situation. If a new form of stress in which no method of escape can be found is again presented, another personality switch is likely to occur. The switch may be either back to the individual's initial personality, or a new personality. In either case, the personality switched to is better equipped to handle the newly presented stressor, and the consequences of stress are avoided.

Multiple Personality Disorder is termed a disorder by the medical profession. In naming and describing the disorder, a condition that requires treatment has been identified. Multiple Personality Disorder, however, does not require any treatment, and is only a symptom of another issue. The most likely issue facing the patient is some form of stress. Personality switching is a far better response to stress than entering the path leading to the exhaustion phase of the General Adaption Syndrome. Non-disordered multiplicity is perhaps the best response possible to stress, and is quite desirable when compared with any path the General Adaption Syndrome has to offer. In fact, persons capable of non-disordered multiplicity are far more capable of handling stress than the general population, and no doubt they are much healthier in comparison.

In most cases, multiplicity does not require any medical treatment because it is not truly a disorder at all. Medical treatment of multiplicity is a form of stress presented to the person capable of multiplicity, therefore further encouraging a personality switch. Multiplicity is, therefore, an adaption to some form of stress that requires, from the viewpoint of the affected individual, an escape from the stress. In escaping from the stress, the physical health and sanity of the person is preserved. What is a disorder, however, is allowing stress to manifest to the point of developing a debilitating chronic disease, or to the point of the proverbial nervous breakdown.

Many other adaptions can be found which occur as a response to stress. The general mechanisms involved in these disorders are also clearly defined. These responses vary from person to person, and are largely determined by developmental factors and environmental issues. Many of these other stress responses are improperly categorized as psychological disorders.

I have a friend who is a doctor on an island of the South Pacific. When you schedule an appointment with her office, you are told to come on a specific day, either in the morning or in the afternoon. That is the greatest resolution of time she will give the patients - the morning or the afternoon. If the patient has to wait an hour, the patient does not care. They just talk and visit with the other patients who are waiting, or read a magazine. Contrast that with the appointments scheduled at five or ten minute intervals with the typical medical doctors office.

Chapter 9
Bipolar Disorder

Bipolar disorder is classically described as a psychiatric condition defined by extreme mood swings. These mood swings can range from severe, debilitating depression to severe, uncontrollable mania. The symptoms associated with bipolar disorder have a tendency, over time, to worsen with or without treatment. Many subclassifications of bipolar have been defined; subclassifications are categorized based upon the duration of the different phases and both the intensity and duration of the accompanied mood swings. Additionally, other types of bipolar behavior are found in several other disorders.

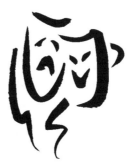

Bipolar disorder was formerly known as Manic-Depressive disorder. Manic-Depressive disorder is a more accurate term, but, in recent times, has become a politically incorrect term. The term *bipolar disorder* sounds like it refers to less severe and more acceptable disorder than does Manic-Depressive disorder. The connotation of being either manic or depressed sounds almost as if the patient is ready to be admitted to a mental health facility. Often unwilling to be diagnosed or labeled with such a condition, the patient is less likely to seek medical care. The newer term, bipolar disorder, does not sound as severe, and, for that reason, is a more acceptable diagnosis for the patient. With a more acceptable term for the condition, the patient is often more willing to accept the diagnosis, and begin taking medication for the disorder. In many cases, however, what is diagnosed to be bipolar disorder is nothing more than a normal response to everyday life. By changing the name of the disorder, the diagnosis rate of the disorder has increased, subsequently resulting more people supposedly needing treatment.

Whereas bipolar disorders have an energetic or euphoric stage and a separate and distinct depressive stage, depression is characterized by only a depressive stage, and is sometimes called unipolar depression. It has been postulated that bipolar disorder and unipolar depression are different expressions of the same disorder. Since neurotransmission and mood are involved in both depression and bipolar disorder, this would lead us to believe that both disorders, at least to some degree, have some common basis. However, the depressive phase of bipolar disorder, when examined closely, has no true resemblance to classical depression. The drugs used in the treatment of depression are often used in the depressive stage of bipolar disorder, and have little long term benefit in correcting the bipolar condition.

Many theories suggest various causes of bipolar disorder. Both physiological and social causes are often cited. No specific laboratory tests lead to the diagnosis of bipolar disorder. Laboratory tests, however, are often performed specifically to identify or rule out any potential illnesses or disorder that may have the same symptoms of bipolar disorder. When no other satisfactory cause can be found, the diagnosis of bipolar disorder is assigned. The diagnosis of bipolar disorder is a diagnosis of exclusion, based purely on patient history and current subjective complaints. A diagnosis of exclusion is often suggestive of another undiagnosed underlying cause.

Bipolar disorder appears to have, to some degree, a genetic basis. Psychological factors also have been shown to play a role. Bipolar disorder is classified based upon the severity of the alternating manic and depressive phases, and the time between episodes. Certain criteria must be present for each classification, and when the criteria are met, a more refined diagnosis is assigned by the physician. In cases when the diagnostic criteria cannot be met, Bipolar Disorder NOS (Not Otherwise Specified) is put forth as the diagnosis. Bipolar Disorder NOS is technically a second level of an exclusionary diagnosis, which is effectively the equivalent of telling the patient that no one has any idea what is wrong.

Specific life events have a tendency to influence the two poles of bipolar disorder. Stressful negative events are often reported to lead toward the depressive stage of bipolar disorder. Major successes and accomplishments, have a tendency to precipitate the manic phase of the disorder. In the initial stages of the disorder, full-blown depression or mania is not usually seen either by the patient, their family, or their acquaintances. Subclinical depression and hypomania are the norms during these initial stages, and are often difficult to recognize even by the skilled general practitioner. At first, symptoms are often dismissed as "just ups and downs." Repeated negative events are reported to provoke progressively deeper depression phases. Likewise, repeated major successes and accomplishments provoke a more intense and energetic manic phase. Over time, these repeated stressful events appear to lower the threshold at which a mood change occurs. If this is allowed to continue unabated, mood changes can occur for no apparent reason.

Why Am I Sick? And What To Do About It

This clearly appears to be some adaptation of the nervous system in response to the psychological events of negative and positive experiences.

Treatment from a traditional psychological approach involves recognizing triggers and alleviating acute symptoms through counseling. Traditional allopathic treatment of bipolar disorder involves long term treatment using mood stabilization drugs. Lithium is the most commonly used drug for this purpose. Although Lithium has been used in bipolar disorder for many years, its exact mechanism of action is unknown. Antipsychotic medications have been used for acute, uncontrollable manic phases. Antidepressants have been used during acute depressive stages, including monoamine oxidase inhibitors (MAOIs) and tricyclic antidepressants. A significant known problem with the use of medications for bipolar disorder is that the dosage needs to be adjusted quite often. Rarely will the same dosage be effective for any extended period. More common is that additional medications must be added periodically to maintain stability of the patient.

Some newer medications prescribed in the treatment of bipolar disorder have serious side effects associated with them. Some of these medications used to treat bipolar disorder are also used in the treatment of schizophrenia. Bipolar disorder and schizophrenia are conditions with different clinical presentations, different etiologies, and different neurotransmitter anomalies; logic therefore suggests different treatments are indicated for each disorder. One must wonder why the medication used to treat one disorder is also expected to be effective in a completely different disorder. The mechanism of action of one such medication involves a multifaceted dopamine D_2 receptor partial agonist, serotonin $5HT_{1A}$ receptor partial agonist, and $5HT_{2A}$ receptor antagonist. Unless the patient specifically has a decreased dopamine D_2 receptor activity, decreased serotonin $5HT_{1A}$ activity, and $5HT_{2A}$ receptor hyperactivity, the drug cannot simply be expected to be a good match for the condition. With hundreds of types of neurotransmitter binding sites, such a specific condition of hyperactivity and hypoactivity is statistically unlikely to occur. The medication, in having such an esoteric mechanism of action, could not go to waste, therefore a condition must be searched for in which it is, at least to some degree, effective. Some evidence exists that these medications can lead to potentially life threatening conditions, such as neuroleptic malignant syndrome, as with any chemical agent modifying the effects of dopamine. These medications have also been shown to carry serious metabolic risk factors. The question arises about whether living with bipolar disorder is better than being dead. If a medication carries a potential side effect of death, it is obviously not correctly targeting the source of the patient's condition. When taking a medication that has these potential side effects, wisdom would suggest careful evaluation of whether a change in medication or treatment plans is in order. A qualified health care provider should be consulted before initiating any changes in medication.

Environmental factors obviously play a role in bipolar disorder. In fact, environmental factors play a role in all disorders involving cognitive function. When an environmental factor, for example sunlight, noise, physical confrontation, or any stimulus for that matter, is presented to the body, a neurological response will occur. The type of response is dependent on many factors. One factor is the current state of neurotransmitter availability in the brain. More specifically, the balance of neurotransmitters in various areas of the brain largely determines the response. Other factors, such as hormone levels, neuronal fatigue, and overall emotional state also play a role.

A question arises of why the same neurons located in the same brain of the same person with bipolar disorder are sometimes in a hyperactive state, yet at other times appear to be in a depressed state. Since neurons are not dynamically created and destroyed on an as needed basis, the answer must lie outside the actual physical neuronal connections of the brain. Since the same neuronal structure is present in both phases of the disorder, the answer will be found in how these neurons communicate to each other. We can conclude that, since neurons communicate with each other through neurotransmitters, some aberration of neurotransmission or imbalance in neurotransmitters must be responsible for the disorder.

Positive accomplishments precipitate the manic phase of the disorder, and negative events are reported to provoke the depressive phase of the disorder. The episodes, over time, appear to increase in intensity, requiring a lesser degree of stimuli to cause the associated mood swing. This gives us another clue regarding the disorder. An inverted tolerance factor is also involved, since diminished intensities of stimuli are required to generate the even greater, more intense mood swings. This appears to be the result of a closed loop positive feedback mechanism by which the associated nerve pathways develop stronger and stronger neurological connections. The medical term for the formation of these stronger connections is *synaptogenesis*. Synaptogenesis subsequently allows for more efficient neurotransmission within the closed loop. In addition, an internal reward mechanism involving the associated neurology clearly seems to be taking place.

Similar closed loop positive feedback mechanisms develop in epilepsy and other seizure disorders. Interestingly, a tonic-clonic (grand mal) epileptic seizure is followed by a short period of great fatigue. With both bipolar and the epileptic seizure, a period of hyperactivity is followed by a refractory period of hypoactivity. Factors such as neurotransmitter imbalances, genetics, fatigue, stress levels, malnutrition, and blood sugar dysregulation are just a few factors implicated in seizure disorders. These factors can affect the excitability of neurons. Certain triggers initiate hyperactivity of the regions associated with seizures, for example, flashing lights or action packed video games. This pattern of closed loop feedback mechanisms appears to be present also in bipolar disorder; the developed feedback loops just affect different areas of the brain. The period of duration of hyperactivity and hypoactivity also varies. In each case, the period of hypoactivity is somewhat proportional to the period of hyperactivity. In either case, periods of relative normalcy can be observed between the hyperactive and hypoactive states.

Anti-seizure medications have been investigated in the treatment of bipolar disorder. Indications are that the medications developed to control seizures also are effective in the manic phase of bipolar disorder. This is not surprising. Anti-seizure medications typically have a direct effect on Gamma-aminobutyric acid (GABA), which is the primary inhibitory neurotransmitter in the brain.

Specifically, anti-seizure medications act by prolonging the action of Gamma-aminobutyric acid at the synaptic junction. One method of accomplishing this is by inhibiting the reuptake of the neurotransmitter. These are referred to as Gamma-aminobutyric acid reuptake inhibitors. When levels of Gamma-aminobutyric acid are low, certain areas of the brain can become hyperactive. Worse yet, if dopamine, norepinephrine and serotonin levels are elevated, and Gamma-aminobutyric acid levels are low, the patient has a very high susceptibility to entering the manic phase of bipolar disorder. The neurotransmitter Gamma-aminobutyric acid is also involved in areas of the brain associated with emotion, stress, and anxiety. Not surprisingly, low levels of Gamma-aminobutyric acid have a high correlation with bipolar disorder.

Low Gamma-aminobutyric acid levels result in greater activity of the neurotransmitters dopamine, serotonin, and norepinephrine. Dopamine is the neurotransmitter involved in the reward system of the brain. Addiction is often found to involve the neurotransmitters dopamine and serotonin. During the manic phase of bipolar disorder, the patient often reports increased energy, feeling good, and overall euphoria. It is the over activity of these neurotransmitters that is responsible for these positive feelings. The increased activity of these neurotransmitters also provides the basis for the reward mechanism of bipolar disorder. The period of high energy and euphoria essentially continues unabated until the patient literally runs out of energy. In a sense, the manic phase of bipolar disorder literally has an addictive quality to it.

The mechanism involved in the manic phase of bipolar disorder is a neurological positive feedback loop within the neurology and biochemistry of the brain that, at least in part, involves the reward centers of the brain. The result of the positive feedback loop is continuous amplification, where the feedback mechanism drives itself to a higher level and, in turn, will continue unabated until biological fatigue of the driving mechanisms finally occurs. Once the neurons are rested, under the proper conditions another cycle is certain to occur.

Antipsychotic medications are typically used during acute, uncontrollable manic phases is quite understandable once the mechanism behind bipolar disorder is examined and understood. If Gamma-aminobutyric acid (GABA) levels are low, increased action of and sensitivity to dopamine results. This increased action, is, in part, responsible for the manic phase. Antipsychotic medications typically target dopamine receptors, specifically inhibiting the action of dopamine. This type of antipsychotic medication is termed a dopamine antagonist. Dopamine, in this case, acts as an excitatory neurotransmitter. The antipsychotic medication, by inhibiting the action of dopamine, reduces the symptoms associated with the manic phase.

If Gamma-aminobutyric acid levels can be restored, the actions of the neurotransmitters dopamine, serotonin, and norepinephrine will be normalized. The medical approach is to prolong the action of Gamma-aminobutyric acid in the synapse. This approach, however, does not restore the level of the neurotransmitter. The holistic approach would be to take a vitamin supplement of Vitamin B6 to aid in the conversion of glutamate in the brain to Gamma-aminobutyric acid. Gamma-aminobutyric acid is synthesized in the brain from alpha ketoglutarate and the Vitamin B6 derivative pyridoxal phosphate in a biochemical reaction known as the GABA shunt. Dietary supplementation with the precursors to Gamma-aminobutyric acid would provide the body with the materials it needs to regulate itself. Dietary supplementation of Gamma-aminobutyric acid itself would most likely prove beneficial. Incidently, seizures often occur in a Vitamin B6 deficient state in susceptible persons.

The Kava Kava herb has been shown to be effective in normalizing Gamma-aminobutyric acid levels, and may be used as an effective treatment of bipolar disorder by the alternative practitioner. Organic chemicals called kavalactones, which are contained in Kava Kava, appear to stimulate the production of more attachment sites in the body for the neurotransmitter Gamma-aminobutyric acid. The resultant increase in number of Gamma-aminobutyric acid receptor sites would lead to increased Gamma-aminobutyric acid activity. Increased numbers of receptor sites leading to increased Gamma-aminobutyric acid activity is the basis for a cure for the disorder. Kava Kava may also prevent reabsorption of norepinephrine, a neurotransmitter undoubtably elevated in the manic phase of bipolar disorder. Since Kava Kava may interact with other medications, use of this herb should be supervised by a qualified health care professional.

The manic phase of bipolar disorder is invariably followed by the depressive phase. The depressive phase of bipolar disorder is not depression in the classical sense. Specifically, the depressive stage is actually a refractory period, or a period of rest, needed by the fatigued neurons that were hyperactive during the manic phase. These fatigued neurons are in a state of neurotransmitter depletion, energy depletion, or any other result from the excessive neurological activity that occurred. Neurons cannot maintain a hyperactive state indefinitely, just like a marathon runner cannot run indefinitely. Periods of hyperactivity will invariably be followed by periods of hypoactivity. Once the neurons have rested, they are then in a state of susceptibility for another manic phase. In other words, whatever goes up, must come down. Since the depressive phase is not depression in the true sense, but is caused by neuronal fatigue, the use of antidepressant medications is generally of no value in bipolar disorder. Herbal supplements with antidepressant properties, such as St. John's Wort, are similarly of no value to those with bipolar disorder.

Bipolar disorder does not have its origin with events that are depressive in nature. Bipolar disorder has its origin exclusively in events associated with the manic phase. This becomes increasingly obvious when the fact that averting the manic phase through either medication, counseling, or both, subsequently prevents the onset of the depressive stage. This is also substantial evidence that the depressive stage is caused by neuronal fatigue, and is not related to classical depression.

Other disorders also have a clearly bipolar characteristic to them. These other disorders, however, are not classically considered bipolar disorders by modern medicine. The only difference found in these other disorders and the classical definition of bipolar disorder are the workings of the internal reward mechanism. Specifically, the area of the brain associated with hyperactive closed loop positive feedback mechanism varies, depending on the type of bipolar disorder in question. The same patterns of hyperactivity, accompanied by some internal reward mechanism, followed by a hypoactive refractory period clearly exist in persons with these other bipolar disorders. The bipolar pattern is the same. The activity and reward system is, however, different.

Hypersexuality, sometimes known as nymphomania, is one such disorder characteristic of bipolar activity. In the case of hypersexuality, the person goes through periods of tremendous swings in sex drive. What constitutes normal sexual activity varies from person to person, just like what constitutes a normal limit of mood swings varies from person to person. The only difference between hypersexuality and classical bipolar disorder is the reward system involved.

Other individuals who are not classically bipolar are also found addicted, in a sense, to the natural high produced by rapidly elevated norepinephrine levels. Skydivers, rock climbers, persons who enjoy the excitement of fast roller coasters, persons who see one thriller movie after another, and anyone else who thrives on high energy excitement may also be addicted to the spike in norepinephrine levels and the subsequent mood elevation that these activities provide. One major difference between the bipolar patient and the thrill and a high energy enjoyment seeker is that, in the bipolar patient, a closed loop positive feedback mechanism affecting the reward center of the brain is found, which serves to reinforce the cycle. In the thrill seeker and high energy enjoyment seeker, the closed loop mechanism affecting the reward center is not found. In the case of the thrill seeker, the spike in norepinephrine levels during these activities promotes an elevated mood, therefore the activities are likely to be repeated. Any sports activity promotes the release of endorphins, contributing to the elevated mood. The *runners high* is an example of an elevated mood due to endorphin release experienced by those who participate in distance running. In the thrill seeker or athlete, no detrimental effects to the persons social life are typically evident, therefore treatment is unnecessary.

Other disorders with a bipolar component are identified in Table 9.1. This list is by no means complete. While dopamine is traditionally thought of as the neurotransmitter associated with the reward centers of the brain, other neurotransmitter systems can carry similar reward effects. The bipolar activity involved gives a definite clue about which neurotransmitter system is likely to be contributing to any chemical imbalance. Other factors, such as personality, are involved as well, and largely determine the bipolar activity of choice of affected individuals. Any pattern of repeated binge-type activity is suspect of bipolar activity. The column entitled *Reward System Involved* identifies the neurotransmitter or other system likely involved in the associated reward mechanism of the indicated disorder. In some cases, multiple neurotransmitter systems are involved. Interestingly, medications used in the treatment of classical bipolar disorder are often used for other binge behaviors as well. Not surprisingly, these medications also target the neurotransmitter Gamma-aminobutyric acid.

Multiple neurotransmitter systems and endorphins are involved in any bipolar disorder to varying degrees. With multiple neurotransmitter systems involved, periods of hyperactivity and hypoactivity can vary from days to months. The refractory period of neurons, or period of hypoactivity following the period of hyperactivity, also varies significantly and is determined by factors such as sleep, nutrition, activity levels, lifestyle, and stress levels. Environmental factors are also involved. With many factors influencing an individual's behavior, is it not surprising that the expression of bipolar characteristics varies greatly from person to person.

What decides, then, when we choose to treat any bipolar disorder? Activity levels that are considered normal for one person would be considered excessive and inappropriate for other individuals. Within certain bipolar classifications, periods of hyperactivity may, in fact, be desirable. When the disorder, whether bipolar disorder as classically described, hypersexuality, or any other binge-type activity causes impaired social functioning, it then moves into the realm of something that should be considered for treatment. The level and scope of any treatment rendered should be directed toward the restoration of proper social function. Particular attention must be given as not to use treatment protocols that overly suppress the personality characteristics of the individual, thus allowing for the unimpaired freedom of expression of the individual. When impaired social function is restored, the bipolar activity is then considered cured.

Bipolar Disorder	Reward System Involved
Classical Bipolar	Norepinephrine, Dopamine
Hypersexuality	Various
Binge Eating	Serotonin
Binge Smoking	Dopamine, Norepinephrine
Binge Shopping	Various
Thrill Seeker	Norepinephrine
Binge Drinking	Various
Binge Exercising	Endorphins

Table 9.1   Disorders of a Bipolar Basis

Bipolar disorders, if required to be treated, are best treated by natural means, and provide the only treatment that can ultimately lead to a cure. The medical approach does not cure the disorder, but instead treats symptoms through medications, allowing the patient to function in society in somewhat of a more normal manner. The natural approach, however, may not be appropriate for everyone who has been diagnosed with a bipolar disorder. Holistic psychology offers treatment that has as an ultimate goal of complete recovery from symptoms of any bipolar disorder. Instead of medication, other techniques and lifestyle changes are utilized in achieving this goal. Changes potentially include maintaining an overall healthy lifestyle, including proper diet and nutrition, meditation, and exercise. Psychological techniques will involve close and detailed monitoring of the patient, with biofeedback, EEG, and changes to cognitive processes (thought patterns). Social support systems are also very valuable in any natural approach.

The holistic approach would most likely involve the use of a Gamma-aminobutyric acid supplement, the neurotransmitter implicated in bipolar disorders. Some research indicates that it is questionable whether Gamma-aminobutyric acid can cross the blood-brain barrier. This research itself is questionable for several reasons. The first reason is that the effects of Gamma-aminobutyric acid supplementation can readily be noticed by many who have used the supplement. The second reason is that the majority of the research is done on rats. Humans are not rats. Thirdly, the results of any research performed generally arrives at the conclusion that "Gamma-aminobutyric acid does not readily cross the blood-brain barrier." The word *readily* constantly appears repeatedly in reference to Gamma-aminobutyric acid crossing the blood-brain barrier. No research, however, boldly claims that Gamma-aminobutyric acid cannot cross the barrier. Finally, the physical size of the Gamma-aminobutyric molecule is often cited as the reason that the molecule has difficulty crossing the barrier. Interestingly, Gamma hydroxybutyric acid (GHB), a common date rape drug with a similar chemical structure and size, crosses the blood-brain barrier very effectively. The size of the molecule, therefore, is not the issue. Evidently, research appears to be directed to prove the ineffectiveness of Gamma-aminobutyric acid for some reason. Commercially available Gamma-aminobutyric acid supplements are formulated at concentrations to ensure that some Gamma-aminobutyric acid is able to pass through the barrier. This amount probably varies from person to person; therefore, obtaining the advice of a natural health practitioner when using this, or any natural supplements, would be advantageous.

Various forms of yoga and meditation to quiet the mind have also been proven effective in controlling the closed loop feedback mechanisms associated with bipolar disorder. Theta waves are thought to be formed by the limbic system, the region of the brain associated with emotions. During Yoga and meditation, theta waves have been shown to increase, while activity in the frontal and other cortical lobes of the brain that originate thought processes is diminished. This would serve to break the feedback loop associated with the manic phase. Yoga and meditation also stimulate the parasympathetic nervous system, particularly the parasympathetic-limbic pathway, resulting in relaxation of the body and mind.

Incidentally, worry and anxiety is another example of a closed loop mechanism. This is not unlike the closed loop positive feedback mechanism found in bipolar disorder and seizures. The only difference is that the closed loop associated with worry affects a different area of the brain, and specifically does not involve the reward centers of the brain. The chronic worrier, in essence, has also developed stronger and stronger neurological connections, increasing neurotransmission efficiency within the closed loop. This increased efficiently within the loop explains why, for some persons, it is difficult to stop worrying. Other repetitive thought processes occur as a result of the same mechanism. With no reward mechanism in place, these neurological closed loop mechanisms are easier to terminate.

If we wanted to precipitate a manic episode in a classically bipolar individual, any activity that raises norepinephrine levels should suffice. For example, strapping a parachute on the bipolar patient and flying them to 14,000 feet, then pushing them out of the plane would raise norepinephrine levels to quite an abnormally high level. This activity would also cause the mind of the chronic worrier or anxiety sufferer to run in circles. The norepinephrine spike from this type activity can also break the bipolar patient out of the depressive stage. Since a manic episode can be forced to occur by certain activities, avoidance of specific activities known to initiate a manic episode must be avoided. These activities include any event or activity that would cause a spike in norepinephrine levels. In other words, activities that lead to an "adrenaline rush" should be avoided.

A high prevalence of undiagnosed and untreated metabolic disease is found to exist in patients with various psychiatric and mental disorders, any bipolar related disorder being no exception. Inadequate or improper nutrition can also cause mood problems even in those who have not been diagnosed with bipolar disorder. Even in a perfectly healthy person, maintaining a healthy diet and adequate nutrition is important for achieving mental stability. The brain is one of the most metabolically active organs of the body. With millions of biochemical processes occurring simultaneously in the body, understanding why either improper or inadequate nutrition will subsequently result in less than optimal function, and in some cases, dysfunction, is easy to see. Research indicates several supplements that have been shown to reduce the severity of the manic and depressive phases of bipolar disorder. Supplementation of the diet with Omega-3 Fatty Acids has been shown to reduce the irritability component of a significant percentage of patients suffering from bipolar disorder. This is further evidence that the family of bipolar disorders has associated dietary factors in addition to possible genetic causes.

In addition to the use of certain dietary supplements, avoidance of certain dietary components also plays a key role in the management of bipolar disorders. Any food or chemical classified as a stimulant or depressant should be avoided. Foods or chemicals with these characteristics have a tendency to change the mood and energy levels even those persons who have not been diagnosed with any type of bipolar disorder. Avoiding refined sugar, caffeine, alcohol, and chocolate should be taken into consideration.

Persons with any bipolar disorder should not use aspartame, an artificial sweetener. Aspartame breaks down in the body into its three components, aspartic acid, phenylalanine, and methanol. In the body, the amino acid phenylalanine is readily converted to the amino acid tyrosine, the precursor amino acid to the neurotransmitters dopamine and norepinephrine. The problem arises because the transport of phenylalanine into brain is mediated by a carrier mechanism shared with other amino acids in the same class. These other amino acids are tyrosine and tryptophan. Excess levels of phenylalanine inhibit the transport of tyrosine and tryptophan into the brain by the carrier mechanism. This is due to the saturation of the carrier mechanism by phenylalanine. Limiting the transport of tyrosine as a result of the presence of excess phenylalanine might sound desirable since it will limit the subsequent conversion to dopamine, but nothing can be further from the truth. If tyrosine availably is limited, the biochemical mechanisms involved in the conversion of phenylalanine to tyrosine will become more efficient. When tyrosine is again available to the brain, the cascade of biochemical reactions involved in the conversion to dopamine or norepinephrine will go into high gear, and a short term surplus of these neurotransmitters will occur. This has a great probability of precipitating a manic episode.

Since the excess amounts of phenylalanine as a result of the breakdown of aspartame also decreases the transport of tryptophan into the brain by the carrier mechanism, conversion of tryptophan to serotonin is subsequently inhibited. Ingestion of aspartame, therefore, can cause an imbalance of the neurotransmitter serotonin. Decreased levels of serotonin can lead to certain types of depression. As with the mechanism involving tyrosine to dopamine conversion, when tryptophan is again available and transported by the carrier mechanism, the cascade of biochemical reactions involved in the conversion to serotonin will occur at a rapid rate.

Interestingly, the high levels of phenylalanine as a result of the breakdown of aspartame can set the stage for seizures in susceptible individuals. Anyone who has had seizures due to this artificial sweetener knows this relationship is more than a casual one. The biochemical mechanisms associated with the aspartame induced manic episode and the aspartame induced seizure are the same. If aspartame was classified as a drug, it would fall into the category of a nonspecific neurological disruptor.

Another component of the breakdown of aspartame is aspartic acid. Aspartate, which is the conjugate base of aspartic acid, acts as an excitatory neurotransmitter. Specifically, aspartate stimulates N-methyl d-aspartate (NMDA) receptors in the brain. This is the same receptor stimulated by the amino acid neurotransmitter glutamate. Glutamate, another excitatory neurotransmitter, is a component of the breakdown of monosodium glutamate. Although aspartate does not stimulate the NMDA receptor as strongly as glutamate, aspartame is metabolized and absorbed very quickly, causing a rapid rise in blood plasma levels. This periodic rapid rise results in transient overstimulation of the receptors many times during the day. Transient overstimulation of any neurotransmitter system can effectually cause mood changes.

The purpose of avoiding various activities and foods that can have a stimulation effect is to break the closed loop positive feedback mechanism that has developed. The causative factors responsible for initiating the closed loop feedback mechanism differ from patient to patient. Factors involved in breaking the loop will also differ from patient to patient. In breaking the cycle associated with the feedback mechanism, the underlying neurological connections responsible for the manic phase will become weaker over time.

This process will take considerable time, and should be supervised by a qualified counselor. Eventually, these connections will return to near normal, at which time certain activities can be reintroduced. This is, in fact the only way in which to cure any type of bipolar disorder.

A Gamma-aminobutyric acid (GABA) supplement and the herb Kava Kava may be purchased from any health food store. Since persons with bipolar disorder are often unaware of the manic phase until it is substantially underway, any change in treatment protocols should be carefully supervised by a qualified practitioner. Periodic adjustments are often made to medications used in the treatment of bipolar disorder. Likewise, any natural product will also require periodic adjustments. The natural health care provider, in many circumstances, may suggest additional regimens in the treatment of any bipolar condition.

Gamma-aminobutyric acid is a very interesting neurotransmitter. Cases of restless leg syndrome and bruxism (nocturnal teeth grinding) often resolve by using such a simple dietary supplement.

Why Am I Sick? And What To Do About It

Chapter 10
Depression

Depression is a state of moderate to intense sadness or melancholia. Sufferers of depression state they feel sad or down for no apparent reason. The effects of depression affect most or all activities of an individual's life. These effects can be mild and transient to debilitating and severe. Depression is often referred to as unipolar depression. All depression has a both a type and cause. Various types and causes of depression have been described, all of which are well documented. In treating only the symptoms of depression, which is the depression itself, the cause has been ignored. The proper treatment of depression should be focused on addressing the actual cause, rather than purely symptomatic relief. If the cause of depression was removed, any depression would resolve on its own.

Depression has many causes. Some causes of depression have a physiological basis, other causes have dietary, environmental, social or psychological factors involved. Psychological factors often play a significant role. In many cases, depression has specific known causes, and is often classified based upon the causative factor(s). Objective evidence is rarely, if ever, present in most forms of depression. Subjective evidence supporting the classification is, on the other hand, almost always present. No specific laboratory tests are diagnostic of depression. Laboratory tests, however, are often performed specifically to identify any potential illnesses or disorder that may be causing the associated symptoms of depression. In some cases, the diagnosis of depression is offered on the basis of exclusion, based purely on patient history and current subjective complaints. A diagnosis of exclusion is issued when no other explanation for the signs and symptoms can be found. In many cases, the cause is not searched for following the diagnosis of depression.

If the cause of depression can be discovered, elimination of the causative factors would cause the depression to cease, and is the only logical treatment leading to a cure. In some cases, multiple causative factors may be present. In essence, having more than one type of depression at the same time is a distinct possibility. While this does not seem fair, it is often the case. A patient can have postpartum depression in conjunction with Seasonal Affective Disorder, which exemplifies this quite well. In identifying the various types of depression, a better understanding of the appropriate treatment is gained.

If the specific type of depression is incorrectly diagnosed, the treatment may provide no benefit. Light therapy, for example, is often prescribed for Seasonal Affective Disorder. One study indicated that light therapy was not found superior to the placebo effect in the treatment of depression. This study obviously did not take into consideration the type of depression suffered by the patient. Other studies indicate great success in the treatment of depression with light therapy. In the latter studies, the lack of exposure to sunlight was a significant causative factor in depression. Exposure to sunlight, therefore, alleviates depression if lack of exposure to sunlight is the cause. The type of depression, therefore, dictates the appropriate treatment. Proper diagnosis and treatment, therefore, are of the utmost importance.

A high prevalence of undiagnosed and untreated metabolic disease is often found in patients diagnosed with depression. Metabolic diseases, also called inborn errors of metabolism, are diseases that affect the energy production at the cellular level. Metabolic diseases, while most often genetic, may also be acquired as a result of the diet, exposure to toxins, or infections. Certain metabolic diseases require a change in diet, most often eliminating something that is not able to be processed due to the presence of the disease. With certain metabolic diseases, the patient often goes through their entire life unaware that the disease is present. Metabolic disease of a genetic origin is usually diagnosed by symptoms and patient history. Genetic testing, although expensive, can be used as well.

Depression can often be linked to scarce or missing nutrients in the diet. One common dietary cause of depression is a reduced level of Omega-3 fatty acids. This is largely due to the lack of these essential fatty acids in the modern day diet. Another dietary cause of depression is a nutritional deficiency of the amino acid tryptophan, which is the precursor to serotonin. If tryptophan levels are low, serotonin levels subsequently decrease. Decreased serotonin levels have long been implicated in depression. Many medications, such as selective serotonin reuptake inhibitors (SSRIs) have been developed to address depression of this type. Tryptophan statistically is the most commonly found deficient amino acid found in essential amino acid profiles. It is not surprising that serotonin-related depression is so common in modern day society.

Genetic factors have been shown to play a significant role in depression. One example of a genetic factor influencing depression has been demonstrated in persons with Celiac disease. Dysfunction of the serotonin system due to impaired availability of tryptophan is implicated in depression among persons with untreated Celiac disease. This correlation is clear evidence of a genetically based nutritional link to this specific type of depression. As is the usual case, a genetic predisposition to a disease also requires an environmental factor. In the case of the patient with genetically based Celiac disease, consuming gluten containing foods is the environmental factor required in order to cause depression. Celiac disease is known to disrupt the integrity of the intestinal lining, leading to malabsorption of nutrients. This subsequently leads to a state of malnutrition, ultimately leading to a long list of other disorders. Treating this type of depression with antidepressants is the worst possible choice. Avoidance of gluten containing foods, and correcting any digestive system issues that may be present, is clearly the best choice.

Seasonal Affective Disorder is a type of depression that occurs in the winter months when the amount of daylight is decreased and weather conditions often prohibit outside activities. When this is the case, the solution is simply to increase exposure to sunlight. Artificial light boxes have been created for this purpose, and provide an excellent alternative to natural sunlight during times of inclement weather. The increased exposure to sunlight alleviates or eliminates depression in individuals diagnosed with Seasonal Affective Disorder. Serotonin is the neurotransmitter implicated in Seasonal Affective Disorder. In addition to light therapy, tryptophan or 5-hydroxytryptophan (5-HTP) supplementation may therefore benefit persons with Seasonal Affective Disorder.

Postpartum depression is another type of depression that has a specific cause, and is primarily due to fluctuating hormone levels. Symptoms typically begin within three months of delivery and generally last for three months or less. This is more of an acute depression with a limited time of occurrence, and typically resolves on its own. Fatigue, an abrupt change in lifestyle, and circadian rhythm changes are all factors that contribute to postpartum depression. Once the new mother has adapted to the lifestyle changes, postpartum depression will usually resolve quickly.

Depression is often found concomitant with other disorders. Certain chronic illnesses, including cardiovascular disease, hepatitis, mononucleosis, hypothyroidism, Parkinson's disease, fibromyalgia, and chronic fatigue syndrome can contribute to depression. Although most chronic disease is reversible, some are not. Whether any specific chronic disease is reversible or not, improving general overall health will greatly improve any symptoms of depression. Treatment of depression that occurs as a result of chronic disease will resolve when the chronic disease is reversed.

Certain prescription medications carry depression as a side effect. If depression results from a medication, careful consideration must be given to whether an alternative medication may be more appropriate.

Patients who are depressed are also most likely suffering from chronic stress. In the General Adaption Syndrome model developed by Hans Selye, patients suffering from depression most likely will fall into either the resistance phase or the exhaustion phase, the exhaustion phase being the most likely. Patients currently in the resistance phase will ultimately enter the exhaustion phase unless the causes of stress are identified and eliminated. When stress is found concurrent with depression, it will be found that the causes of both stress and depression are the same. In eliminating the causes of stress, the causes of depression are also eliminated. This is why making any change necessary involving those facets of the patient's life contributing to depression is very important. Furthermore, as the General Adaption Syndrome model suggests, the long term use of pharmaceutical agents to treat depression will most likely hasten the onset of the exhaustion phase by adding yet another source of chemical stress with which the body must contend. If stress is a factor in the cause of depression, viable treatment protocols must include addressing reversal of the General Adaption Syndrome.

Cortisol is produced by the adrenal glands when the body is under stress. Biochemically and physiologically, the body does not see any difference between chemical, physical, or emotional stress. Cortisol is released as a response to chronic stress, no matter the source of the stress. Cortisol is known to be elevated in depression and sleep disturbances. An elevated cortisol level activates a liver enzyme called *tryptophan pyrrolase*, which breaks down the amino acid tryptophan, decreasing the amount available by the body to make serotonin. Chronic stress therefore leads to reduced serotonin levels because of the tryptophan limiting effect of cortisol. Decreased serotonin levels are highly implicated in depression.

If the cause of depression does not fall into any known category, Depressive Disorder, NOS (Not Otherwise Specified) is put forth as the diagnosis. This diagnosis is a diagnosis of exclusion. When any diagnosis of exclusion is offered, it would always be most beneficial to continue searching for the underlying cause of the disorder. This applies to depression, as with any Not Otherwise Specified diagnosis. The type of depression and the cause must be specifically identified, and steps must be taken to change whatever situation is contributing or causing the depression.

It is not surprising that many people in modern day society are depressed. In a society where most people spend little time in the outdoors, consume artificial sweeteners such as aspartame, are under chronic stress due to any number of reasons, and have a diet of highly processed food, it is quite understandable why depression is occurring at record levels. In some cases, depression can occur as a result of the presence of chronic disease. Likewise, chronic diseases can also cause depression. Considering the possibility that a chronic disease may be present in depression is important, even though the chronic disease may be yet undiagnosed. Regardless of why depression exists, certain lifestyle characteristics and environmental factors appear repeatedly in cases of depression. Any lifestyle issues that are known to precipitate depression must consequently be addressed. Environmental factors contributing to depression must also be identified and appropriate adjustments must be made.

The traditional allopathic treatment of depression is antidepressant medication. The type of medication is selected based upon the neurotransmitter system most likely involved. In some cases, medications are prescribed that act on multiple neurotransmitter systems. Serotonin, dopamine and norepinephrine are the most commonly implicated neurotransmitters in depression. By various mechanisms of action, the antidepressant medication attempts to restore normal neurotransmission. In other words, the intent of these medications is to restore neurological balance. The mechanism of action of one class of antidepressant drug used to treat depression is to prolong the action of the neurotransmitter at the synaptic junction. Medications of this type are commonly called reuptake inhibitors. If a specific type of medication does not alleviate the depression, one with a different mechanism of action is often tried. Another class of drug commonly used inhibits the breakdown of the neurotransmitter at the synaptic junction, thus prolonging its effect. Monoamine oxidase inhibitors (MAOIs) are an example of this class of antidepressant.

At times, the symptoms associated with depression disappear spontaneously. The medical community calls this remission. If we look at it from another perspective, the lack of the symptoms of the disorder is the normal state of the patient, as opposed to being remission. When this happens, the disorder actually ceases to exist, rather than being in remission. If depression is in remission, it simply suggests that the cause of depression was eliminated and the patient is now normal again. If the patient gets well, and is no longer depressed, some outside influence, such as the diet, social circumstances, or medications, could have changed. These changes satisfactorily explain why the patient has improved, but are often overlooked or dismissed as irrelevant by the medical professional. Perhaps some internal influence, such as thought processes, could have also changed, again explaining any improvements realized. The effect of these influences, whether internal or external, may not be realized until several weeks or several months later. For this reason, linking external factors to the mental state of the patient is sometimes difficult.

Antidepressants are reported to have many side effects. Many of these side effects are quite serious, and for some reason, appear to be downplayed by the proponents of antidepressant therapy. Side effects of antidepressant medications include sexual impotence, loss of libido, uncontrollable anger, anxiety, weight gain, weight loss, sleep disruption, nausea, abdominal pain, agitation, constipation, dry mouth, and so on. If the medication treated and corrected the actual problem, no side effects would be present. If the antidepressant medication actually cured anything, the medication would, at some point, no longer be needed. In treating depression with medication, more problems are created, some of which must be treated by even more medications, with even more side effects. Medication, when used in treating depression, is covering up a symptom most likely as a result from another underlying issue.

If we can find the cause of the depression and address the problem at the root cause, it logically follows the disorder will cease to exist. The problem lies in identifying the root cause. In some cases the solution is simple, yet in other cases a more complex scenario exists requiring a more complicated, yet doable, solution. Finding the cause of depression is perhaps easier than one thinks. The usual causes are stress, employment, unemployment, lack of physical activity, poor nutrition, the use of various medications, and the presence of chronic diseases. Once the cause or causes of depression are found, action must be taken to eliminate the cause. Failure to address the cause will only result in continuance of depression, which is generally observed to worsen over time.

Several characteristic types of depression are known to exist. These types of depression are not to be confused with the causes of depression. The different types of depression are specifically linked to different neurotransmitters of the brain. Antidepressant medications specifically target these different neurotransmitters, which is why many different types of medications to treat depression are found to exist. Neurotransmitters have a delicate balance, and when they get out of balance, it is quite predictable what effects the imbalance will have. If the neurotransmitter system associated with the depression can be identified, steps can be taken to correct any imbalances that may have occurred.

One type of depression is where the patient is anxious and agitated, and often feels as if they are under stress for no reason at all. Depression as a result of chronic worry falls into this category. If this is the case, the neurotransmitter serotonin is most likely implicated. When this type of depression is present, the patient often consumes significant amounts of refined sugar because of the serotonin releasing effect sugar has. The patient with this type of depression may be found using alcohol or tranquilizers to alleviate the symptoms of the depression. Gamma-aminobutyric acid may also be implicated in this type depression and is commonly overlooked by the general practitioner. Specifically, low levels of Gamma-aminobutyric acid will allow imbalances in other neurotransmitters to be more pronounced.

Another type of depression, which is more common, is where the depressed individual is in more of a classical depressed state. This type of depression is found to include symptoms of melancholy, passiveness, apathy, and social inhibition. In this type of depression, one or more of the neurotransmitters serotonin, dopamine, phenylethylamine or norepinephrine are generally implicated. The patient with this type of depression often uses caffeine, narcotic medications, or stimulants to reduce the symptoms of the depression. The type of narcotic or stimulant used will give the natural health practitioner insight into the specific neurotransmitters involved. In these cases, supplementation of the diet with the appropriate precursor amino acid of the implicated neurotransmitter is usually indicated.

A third type of depression could conceivably be a combination of the anxious and agitated type and the classically depressed type. This can easily be mistaken for bipolar disorder. In the case of this patient, imbalances in any combination of the dopamine, norepinephrine, serotonin, or Gamma-aminobutyric acid neurotransmitters might be involved. When this is the case, underlying dietary or nutritional issues may be a contributing factor.

Certain amino acid deficiencies can lead to specific neurotransmitter imbalances. In some cases, specific amino acids are the precursors to neurotransmitters, meaning that the amino acid is converted through several biochemical steps to the neurotransmitter. Other amino acids, specifically glycine, taurine, glutamate, and aspartate, act as neurotransmitters themselves, and do not require biochemical conversion. Other neurotransmitters are amino acid derivatives, such as Gamma-aminobutyric acid (GABA). Some neurotransmitters are excitatory, others are inhibitory, and yet others can act as either excitatory or inhibitory. Table 10.1 identifies several common neurotransmitters, their precursors, and the general role they play.

Neurotransmitters act by binding to specific receptors on the neuronal synapse. A neurotransmitter can either excite the adjacent neuron or inhibit the adjacent neuron. The determining factor of the activity of a neurotransmitter depends on the balance between the number of excitatory and inhibitory processes affecting the neuron, and, of course, the receptor type. This is why some neurotransmitters can act in both an excitatory or inhibitory role.

The class of neurotransmitters, termed the monoamines, is often implicated in depression. Dopamine, norepinephrine, adrenaline and serotonin are the classic examples of neurotransmitters in this class. Monoamine oxidase inhibitors (MAOIs) are a class of antidepressants that target these neurotransmitters. The mechanism of action of a monoamine oxidase inhibitor is to inhibit the breakdown of the monoamine neurotransmitter in the synaptic junction. A monoamine oxidase inhibitor is a nonspecific drug, affecting all monoamine neurotransmitters in the various types of synaptic junctions. Monoamine oxidase inhibitors have potentially serious side effects associated with them. With such a broad scope of neurotransmitters associated with the mechanism of action, a monoamine oxidase inhibitor is, perhaps, the worst possible treatment choice for depression.

One specific neurotransmitter, phenylethylamine, may also be involved in certain types of depression. The amino acid phenylalanine is the precursor to phenylethylamine, a neurotransmitter involved in sexual attraction and emotional infatuation. Classical antidepressant medications do little to restore phenylethylamine levels. This explains, in part, why antidepressant medications have been frequently associated with sexual side effects, such as impotence or loss of sex drive. Chocolate, incidently, contains phenylethylamine, explaining why, when certain persons are depressed, eating chocolate alleviates the depression. If eating chocolate alleviates the depression, the amino acid phenylalanine or its metabolic pathways are likely to be involved.

Depression, then, has both a type and a cause. The type refers to any specific imbalances in the biochemistry of the associated neurology. The type of depression is determined by the presence of any nutritional issues, neurotransmitter imbalances, hormone balance, and any other biochemical variable that may be present. Causes of depression, not to be confused with the types of depression, involve environmental factors, dietary factors, social factors, and other factors of a non-organic basis. Specifically, the causes of depression often include emotional issues, thought patterns, nutritional issues, or any restrictions placed on life due to any reason. In some cases, the cause of depression is what lead to the specific type of depression. In other words, the external factor influences the internal factor. In other cases, the type of depression can exist without a social, emotional or mental cause, as often happens with malnutrition.

Neurotransmitter	Precursor	Action
Dopamine	Tyrosine	Excitatory or Inhibitory
Serotonin	Tryptophan	Excitatory or Inhibitory
Norepinephrine	Tyrosine	Excitatory
Epinephrine	Tyrosine	Excitatory
GABA	Glutamine	Inhibitory
Phenylethylamine	Phenylalanine	Excitatory
Glycine		Inhibitory
Glutamate		Excitatory
Aspartate		Excitatory
Acetylcholine		Excitatory

Table 10.1   Neurotransmitters

The first step in the treatment of any depressive disorder is to identify the type and causes of depression. If the proper type and cause of depression are identified, the appropriate treatment will succeed. If the type or cause of depression is incorrectly identified, inappropriate treatment is likely to have little or no positive results.

Once the type of depression has been identified, steps should be taken to correct any potential amino acid deficiencies that can result in any associated neurotransmitter imbalances. Correction of neurotransmitter levels may require several weeks of amino acid supplementation. Once neurotransmitter levels return to normal, continued amino acid supplementation is usually not required.

Obtaining proper overall nutrition is an imperative part of treating depression. Certain foods that can contribute to depression should be avoided. These are usually identified as "comfort foods" that one eats when they are depressed. Chocolate appears to be high on the list, along with sweets and other non-nutritious highly processed foods. These foods invariably cause an upward swing in blood sugar, which temporarily relieves the symptoms associated with depression. The problem is that refined sugar overloads the digestive and endocrine system, and a subsequent drop in blood sugar levels is inevitable a short time later. The drop in blood sugar will increase any symptoms associated with depression. As much as the depressed patient wants to eat sweets to feel a little better, doing so will not be beneficial in any long term relief. Maintaining healthy blood sugar levels by consuming foods with a low glycemic index is very important in treatment of depression.

Persons with depression or any depression related disorder should not consume the artificial sweetener aspartame. Aspartame breaks down in the body into its three components, aspartic acid, phenylalanine, and methanol. The transport of the amino acid phenylalanine into the brain is mediated by a carrier mechanism shared with other amino acids, specifically tyrosine and tryptophan. Excessively high levels of phenylalanine will inhibit the transport of tyrosine and tryptophan by the carrier mechanism into the brain. Since the neurotransmitters dopamine and norepinephrine are synthesized from tyrosine, and the neurotransmitter serotonin is synthesized from tryptophan, limiting the transport of these amino acids into the brain can subsequently limit the levels of these neurotransmitters in the brain. This can lead to depression. It is no surprise, then, that a population consuming vast quantities of aspartame found in diet foods also are enormous consumers of antidepressant medications.

In a world where dieting, the widespread use of artificial chemicals such as aspartame, the use of antacids and medications to suppress hydrochloric acid production, and high stress levels are the norms, understanding why the prevalence of depression is at an all-time high is very easy. Worse yet is the fact that, just because someone stops using these chemicals, it does not necessarily imply that the biochemistry of the brain will immediately return to normal. Restoration of health requires both time and effort. While the antidepressant pill often seems like the easy way out for depression, in most cases it is the worst possible treatment choice. The only thing the pill accomplishes is to hide the depression to enable the person to function within society better. Worst of all, the pill does not address any psychological contributors of depression. Using medication in the form of a pharmaceutical to treat depression is about as effective as hiding from a fire in a closet. Overall health must be restored and the underlying causes of depression must be treated if a person is truly to be healthy.

All causes of depression must be identified and treated, not only a few of the causes, or the ones to that are easy to address. Once any biochemical or nutritional issues are addressed, other areas of a person's life must be seriously examined as well. The question always arises of whether a neurotransmitter imbalance caused the depression or a depressed state caused the neurotransmitter imbalance. Either scenario is quite plausible. More plausible, however, is that the depression can have both a psychological and biochemical basis. In the case of depression originating from psychological causes, any treatment must consist of taking steps to improve overall quality of life, or the depression is unlikely to resolve. This involves identification of what facets of a person's life is contributing to the depression. Not as obvious is what is absent from a person's life that is also contributing to depression. Specifically, what is the person not doing that they want to be doing, or, more specifically, what activities and relationships leading to the enjoyment, satisfaction, and fulfilment of life are missing. The psychological component of depression is much more difficult to address than the biochemical and nutritional issues. Psychological factors involved in depression cannot be ignored, and certain issues must be resolved to eliminate depression.

One characteristic is very common with the vast majority of depressed patients. At times this characteristic is clearly evident, at other times it is not so evident, even possibly partially repressed. This characteristic is the patient suffering from depression is not doing what they really want to do in life. This encompasses a significant portion of their life, and is not limited to simply employment or the person's social situation. When we were all younger, we had at least some vision of what our life would be like when we got older. Often, however, what has happened and what we wanted to happen are two different things. Dreams remained dreams, and have faded into the darkness. Stress and anxiety have taken center stage, brightly lit by the spotlight. It logically follows that if a person is doing what they really want, fulfilling their life's dreams, they would not be depressed at all. It is never too late to begin anew, whether happiness is found in the dreams of our earlier years or new dreams discovered in more recent years.

What steps do we then take to resolve any psychological contributors to depression? Society tells us one thing, family tells us another thing, employers tell us something else, and we are often caught between the proverbial rock and a hard place. In other words, being confined and boxed in leads to the suppression of any personal expression, which, in turn, leads to the inability to experience pleasure. In fact, depression may as well be defined as the inability to experience pleasure. This constant suppression of inner desires can easily lead to depression. Depression, in turn, can lead to other chronic diseases. In order to break the cycle of depression, a person must then choose a path that is more in line with what they really want out of life, as opposed to what everyone else wants for us or from us. When someone is doing the things they want to do, the ability to experience pleasure returns, and depression resolves.

Just how does someone make changes to those areas of their life that are causing a problem? Certain things must be eliminated from the daily routine, and yet other activities would be quite beneficial to add. Undertaking the goal of completely changing one's life would be adding even more stress on top of the already stressful lifestyle that initially was a factor in causing the depression. Nevertheless, if the depression is to be eliminated, something is going to have to change. The number of ways to incorporate any changes into life is as many as the number of people who are in need of making the change. What works for one person, may, in fact, work for another person, but this is usually not the case. In most instances, that book outlining the five step program to happiness will not work either, and will end up at the garage sale with the countless diet books that also did not work.

Identifying the causes of depression is often quite simple for the person who is depressed. Likewise, for that same person, identifying anything that will lead to happiness is also quite easy. The significant others and close friends of the depressed person often have a fairly clear idea of what is beneficial or detrimental to the person's life. Carrying out of any changes required, however, is where the difficulty often lies. Perhaps the best advice on this subject is found on a popular bumper sticker, and reads *Just Do It*. So, are we then saying that a depressed person should just quit that tremendously stressful job that is likely a significant cause of the depression? The answer is yes, we most certainly are. However, if money is an issue, a new position may need to be secured first before resigning from the old position. Any step in the right direction gives a brighter outlook for the future.

Socially related factors contributing to depression are often easy to change. At times, breaking a relationship with a friend is necessary if that friend is a significant contributor to any depression that may exist. Since unhealthy relationships are a common problem, this scenario will be used as an example. Someone who continually exports all their emotional problems and strife to everyone around them is in need of professional help, but instead, uses all of their friends as a free psychologist. Recall our definition of health, which reads:

> *Health is the perfect harmony of the whole person in body, mind, and spirit, and perfect harmony of that person with respect to their social and physical environment.*

A continual disharmonious relationship, therefore, has no place in health. In the case of the friend who is the master exporter of every emotional problem ever known, recalling the three principles leading to an unhealthy state would be wise. These principles are:

1. *Something enters into the mind that should not be in the mind,*

2. *Something that should be in the mind is not in the mind,*

3. *Something enters into the mind, but, for some reason, the mind can no longer process it correctly.*

The exporter of strife is a clear example of the first principle. In exporting all of their emotional problems, they are filling the minds of the people around them with enormous amounts of their emotional baggage that most likely requires some type of professional attention. In satisfying the first principle, the exporter of strife also denies all of their friends an opportunity of a normal and healthy relationship, therefore satisfying principle number two. Over time, when a person hears the same complaining repeatedly, principle number three is eventually satisfied. Such a relationship cannot be healthy, unless, of course, the emotional exporter changes their ways. Until then, if the relationship is allowed to continue, the three principles will continue to be satisfied, and the chance of obtaining harmony within the social environment has moved into the realm of pure fantasy. If, however, unhealthy relationships are replaced with healthy relationships, harmony is created, and health is restored.

In examining the definition of health and the three principles leading to disharmony of the mind, what needs to be changed to eliminate depression becomes clear. Anything found satisfying even one of the three principles leading to an unhealthy state should be subject to evaluation. If a change is determined to be required, any action taken will depend on many factors. Again, these factors are as seemingly as numerous as the number of problems that exist. This is exactly why the book outlining the five step program to happiness is so utterly useless. Such a book tells someone exactly what to do, why to do it, but, for some reason, never leads to any lasting results. Life cannot be reduced to an assembly manual for happiness. What is needed is a method to evaluate what is leading to an unhealthy state of the mind. Having a method of analysis that can be applied to any personal situation makes much more sense when compared to the five steps to happiness program. The definition of health, and the three principles leading to an unhealthy state, is to be used as a sounding board for any potential problem that may arise. In knowing the goal, removal of roadblocks to the goal is the key.

In addition to removing the roadblocks to happiness, developing desirable relationships and adding enjoyable activities to the daily lifestyle will also help in the elimination of depression. How does one accomplish this goal? Simply put, the answer is that a person needs to decide what they truly want to do, and then do it. Some things may take a day to change, and other things may take years to change. If a change is being made to attain the goal of health, every step toward that goal, however minor it may seem, is one step out of the current undesirable situation and one step into a better situation. Remaining in a situation where freedom of expression is limited is not supportive of health. Moving into a situation that allows greater freedom of expression will lead to a happier and healthier life.

In the depressed individual, elimination of depression is not the goal. To eliminate depression, fulfilling the definition of health is the true goal. In moving toward the goal of true health, health problems, including depression, are left in the wake. If one can obtain perfect harmony of the whole person in body, mind, and spirit, and perfect harmony within the social and physical environment, depression simply would not exist. If any prior depression did exist, it would be long gone when perfect harmony is attained.

I had a friend in high school who figured out life quite early. While we were walking to school one day, I said "I don't want to go to school today." He quickly replied "so don't go." That is simple enough, just don't go. Now why didn't I think of that? He wanted to learn about Zen, so he spent some time at Dai Bosatsu Zendo, in New York, learning from Zen master Soen Nakagawa. Later, he wanted to learn more about automobiles, so he became a Diesel engine mechanic. He became interested in computers, and, sure enough, now he works with computers. He enjoys music, so takes voice lessons and sings in a choir. As an avid bicycler, he still rides well into his 40s. The point is that this person is doing exactly what he wants to do in life, living life to its fullest. Not surprisingly, this person is also not depressed.

Chapter 11
Obsessive – Compulsive Disorder

Obsessive-compulsive disorder is characterized by a patient's obsessive, distressing, and intrusive thoughts leading to related compulsions done in an attempt to neutralize the obsessions. Obsessive thoughts associated with obsessive-compulsive disorder are chronic in nature, and the patient clearly recognizes that the obsessional thoughts are a product of his or her own cognitive thought processes, and not from any outside influence. The patient often recognizes that the obsessive and intrusive thoughts are not based on any sound logic. Obsessive thoughts often lead to marked anxiety or distress. To relieve the associated anxiety, the patient feels driven to perform some act or ritual in response to the obsession. The disorder invariably leads to a diminished quality of life.

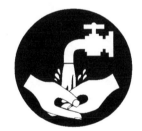

The obsessive-compulsive patient fully realizes that their obsessions and compulsions are unreasonable. The patient often adapts rules that must be applied rigidly to any repetitive behavior or rituals used in response to the obsession. These rules and rituals, which vary from patient to patient, evolve because of their anxiety decreasing effect. The result, over time, is a rigid set of rules for creating order that are followed for the sole purpose of reducing anxiety.

Patients diagnosed with obsessive-compulsive disorder often experience very similar patterns of compulsive behavior resulting from the associated obsessions. Repeated hand washing at regular intervals throughout the day, arranging objects at right angles, perfectly aligning objects in straight lines, counting steps to or from a destination, meticulously cleaning the home, and canceling out bad thoughts with good thoughts are a just few of the common patterns of behavior of the obsessive-compulsive patient. Obsessive-compulsive disorder can also incorporate fears, such as the fear of contamination by sweat, urine, saliva, tears, or feces, resulting in the inability to use public restroom facilities.

Any compulsive actions performed because of obsessive-compulsive disorder are done for the reduction of anxiety. Compulsive cleaning is one example of an activity commonly performed by sufferers of obsessive-compulsive disorder. The act of cleaning is presumably done to create cleanliness of the surroundings and order in the environment. Any microbiologist can inspect the newly cleaned environment of the obsessive-compulsive patient, and uncover any number of pathogens, including viruses, bacteria, mold, and other bugs. The heating and air condition duct work remain uncleaned. Mold or fungus most likely exists under the carpet or in hidden locations. Pathogens will be revealed in the refrigerator and on most every surface of the home. Another compulsive behavior is to line objects up in straight lines and at right angles. A physicist can come along and inspect the lined up objects with lasers and other highly technological measuring equipment and prove to the obsessive-compulsive patient that nothing is even remotely lined up. Great disorder still exists despite the efforts made by the obsessive-compulsive patient to create order. None of this inspection and analysis, however, matters much to the obsessive-compulsive patient. What is important to the obsessive-compulsive patient is that, in their own mind, they have created order to their own level of satisfaction. In creating order, anxiety is temporarily reduced. It is therefore the act of creating order that is the issue, not the actual level of order created.

Many different theories regarding the cause of obsessive-compulsive disorder exist. The majority of research supports the belief that there is some type of abnormality in the serotonin system of the brain. Environmental factors, as in many mental disorders, are reported to play a role. The notion that environmental factors actually play a role in obsessive-compulsive disorder, however, is difficult to understand. Neuropsychiatrists have identified certain regions of the brain associated with obsessive-compulsive disorder. Aberrant activity of a wide variety of certain neurotransmitter receptor sites has been positively correlated with obsessive-compulsive disorder. If any aberration of the brain or neurotransmitter system is involved in obsessive-compulsive disorder, it is more likely that the aberration occurs as a result of obsessive-compulsive disorder rather than actually being caused by the disorder.

The typical treatment of obsessive-compulsive disorder involves either psychological treatment, medication, or both. Medications commonly include selective serotonin reuptake inhibitors (SSRIs), Gamma-aminobutyric acid reuptake inhibitors, tricyclic antidepressants, and, in some cases, antipsychotic drugs. These drugs have a limited effect, and do not cure the disorder. Psychological treatment of obsessive-compulsive disorder involves either behavioral therapy or cognitive therapy, or both. These types of therapy primarily focus on the patient's behavior, and, through various means, attempts to make modifications to the behavior. While voluminous amounts of information exist documenting obsessive-compulsive disorder, little, if any, progress has been made in curing the disorder.

The modern treatment protocol of obsessive-compulsive disorder fails to provide a cure. When the treatment fails to provide a cure, it is likely that the cause of the disorder has not been found. When the cause of the disorder is not addressed, any treatment offered is focused upon symptom suppression. Symptom suppression through medication and behavior modification through psychological counseling does not address the true cause, and therefore cannot provide the cure.

Just what, then, is the cause of obsessive-compulsive disorder? The classical medical modus operandi of complicating a disorder through classification and analysis ad infinitum has made it difficult to come to an understanding of what medicine is actually attempting to treat. If the treatment consistently fails, the treatment is therefore inappropriate for the disease, and another treatment must be found. Before the appropriate treatment can be found, the cause must be identified, In addition, the obsessive-compulsive patient must be able to accept the cause of their obsessive-compulsive behavior before any treatment will prove effective.

Psychotherapy is often not a primary treatment of obsessive-compulsive disorder, but may actually prove to provide the most benefit. This is because the underlying issue causing obsessive-compulsive behavior is left untreated by any modern treatment protocol. The underlying issue is that the obsessive-compulsive patient is attempting to create order in one area of their life as a compensation for unresolved disorder in another area of their life. Once the underlying unresolved disorder is identified, resolution of the conflict will cause the obsessive-compulsive disorder to be cured.

The obsessive-compulsive patient is most likely unaware of any underlying areas of disorder affecting their life. Areas of disorder, however, may be readily apparent to the friends and family of the patient. Unresolved disorder, in some cases, may be deeply repressed, requiring potentially painful counseling sessions to uncover or identify. Many months, or perhaps years, of counseling may be required to identify, treat, and fully resolve the underlying condition. The issue of denial of any area of disorder may also become a factor, but once denial is resolved, the cure is on the horizon. Hypnotherapy may prove beneficial for some patients, and may provide valuable diagnostic information to the professional counselor regarding the origin of the disorder. Applied Kinesiology, as practiced by a qualified practitioner, may also prove beneficial in determining the time at which the disorder began and uncover other issues surrounding the disorder that may be unknown to the patient. The kinesiologist, in conjunction with the professional counselor, would prove valuable in discovering the origins of the patient's obsessive-compulsive behavior.

Underlying issues surrounding obsessive-compulsive disorder may originate at either the spiritual level, the mental level, or both. The unresolved internal conflict will most likely be identified as either a mental-mental conflict or a spiritual-mental conflict. Any combinations of conflict involving the body, mind or spirit may, however, exist. If the spiritual level is involved, spiritual counseling cannot be overlooked. No matter the origin of the conflict, proper treatment would involve any level affected. In eliminating internal conflict, internal harmony is created, and health restored.

As with many diseases, anything affecting the body, mind or the spirit will eventually affect all three. In obsessive-compulsive disorder, this will eventually include the physical body as well, especially when any repetitive compulsive activities lead to tissue damage. Excessive cleaning using ammonia, bleach, antibacterial soaps, and other household chemicals can subsequently cause any number of physical problems leading to any number of other diseases. Constant exposure to pesticides to eliminate household pathogens can also cause other toxic effects in the body. Whatever the compulsive activity, the physical body will most likely eventually be affected. Paradoxically, in an attempt to create order in one area of life, the obsessive-compulsive patient often finds him or herself creating disorder in many other areas of life.

Modern medicine has not provided the answer to obsessive-compulsive disorder. This is evident simply because the treatment is not addressing the true cause of the disorder. As with any disease or disorder, the true cause must be identified and corrected before resolution of the disease or disorder is possible. This not only applies to nutritional issues, chronic diseases, but disorders of mental origin as well. In identifying the true areas of disorder in the obsessive-compulsive patient's life, and providing appropriate counseling to address the issues, the cure for obsessive-compulsive disorder becomes evident.

A frequent visitor to our home appeared to suffer from obsessive-compulsive disorder. This person was driven to clean the home meticulously. Obsessive-compulsive disorder does have its advantages when it is someone else's disorder. When she came to visit, she cleaned everything in sight.

Chapter 12
Fibromyalgia / Chronic Fatigue Syndrome

Fibromyalgia syndrome, formerly called muscular rheumatism and fibrositis, is a syndrome of chronic, widespread pain accompanied by some degree of fatigue. In addition, persons suffering with fibromyalgia often have a wide spectrum of health complaints. Since fibromyalgia is a syndrome, it is defined by a collection of symptoms common to its sufferers. Not all symptoms appear in everyone with the syndrome. Some symptoms associated with fibromyalgia syndrome include sleep disturbances, cognitive dysfunction, paresthesia, headaches, muscle spasms, muscle twitches, depression, fatigue, hypoglycemia, Temporomandibular joint dysfunction, and irritable bowel syndrome to name a few.

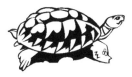

Eighteen designated points are evaluated for tenderness when a patient is checked for fibromyalgia. During the examination, four kilograms of pressure is applied to each of the eighteen points. If the patient feels pain at eleven or more of these points, the diagnosis of fibromyalgia is issued, providing there is an absence of any other underlying disease processes that can account for the symptoms.

Recent studies have suggested that certain neurotransmitters may play a role in fibromyalgia syndrome. Dopamine, norepinephrine, and serotonin appear suspect to varying degrees. Dysregulation of neurotransmitters has been known to cause sleep disturbances, mood disturbances, cognitive disturbances, and digestive disorders. Additional studies show physiological abnormalities in the fibromyalgia patient. One abnormality found is increased levels of substance P, a neurotransmitter involved in pain transmission in the spinal cord. A dysfunction of the hypothalamus, which is the link between the brain and endocrine system, has also been identified as a potential problem. A dysfunction of the thalamus, an area of the brain involved in sensory integration, has been identified as another potential problem in fibromyalgia. It is unclear, however, whether these changes cause fibromyalgia, or represent physiologic changes resulting from fibromyalgia.

Chronic fatigue syndrome is a name given to a disorder characteristic of severe, chronic physical exhaustion, often accompanied with mental exhaustion. The fatigue is often reported as incapacitating, disrupting every facet of a person's life. The onset can be abrupt, or occur over a long time. In addition, the person suffering from chronic fatigue syndrome will likely experience cognitive dysfunction, muscle pain, inflammation of lymph nodes, headaches, joint pain, and sleep disturbances. Not all the symptoms appear in everyone diagnosed with chronic fatigue syndrome.

No identifiable specific cause of chronic fatigue syndrome is known, subsequently, no one treatment protocol is directed toward a cure. Treatment is often consisting of purely palliative measures, or, as often happens, no treatment whatever is offered to the patient. Antidepressants have been used to treat the chronic fatigue syndrome patient, and have been shown to reduce some symptoms to a limited degree. Since antidepressants have their mechanism of action on neurotransmitter receptors, some degree of evidence suggests that dopamine, norepinephrine, and serotonin all may play a role. Neurotransmitter involvement may also implicate the hypothalamus, which is the link between the nervous system and endocrine system. When examining literature and research on chronic fatigue syndrome, every system of the body, to some degree, is clearly affected. For a syndrome that has markedly severe symptoms, surprisingly, no direct causative factor is evident.

No objective criteria, consistent subjective criteria, or pathological evidence is considered diagnostic of fibromyalgia or chronic fatigue syndrome. When a patient presents with the classical myriad of symptoms, diagnostic tests are performed to rule in or rule out certain diseases or conditions. With the chronic fatigue or fibromyalgia patient, laboratory tests are often proved normal, physiological function is generally within normal limits, and no underlying cause supporting the reported symptoms can be found. No correlation between documented examination results, laboratory tests and the patient's complaint can be found. Exhausting the list of potential differential diagnoses, the diagnosis of chronic fatigue syndrome or fibromyalgia syndrome is put forth by the medical doctor. Both chronic fatigue syndrome and fibromyalgia are a diagnosis of exclusion, offered purely on the basis of patient history and subjective symptomatic complaints.

The vast number and nature of the symptoms reported by chronic fatigue syndrome and fibromyalgia sufferers introduce other concerns that must be addressed. Specifically, the question arises of which symptoms are related directly to the condition and which symptoms appear later because of the changed lifestyle and decreased physical activity of the patient. The longer a chronic disease of any type is left untreated, the longer the list of symptoms and complaints gets. Assuming that the sufferers of a particular chronic disease will all follow a similar path in both lifestyle changes and symptoms experienced is not unreasonable. Further complicating the matter is the fact that most chronic diseases have symptoms of an insidious onset, meaning they are slow to occur. By the time the chronic disease or syndrome is diagnosed, the disease has usually progressed to the level that multiple symptoms are present. Many of these symptoms are likely due to other factors that occurred as a result of a chronic disorder, such as a modified lifestyle, a changed diet, and decreased activity levels.

Depression is an example of an ambiguous symptom of chronic fatigue syndrome and fibromyalgia. If depression is reported as a symptom, the question arises of whether the depression was caused by the syndrome, or whether the syndrome was caused by the depression in conjunction with any number of possible other factors. It can easily be argued that depression is often a result of any chronic ailment, and that the depression is not an independent condition that has arisen on its own. It can just as easily be argued that depression can cause a dysfunction of neurotransmitter regulation, and in doing so leads to dysfunction of other systems of the body. When this is the case, the depression worsens, and other symptoms associated with the affected systems of the body worsen as well. In other words, the patient is caught in a downward spiral. Finally, the patient gets to the point where they are depressed, hurting, and a sense of despair looms over them because they have been labeled with a disease for which there is no cure.

Muscle spasms and muscle hypertonicity are yet another example of a condition that either can contribute to chronic disease or be caused by chronic disease. Muscle spasms are involuntary contractions of a muscle. Muscle hypertonicity is the increased overall tension of a muscle. Tight muscles, cramps, trigger points, and painful muscles are all signs of muscle spasms. When a muscle is in spasm, the metabolic rate of that muscle is greatly elevated. The hypertonic muscle or the muscle in spasm is producing the by-products of metabolism, most notably lactic acid, at an alarming rate. Lactic acid, incidently, is very irritating to nerve endings. Lactic acid is what is responsible for the soreness of the muscles following a strenuous workout. If the by-products accumulate in the muscle tissue faster than the body can eliminate them, over time the muscle tissue is not only in spasm, but very hypersensitive to touch due to the accumulation of toxins that are now irritating the sensory nerve endings. In addition, the lactic acid is irritating the motor nerve where it attaches to the muscle, and causes the muscle to remain in spasm. This attachment point of the nerve to the muscle is called the motor point. If lactic acid accumulates at the motor point, it is very painful. A motor point with a build up of lactic acid is commonly termed a trigger point. The classical eighteen points referred to during a fibromyalgia examination are trigger points resulting from muscle spasms. The diagnosis of fibromyalgia by the medical doctor, therefore, is technically nothing more than a diagnosis of eleven or more muscle spasms.

Muscle spasms and muscular hypertonicity are well documented in the fibromyalgia patient. The chronic fatigue syndrome patient also experiences muscle spasms and muscular hypertonicity. Any muscle contraction requires energy to occur, whether the contraction is voluntary or involuntary. When a muscle is in spasm, it is consuming energy at an enormous rate. If muscles throughout the body are in spasm, the body is being depleted of energy that would normally be used for other purposes, such as work, recreational activities, or going to the mall. The muscle in spasm is also producing by-products of metabolism at an enormous rate. When muscles are in spasm throughout the body, toxins are accumulating faster than the body can readily eliminate them. In the chronic fatigue syndrome patient, the most evident symptom is fatigue. A major contributor to this fatigue is muscle spasm. In the fibromyalgia patient, the most evident symptom is pain. The pain is largely due to the accumulations of toxins in the muscle and interstitial tissues of the body. If both muscle pain and severe fatigue are reported by the patient, the patient is medically diagnosed with both fibromyalgia and chronic fatigue syndrome.

Bone pain is commonly reported in fibromyalgia patients. Bone and joint pain are also common in the chronic fatigue syndrome patient. The outer covering of the bone, called the periosteum, is one of the most pain sensitive structures in the body. The periosteum covers the non-articular surfaces of all bones. Tendons attach to this outer layer of bone tissue. A muscle in spasm is exerting constant force on the tendon, and the tendon exerts constant force on the very pain sensitive periosteum. Multiply the force of hundreds of muscles on 206 bones, and the understanding of why both bone and joint is a common complaint in fibromyalgia and chronic fatigue syndrome becomes clear.

Sleep disturbances are common among fibromyalgia and chronic fatigue syndrome patients. The reticular activating system is the area of the brain that initiates and terminates sleep and wake cycles. Pain has a strong influence on the reticular activating system. If the pain stimulus is above a certain threshold, the reticular activating system terminates the sleep cycle and the patient will wake up. Constant stimulation to this area is not conducive to adequate and restful sleep. It is therefore not surprising that the chronic pain patient has difficulty sleeping. Lack of adequate and restful sleep further contributes to the symptoms associated with the fibromyalgia and chronic fatigue syndrome. Lack of adequate sleep also leads to the dysregulation of neurotransmitters, which has also been implicated in fibromyalgia and chronic fatigue syndrome.

Cognitive dysfunction is a common complaint shared by both fibromyalgia and chronic fatigue syndrome patients. Cognitive dysfunction refers to the various aspects of the mind functioning in a compromised manner. Thought, memory, perception, emotion, and imagination can all be affected to various degrees. Cognitive dysfunction is also a complaint of sufferers of Multiple Sclerosis, depression, anemia, hypoglycemia, tumors, Polyarteritis Nodosa, sleep deprivation, sleep apnea, Systemic Lupus Erythematosus, and Vitamin B-12 deficiency to name just a few. Since thought processes involve neurotransmission in the brain, again neurotransmitters are implicated. Neuronal fatigue can also result in a significant degree of cognitive dysfunction. Neuronal fatigue has many causes, with lack of restful, restorative sleep leading the list.

Some fibromyalgia and chronic fatigue patients also suffer from a condition called Neurally-Mediated Hypotension. Neurally-Mediated Hypotension is a condition in which a neurological component is responsible for low blood pressure. This results in disrupted communication between the brain and the heart, resulting in vague symptoms including dizziness, weakness, fatigue, nausea, mental confusion, feelings of lightheadedness, frequent headaches, muscle pain and occasional profuse sweating. Specifically, the arteries of the extremities dilate, limiting blood flow to the brain, ultimately affecting neurotransmission in the brain. This is substantial evidence that regulation of the body's systems has been extensively impaired in both the chronic fatigue and fibromyalgia patient. Neurally-Mediated Hypotension is an effect, not a cause, of either fibromyalgia or chronic fatigue syndrome. Neurally-Mediated Hypotension is clear evidence that the patient has entered the exhaustion phase of the General Adaption Syndrome.

Chronic fatigue syndrome and fibromyalgia go hand in hand. The sufferers of one disorder have, at least to some degree, some symptoms of the other disorder. This would lead us to believe that chronic fatigue syndrome and fibromyalgia are really both the same disorder, or at least have the same basis. Medicine, however, has divided this disorder into two distinctly named syndromes. Recall that a syndrome is really defined by symptoms common to sufferers of some disorder. In the case of chronic fatigue syndrome and fibromyalgia, the predominant symptom is used to name the syndrome. Oddly, each syndrome is given a name, which, in fact, simply renames the predominant symptom. This is analogous to giving the name "pain syndrome" to any disease that causes pain, or "sleepy head syndrome" to any disorder that causes sleepiness. On the surface, naming a syndrome "sleepy head syndrome" sounds, to be frank, quite stupid. Why, then, would we accept any medical diagnosis that likewise simply renames the symptom? Logic would dictate that more exists to the disease process than symptoms appearing for no apparent reason.

If we examine the concept of a syndrome, we have what is nothing more than a collection of casually related symptoms. In assigning a name to a collection of symptoms, we have done nothing more than bring a Chupacabra into the health care system. To claim that the symptoms are casually related is nothing more than an admission that the cause has not been found. The problem arises when we believe a casual relation exists. The specific symptoms are not casually related at all. Symptoms are very specific, and complaints offered by patients reflect this high specificity with great reliability. Logic will not allow us to conclude that we have a syndrome in which a collection of separate but distinct symptoms are developing independently for no reason at all. These specific symptoms, which have been defined to be casually related, were, in fact, really all parts of the same disorder.

If the concept of fibromyalgia and chronic fatigue syndrome were discarded, and the symptoms experienced by the patient were examined in an objective manner, the true cause might actually become apparent. Once we have identified a cause, the cure also becomes evident. We can then work on reversing the causative factors that allowed the issues of fibromyalgia and chronic fatigue syndrome to manifest. The other choice is to wait for some miraculous cure, but that is simply not going to happen.

Rather than inventing a new name for these health conditions called fibromyalgia and chronic fatigue syndrome, considering what these disorders really are would be more appropriate, which is a generalized diminished capacity of the body to attain health. This would make much more sense than any theories put forth so far by modern medicine. If the body had the capacity to attain health, health would be the inevitable outcome. If the ability to attain health was somehow impaired, the list of symptoms grows longer and longer year after year. In order for reversal of the conditions to occur, increasing the body's capacity to attain health would be the ultimate goal. So, while we will still refer to the classical names given to these disorders, we are really treating the body with various methods to address the reduced capacity to attain health. The methods chosen, therefore, are focused upon increasing the body's capacity to attain, and maintain, health.

One important consideration that cannot be overlooked is that patients who have fibromyalgia or chronic fatigue syndrome are also suffering from chronic stress. In the General Adaption Syndrome model developed by Hans Selye, patients suffering from either fibromyalgia or chronic fatigue syndrome clearly fall into the category of the exhaustion phase. The General Adaption Syndrome model suggests that pharmaceutical compounds used in treating these disorders are adding more sources of chemical stress with which the body must now contend. This additional chemical stress will have the inevitable outcome of causing fibromyalgia or chronic fatigue syndrome to get worse. This is precisely why a chemical compound, herb, or other pill developed to cure either fibromyalgia or chronic fatigue syndrome will never be found. In order to reverse fibromyalgia or chronic fatigue syndrome, specific steps must be taken not only to address the exhaustion phase of the General Adaption Syndrome, but the extensive dysfunction of the systems of the body as well.

The onset of either fibromyalgia or chronic fatigue syndrome generally begins once the ability of the body to recover from stress has been breached. This breach could have been of an insidious or sudden onset. Once the line has been crossed, toxic metabolic waste accumulates faster than it can be eliminated by the body. This breach can be physical, emotional, or chemical stress, or, more likely as a combination of all three types of stress. As a result, multiple adaptations of the body occur, subsequently leading to any number of pathological changes, resulting in a further decreased capacity of the body to function normally. Symptoms, however, do not necessarily appear until some time later. Unaware of any symptoms, the patient continues to operate in a high stress environment, during which time symptoms appear gradually.

Where, then, do we begin? Several factors must be considered in the treatment of any chronic disorder. Fibromyalgia and chronic fatigue syndrome are no exception. The first factor is that if any person suffering from chronic disease and ailments continues to do what they are doing now, the problems will only get worse. Change, therefore, is mandatory. Identifying what must change is the challenge.

Restoration of the digestive tract is a good first place to start. The importance of a properly working digestive system cannot be overemphasized, which is why an entire chapter has been devoted to this topic. In addition, during the advanced phases of the General Adaption Syndrome model, the digestive system is invariably affected. In reversal of fibromyalgia and chronic fatigue syndrome, correction of any existing digestive system issues is mandatory.

Since metabolic by-products have built up in the muscle and interstitial tissue, elimination of this build up of toxins is essential. In both the fibromyalgia and chronic fatigue patient, the rate at which toxins accumulate in the body is faster than the rate at which the body can eliminate these toxins. One of the best methods for accelerating the elimination of these toxins is deep tissue massage therapy. Reduction of muscle spasms will restore the proper function of the muscle. In restoring the function of the muscle, stress involving the joints is reduced. As a result, the range of motion of the joints is increased, and pain and inflammation of the surrounding tissue is decreased. Trigger point therapy is also very useful for reduction of muscle spasms. These treatments are best accomplished by a professional massage therapist because they are quite familiar with lymphatic drainage and the role of soft tissue therapy in the detoxification of the body and in the reduction of muscle spasms. Obtaining a therapeutic massage focused on these goals will provide the best results. A spa massage, which is more for relaxation, will not provide the same therapeutic benefit.

Massage should initially be performed for only one-half hour for the first few sessions. This is because many toxins will be released from the tissues into the bloodstream, which must be broken down by the liver and eliminated by the kidneys. Consequently, increasing the intake of water both before and after a massage will help in elimination of these toxins. It is very likely that the chronic fatigue or fibromyalgia patient will feel worse following massage therapy, especially during the first few massages. This is a positive sign, indicating that the body is detoxifying. After the first few sessions, a one hour massage should be performed once or twice weekly. The massage therapist will offer recommendations, based upon progress, about when to increase the session length.

Muscles that are chronically found in spasm are also found in a shortened state. This significantly decreases the range of motion of the joints that they control. The constant force exerted by muscle spasms on the bones causes joint pain. Chronic muscle spasms also are related to decrease lymph flow. Decreased lymph flow slows detoxification of the bodily tissues. For these reasons, muscles must be stretched to restore their normal tension. Yoga is an excellent way to stretch muscles and restore normal muscle tension. Yoga classes can be taken in the local yoga center, gyms, and by private instructors. Attending a class has many benefits. The class meets at set times every week, individual attention is available, not to mention the social aspects of being with other people. Yoga videos can also be purchased to practice at home. A good massage therapist or chiropractor can also provide instruction on stretching muscles.

When beginning any stretching program, remembering to increase gradually the duration and intensity is important. Some soreness is to be expected during the beginning of the program, but this should gradually decrease over time. The stretching program should be performed three to four times a week for approximately thirty minutes or more per session. If a class is attended that meets on a less frequent basis, home sessions should be added to supplement the class. When stretching is done at home, breaking the stretching session into two 15 minute sessions may be advantageous, one in the morning, and one in the afternoon or evening.

Whenever abnormal muscular stress is exerted upon the bones, the skeleton deviates from its normal biomechanical position. Muscles that are shortened and are in spasm exert unnatural and inordinate forces upon the joints. Continuous skeletal stress can lead to osteoarthritis, bursitis, tendinitis, degenerative disc disease, and even worse muscle spasms than those that already exist. This ever increasing muscular stress is responsible for both the increasing levels of pain and decreased level of energy during each passing year. Massage therapy and stretching will alleviate the muscle spasms responsible for skeletal deviations. Chronic muscle spasms, as found in the fibromyalgia or chronic fatigue patient, have undoubtably caused deviations to the skeleton. Chiropractic care will realign the skeleton, further decreasing stress placed on the joints and muscles.

Chiropractic is founded on the principle that elimination of nerve interference will allow the body to perform at its optimum. A chiropractor can identify any biomechanical abnormalities of the skeleton, and, through a series of chiropractic adjustments, restore the normal alignment and biomechanics of the skeleton. In addition, chiropractic care reduces stress of the nervous system. Thirty-one pairs of nerves exit the spinal cord that connects and controls the entire body. Any interference with the transmission of nerve messages to a particular muscle or organ will result in it not functioning normally or at full capacity. The chiropractor, by removing interference and stress from the nervous system, opens the path for the body to perform at its maximum potential.

Chiropractic specifically addresses a condition known as a vertebral subluxation. A subluxation is the malposition of a vertebra with an adjacent vertebra that subsequently causes pressure on the nerve roots exiting from the spinal column. When a subluxation occurs, nerve impulses are interfered with. If enough pressure is exerted on a nerve, the nerve ceases to function altogether. When a subluxation exists, the normal range of motion of the spinal joints is also lost, resulting in decreased freedom of movement. Inflammation of the disc and facet joints of the spine can occur, causing additional pressure on the nerves. The muscles attached to the affected vertebra can go into spasm, and may result in the development of trigger points. Left untreated, a subluxation can lead to osteoarthritis and permanent disc damage. Nerve pressure or impingement results in a decrease in function of the end organ controlled by the nerve. If a nerve going to a muscle is impinged upon, weakness develops. If a sensory nerve is impinged upon, numbness, tingling, or other altered sensation will occur. When the nerves going to the heart, liver or kidney, are interfered with, no physical symptoms may be present, but nonetheless a decrease in function of the organ will be evident. The good news is that chiropractic adjustments can correct vertebral subluxations, thus restoring neurological function.

Restoring the normal biomechanics of the skeleton will drastically aid in reducing the stress exerted on the joints by this tremendous muscle tension. Massage will help to relax the muscles and eliminate toxins, stretching will help restore normal muscle tension, and chiropractic care will restore the proper biomechanics of the skeleton. Perhaps one of the best kept secrets of chiropractic care is prevention of future illnesses. A skeleton with proper alignment and a body free of nerve interference is part of the foundation of good health.

If someone experiences numbness, tingling, pain, or "pins and needles" in their hands or feet, a very strong possibility exists that the cause is a vertebral subluxation. Pressure exerted on a sensory nerve will result in a symptom, which is some form of altered or varied sensation. The symptom, in this case, is obvious. The symptom is an alarm that something is wrong. However, if any interference is found to the nerves going to the liver, no obvious symptoms are evident. Likewise, if interference to the nerves going to the kidneys is found, again, no obvious symptoms are reported. This is true for nearly every internal organ found in the body. No one has ever walked into a doctor's office and said "I believe the parasympathetic nerve supply to the right side of my heart is being interfered with." This a good reason why it is important for anyone who has a chronic disease to see a chiropractor. Interference to the nerve supply to any of the body's organs can impair the function of that organ. Since nerves are found going to every organ, the nerves must obviously have some function. A nerve connects the brain and an organ for a reason, that reason is to facilitate communication. If the nerve supply to the organ is interfered with, the organ can no longer effectively communicate with the nervous system. If that organ is involved in detoxification of the body, the detoxification process can be impaired. One cannot expect to be in good health with a nervous system that is unable to communicate effectively with the rest of the body.

Proper sleep and rest are imperative during the healing process of the body. Often, the fibromyalgia or chronic fatigue patient complains of sleep disturbances. Most sleep disturbances result from imbalanced neurotransmitters. Neurotransmitter imbalances result from stress. Correcting neurotransmitter levels and reducing stress is important if a person is to experience normal and restful sleep. Correction of neurotransmitter levels is a long term process, and does not occur overnight. The process could take several months, especially if other disorders linked to neurotransmitters are present, such as depression or anxiety. Psychological factors are also involved in sleep disturbances. Stress and anxiety are the most common complaints. These issues must be addressed as well. Since the chronic fatigue and fibromyalgia patient are often found in the latent phases of the General Adaption Syndrome, and under stress, recommendations found in the chapter discussing stress would apply.

Melatonin is a hormone found in the brain that plays a part in regulating sleep. Both melatonin and serotonin are synthesized through biochemical pathways involving the essential amino acid tryptophan. Serotonin is a neurotransmitter that affects the mood, and is often referred to as the "feel good" neurotransmitter because of its antidepressant action. Serotonin is also a neurotransmitter found in the intestinal tract, where it increases motility of the small intestine. If tryptophan levels are very low, the conversion to serotonin and melatonin cannot simply occur. With low levels of melatonin, restful sleep becomes very elusive.

Since tryptophan is an essential amino acid and cannot be synthesized by the body, it must be obtained through the diet. When significantly low levels of tryptophan are found to exist, dietary sources of tryptophan are typically insufficient to restore normal levels in the body. For this reason, a dietary supplement of tryptophan is beneficial in restoration of serotonin and melatonin levels. When selecting a tryptophan supplement, be sure to purchase one that does not contain any added herbs. Some herbs, which are often added to a tryptophan supplement, such as Valerian Root, can cause depression in susceptible individuals. Occasionally, Vitamin B-6 is added to the supplement, which facilitates the conversion of tryptophan to serotonin. Other vitamins may also be added in small amounts by the manufacturer that play a role in the conversion. The added vitamins to a tryptophan supplement are therefore beneficial.

Do not purchase a melatonin supplement. Melatonin is a hormone. Taking a melatonin supplement will interfere with the feedback mechanisms of the brain involving the synthesis of melatonin. Allowing the body to regulate the production of melatonin naturally is far superior to taking the hormone melatonin in supplement form. Using the precursor to melatonin, either tryptophan or 5-hydroxytryptophan (5HTP), is a better choice.

A tryptophan supplement will also aid in reducing depression. The lowest effective dose that eliminates depression and corrects sleep disturbances is the most efficacious. Since many biochemical reactions in the body compete for tryptophan and only a small percentage of ingested tryptophan makes it to the brain, therapeutic levels of supplementation should typically be between one thousand and three thousand milligrams (1000-3000 mg.) daily. Overloading the body with higher doses of tryptophan is counterproductive. This is because a liver enzyme, *tryptophan pyrrolase*, breaks down any excessive amounts of tryptophan, adding metabolic by-products that must be eliminated by the body. A natural health care provider should be consulted prior to beginning any program using supplements to restore health.

Exercise is an excellent way not only to improve physical fitness, but improve mental attitude as well. Exercise has been shown to reduce the symptoms associated with depression, a frequent complaint of patients with chronic diseases. Likewise, exercise also reduces stress levels. The physical benefits of exercise include improved cardiovascular health, improved muscle strength, and greater flexibility. Exercise also improves circulation, and helps lower blood pressure.

Perhaps the most important class in high school was gym class. When one contemplates it, any information memorized in history class can be found in a book or on the internet. If someone was not good at math, they can always hire an accountant to balance their checkbook. Anyone bad at English can still communicate with their friends and co-workers, and, after all, many are reading this book. In science class everyone cut open frogs, and down the hall in psychology class they were taught cutting open frogs is cruel and unusual behavior. But, in gym class, everyone exercised, and the truth is that no one can exercise for someone else. Exercise is something that everyone must do for him or herself. Gym class also instilled the concept of competition, whether the competition is with others or with our self. Anyone found exercising in the gym, running, or participating in sports is always trying to improve upon their best personal performance.

When the word exercise comes to mind, we most often think of weightlifting or running. Exercise, however, encompasses far more than just these two activities. Examples of other types of exercise are speed walking, bicycling, jogging, swimming, kayaking, dance, tennis, basketball, Pilates, Yoga, and martial arts. Martial arts is an excellent type of exercise program because it encompasses strength training, coordination, balance, and aerobics. Varying any exercise programs over time is important so that the body does not adapt to the same routine. Joining an exercise class is also beneficial because of the personal instruction available and consistency factor of the class meeting at set times during the week.

Since the fibromyalgia and chronic fatigue patient have entered the exhaustion phase of the General Adaption Syndrome, high intensity exercise will initially be counterproductive. Exercise is often avoided by patients with fibromyalgia or chronic fatigue syndrome because the symptoms associated with these disorders typically get worse following any physical activity or exercise. The intensity of any exercise program should be increased gradually according to patient progression. Some exacerbation of symptoms is likely to occur from time to time and is only temporary. Exercise will increase the metabolic rate of the body, which would typically cause more toxins to accumulate in the tissues. Massage therapy, proper nutrition, stretching, and adequate rest, however, will increase the body's ability to detoxify.

Exposure to sunlight has many health benefits. Exposure to sunlight in the warmer months is actually a form of dry heat. Dry heat is used for detoxification of the body. Sunlight has also been shown to have antidepressant properties. This is most notable in persons with Seasonal Affective Disorder, a type of depression that results from decreased exposure to sunlight. People with Seasonal Affective Disorder are more prone to depression during the Winter months when weather conditions and shorter days prohibit outdoor activities. Many people, although they have not been diagnosed with Seasonal Affective Disorder, report an elevated mood when exposed to sunlight. Taking time to be outside in the Sun is sure to benefit everyone, not only those who have Seasonal Affective Disorder. During inclement weather, an artificial light box can be used to simulate natural sunlight. Research indicates that, when exposed to artificial light in a controlled manner, such as the light provided by a light box, the symptoms associated with Seasonal Affective Disorder are alleviated.

A modern belief exists that the Sun is some big evil disc in the sky that is going to give everyone skin cancer. Recently, this has been disproved, which really means that it was never really proven at all. Believing that a repetitive sunburn year after year can cause skin damage is realistic. This type of Sun exposure is what typically leads to skin cancer later in life. Light to moderate sun exposure, however, can hardly be implicated in skin cancer, except in the rare cases of persons who are genetically incapable of producing adequate amounts of melanin.

When sunlight enters the eyes, the optic nerve is stimulated in proportion to the intensity of sunlight. Above a certain threshold, the stimulation of the optic nerve also causes stimulation to both the hypothalamus and pineal glands. The primary neurotransmitter associated with the Hypothalamus is serotonin. Serotonin is also a neurotransmitter often implicated in depression. Stimulation of this area of the brain has been shown to reduce depression, without any of the side effects common with antidepressant medications. In the Pineal gland, Melatonin is a hormone associated with sleep and wake patterns. Above a certain threshold, sunlight exposure can inhibit Melatonin production, thus inhibiting sleep. This inhibition of sleep is what is expected during the day. Conversely, when a person is not exposed to sunlight, Melatonin levels remain elevated during the day, and the person often feels tired and has a lack of energy. As a result, circadian rhythms are disrupted, and the person ends up wanting to take a nap during the day and is unable to sleep at night. Exposure to bright sunlight would be quite beneficial to anyone who lacks the energy to carry out daily activities or unable to sleep at night.

Most people can remember quite well the days they spent on the beach years ago. Those were generally good times, everyone had fun, and the memories are often very vivid and clear. People who have enjoyed the beach before often cannot wait to return. The same excitement can often be found surrounding a vacation at a ski resort. The reflection of the sun on the snow greatly increases the intensity of the sunlight we perceive. In some cases, when people return from the beach or ski slopes, they are immediately planning their next vacation so they can return in a few weeks or months. The elevated mood from the exposure to bright sunlight creates such a good feeling, making people want to return. This is perhaps the reason that the beaches, ski slopes, and the tropics are common vacation destinations.

If getting it out in the sun is not possible, purchasing an artificial light box will help alleviate some symptoms of depression. Traditional indoor lighting does not emit sufficient light to surpass the threshold needed to stimulate the Hypothalamus and Pineal glands. The better light boxes are engineered with this threshold in mind. Light therapy devices are rated in lux, and the light intensity rating is measured at a specific distance away from the light box. Ten thousand (10,000) lux is a generally accepted standard for therapeutic light boxes. Sources of quality therapeutic light boxes can be found in Appendix I.

Maintaining correct body weight is imperative in reduction of the symptoms associated with fibromyalgia and chronic fatigue syndrome. Maintaining an appropriate weight can also decrease the likelihood of developing certain other diseases such as diabetes, heart disease, and high blood pressure. Any additional weight carried is placing additional stress on the already fatigued muscles of the fibromyalgia and chronic fatigue patient. The truth of the matter is that most people who suffer with chronic diseases are typically overweight. Adjustments to activity levels, diet, and stress levels to maintain an ideal weight would therefore be beneficial to any chronic disease sufferer.

If someone was to fill a backpack with 30 pounds of weight and carries it around for a few hours, they would begin to fatigue quite easily. Fatigue would come a lot faster if activities such as cutting the lawn, cleaning the house, or washing the car was done while wearing the 30-pound backpack. Carrying around an extra 30 pounds of fat is not much different. The only difference is the fat accumulated slowly. If the fat were suddenly gone, the same relief would be felt as in removing the 30-pound backpack. Weight loss, however, is inherently slower, but the same effect will be realized.

Weight gain occurs when a person consumes more calories from food than is expended. To maintain constant weight, the number of calories consumed should equal the number of calories expended. When a person eats more calories than is expended, the energy balance is tipped toward weight gain. When a person eats fewer calories than is expended, the energy balance is tipped toward weight loss. Many other issues are also involved when it comes to caloric balance, such as genetic and environmental factors.

No miracle weight loss method has ever been found. Losing weight is simply a matter of tipping the energy balance toward expending more calories than are consumed. Increasing the activities that expend calories, such as exercise, will eventually lead to weight loss, all other factors being equal. Decreasing the number of calories consumed will also lead to weight loss. A combination of increased activity in conjunction with decreasing the number of calories consumed daily proves most beneficial. This is because exercise increases the basal metabolic rate (BMR) of the body. The basal metabolic rate is the rate at which the body burns calories while at rest. When exercise is part of any weight loss program, the basal metabolic rate increases, so, even at rest, the body is burning more calories.

The basal metabolic rate (BMR) decreases about ten calories per day each year after about the age of 25. At the age of 35, the BMR is therefore 100 calories per day less than at the age of 25. This means that at 35 years old, the caloric requirements of the body have decreased by 100 calories per day. At 45 years old, the caloric requirement of the body is now 200 calories less than at the age of 25. One pound of body fat is the equivalent of 3,500 calories. If someone continues to eat the same amount of food at the age of 35 as they did at 25, every 35 days they would theoretically gain one pound of fat, all other factors being equal. Seeing where all the extra pounds came from over the years is not difficult.

Since the body does not burn fat exclusively during exercise, expending 3,500 calories will not result in a loss of one pound of fat. During exercise, the body burns carbohydrate and fat at approximately a 50:50 ratio. After about an hour of heavy exercise, the percentage of fat burned increases as carbohydrate reserves get depleted. Using the 50:50 ratio, approximately 7,000 calories must be expended to lose one pound of fat.

Avoidance of the consumption of "empty calories" when trying to lose weight is highly recommended. Empty calories, which carry little nutritional benefit, include refined sugar, refined flour, and other highly processed foods. Rather than drinking a soft drink, having a piece of fruit would be a better choice. Eating bread with meals is unnecessary, especially when covered with butter. While bread and soft drinks have calories, they will essentially be converted to fat which must be burned off later by even more exercise. No benefit can be found in eating foods that will contribute to the fat reserves of the body when someone is trying to lose weight.

Other important considerations are proper nutrition, elimination of stress, and avoidance of environmental toxins. The importance of these factors cannot be overemphasized; therefore, an entire chapter has been devoted to each of these topics. The advice offered in these chapters must also be followed if the fibromyalgia or chronic fatigue syndrome patient is to improve.

To summarize the treatment protocol for fibromyalgia and chronic fatigue syndrome disorders, we begin by:

1.   Restore the digestive system,
2.   Obtain frequent massages,
3.   Stretch tight muscles,
4.   See a chiropractor,
5.   Obtain adequate rest,
6.   Balance and stabilize neurotransmitters,
7.   Exercise regularly,
8.   Get plenty of sunlight,
9.   Lose any extra weight,
10.   Obtain adequate nutrition,
11.   Avoid environmental toxins,
12.   Eliminate stress.

In eliminating the classical symptoms of fibromyalgia and chronic fatigue syndrome, we are primarily concerned with eliminating stress and the accumulated effects of stress. Three types of stress exist that affect the body. They are chemical stress, emotional stress, and physical stress. In eliminating stress, we eliminate the cause of many symptoms. Stress, however, leads to even more stress, and this poses a problem. Specifically, physical stress, such as stress caused by a muscle spasm, eventually leads to chemical stress, in the form of accumulated toxins. Accumulated toxins within the muscles cause pain, eventually contributing to emotional stress. This certainly does not include all the other sources of stress an individual may have. A major consideration of reversing fibromyalgia or chronic fatigue syndrome is to exit the exhaustion phase of the General Adaption Syndrome model described by

Hans Selye. The key, then, is to eliminate all sources of stress, thus restoring balance and the body's ability to detoxify itself. In doing so, we further restore the ability of the body to attain health, which reflects our original goal.

The program for reversal of these chronic conditions is undoubtably a significant change in the lifestyle for many affected people. The changes discussed are, for the most part, mandatory, and not a list to pick and choose those items that are convenient or fit into the daily schedule. If this sounds difficult, it is because it is. Any change is difficult, but a time will occur when a change is needed. Going for two massages a week, seeing a chiropractor, taking an exercise class, stretching at home, going to Yoga class, and so on, appears as if a large amount of time and effort are required. If the activities suggested may appear as if they will take one or two hours a day on average to accomplish, it is because they will. What is being asked is to replace unhealthy activities with healthy ones. The decision must be made of whether to be tired and in pain 24 hours a day or make the required changes.

Many people are already living a lifestyle very similar to the changes suggested. They are among the healthiest people in the community. It is no secret how they got that healthy. Their health is a result of their lifestyle. If they continue with their healthy lifestyle, they will not get fibromyalgia or chronic fatigue syndrome. While the changes suggested may seem monumental at the onset, after living a lifestyle conducive to health for a year or two, one would dread going back to the old way of life.

A 32-year-old female patient came into the office with back and neck pain. She stated on the entrance form that she was recently diagnosed with fibromyalgia. The patient was distraught by the diagnosis offered by the medical doctor, believing that she is destined to live a lifetime of pain. I told the patient there was no such thing as fibromyalgia, and that fibromyalgia is nothing more than a "garbage can" diagnosis that the medical doctor gives when they have no other answer for you. A few adjustments and massages were performed over a period of a few weeks. A few suggestions regarding lifestyle changes, such as exercise and dietary changes, were given to the patient. The patient leads a physically active life today, totally pain free.

Chapter 13
Multiplicity

Multiplicity is perhaps the most interesting personality variation known of all conditions that have a primarily psychological basis. Multiplicity has been called Multiple Personality Disorder, and has most recently been known as Dissociative Identity Disorder. For purposes of discussion in this chapter, we will refer to the condition using the medical term *Multiple Personality Disorder* when referring to the condition from the viewpoint of the medical profession. Otherwise, the more accurate term *multiplicity* will be used. The newer term, Dissociative Identity Disorder, is a meaningless term and misrepresents what the condition actually is.

Multiple Personality Disorder is considered a mental condition in which two or more distinctly identifiable personalities exist within the same person. Each personality is expressed at different times, but not simultaneously. The defining feature is a significant

$$1+1=1$$

degree of identity alteration. When a personality switch occurs, the person will exhibit different behaviors, personality traits, thought patterns, and cognitive abilities. Mutual exclusion of the characteristic personality traits of each identity is also seen in Multiple Personality Disorder. Distinct memories associated with each personality are also characteristic of Multiple Personality Disorder. This mutual exclusion of memories is seen to varying degrees in both the long term and short term memory of the affected person. The person, therefore, often will not remember what transpired when another personality was in control. As a result of different memory sets, the person with Multiple Personality Disorder will have separate sets of life experiences.

The question of whether multiplicity is an actual disorder or an invented one has been under question in recent times. Enormous amounts of medical research support the existence of Multiple Personality Disorder. Electroencephalogram (EEG) studies support the theory of the potential existence of multiple personalities in one person. Sufficient objective and subjective evidence is submitted by researchers that clearly support the existence of the condition. The opinions put forth by decades of research, for some reason, have been ignored in favor of the unsubstantiated opinion that the disorder is of a questionable existence. Since no medical treatment for Multiple Personality Disorder can be offered, the physician who diagnoses the condition has essentially put forth a dead end diagnosis. The medical profession has no pill to prescribe, no body part to extract, and no brain surgery that can cure the condition. Any treatment, therefore, is limited to non-medical protocols. With no medical treatment available, it is easily understood why the existence of the condition is under question.

Both of the terms Multiple Personality Disorder and Dissociative Identity Disorder imply that an actual disorder exists. The existence of something termed a disorder implies that some consideration should be given to the treatment of whatever the disorder is. Recently, consideration has also been given to the possibility that the disorder does not even exist. No consideration, however, has been given to the possibility that multiplicity is a normal condition. Perhaps what has been called a disorder for decades is not really a disorder at all. If this is the case, multiplicity would fall into the category termed a *normal variant*. When a condition is termed a normal variant, the condition is considered a normal condition, but occurs at a much decreased frequency than is found in the general population. Hundreds, if not thousands, of conditions considered normal variants are found in medicine. Placing multiplicity in the category of a normal variant would be an appropriate step in reclassifying the condition. In doing so, however, we open the door to placing nearly every psychological disorder into the category of a normal variant. Attention deficit disorder, disorders involving teenage behavior, many learning disorders, social anxiety disorder, and separation anxiety disorder, are just a few so-called disorders that would be considered normal variants. Treatment of a normal variant is not normally necessary, and therefore is not eligible for insurance reimbursement. Consequently, the reclassification of multiplicity as a normal variant is not likely to occur.

If we examine the concept of multiplicity, we have a well-defined collection of clearly related personality characteristics. Clearly identifiable characteristics associated with the same condition, which are observed to occur in a definable segment of the population, simply does not occur by chance. When something does not occur by chance, yet cannot be clearly proven, it is nothing more than concrete evidence the cause has not been found. A problem arises, however, when we believe that a cause, in every case, must exist. No consideration is given to the possibility that multiplicity is a natural condition and therefore has no cause. The characteristics associated with multiplicity are very specific. Furthermore, the experiences described by patients reflect high specificity and great reliability. The condition cannot be simulated or faked even by the most knowledgeable individual. Logic, therefore, must lead us to conclude that we have a clearly defined condition. If we have a clearly defined condition, it cannot be simply dismissed as nonexistent.

Some researchers attempt to link Multiple Personality Disorder to some form of epilepsy or seizure disorder. In effect, this theory states that a seizure of some sort has occurred, thus altering cognitive processes to some degree. A seizure is an aberrant form of uncontrolled neurotransmission generally characterized by the presence of a closed neuronal circuit. In contrast, the neuronal switching involved in Multiple Personality Disorder is very specific, repeatable, and in some instances, controllable. If Multiple Personality Disorder was, in fact, a seizure related condition, one would expect that the uncontrolled neurotransmission characteristic of a seizure would leave, in its wake, a different personality following each instance. In addition, medications in the class of Gamma-aminobutyric acid reuptake inhibitors commonly used in the control of seizures would be expected to have some effect on Multiple Personality Disorder. This effect of a Gamma-aminobutyric acid reuptake inhibitor has not been demonstrated clinically. It is doubtful that Multiple Personality Disorder has anything to do with any type of seizure disorder. Any objectively demonstrated changes in neuronal activity or patterns are most likely an effect of the personality switch, not the cause of the switch.

Religious entities have long equated Multiple Personality Disorder with demon possession. Certain religious groups, particularly the Roman Catholic Church, appear to relate any potential disorder of the mind to demon possession. The Roman Catholic Church is always found to be at least 100 years behind science. This is clearly demonstrated throughout history. For example, the Roman Catholic Church had taught for centuries that the Earth was positioned at the center of the universe, and the planets and the Sun revolved around the Earth. In developing the Sun-centered theory of the solar system, Copernicus was condemned by the Roman Catholic Church, and the theory was declared as heresy. No Pope can solve a third-order differential equation, solve a triple integral, much less understand calculus of variations. For some reason, however, the opinion of the man holding this office is treated as if he actually knows something regarding the advanced mathematics required to understand astronomy. The Pope has about the same level of medical knowledge as he does advanced mathematics. The Roman Catholic position on Multiple Personality Disorder, or any other mental disorder, must be dismissed on the basis of ignorance alone.

Someone may ask or wonder what it is like to have Multiple Personality Disorder or be capable of any form of multiplicity. A researcher may examine many cases of patients diagnosed with Multiple Personality Disorder, intensely study the disorder from every angle, and carefully document any characteristics of the disorder. None of this work, however, gives any true meaning about what it is like to have Multiple Personality Disorder. Even more incomprehensible to the researcher is the notion of non-disordered multiplicity. To the non-disordered multiple, it is equally incomprehensible to claim that multiplicity does not exist. The only answer to truly understanding multiplicity is, therefore, to experience multiplicity. Unless one experiences multiplicity first hand, no written words or verbal explanation can adequately describe the experience. Any medical professional, religious figure, or skeptic, who doubts the ability of someone capable of multiplicity to switch at will should perhaps study the chapter on Zen. In understanding Zen, even minimal enlightenment will reveal the mechanism behind multiplicity, clarifying any doubt.

Multiplicity was a relatively unknown condition until 1980. Before that year, approximately 200 cases of Multiple Personality Disorder were reported. After 1980, the number of reported cases is found in the tens of thousands. This figure does not take into account any undiagnosed cases. Multiplicity appears to be more prevalent in the United States of America. The question arises, then, what has changed since 1980 to cause such a dramatic increase in persons capable of multiplicity. In addition, the question arises about what is unique to the United States of America to account for the disproportionate number of cases when compared with the rest of the world.

Several changes in society can be identified that occurred around the year 1980. The changes around that time began with the arrival of the personal computer. As a device marketed to increase productivity, additional workplace stress came bundled at no charge with the package. Computers can be now found in nearly every home, in the workplace, and in every school. The personal computer is no longer exclusively found in the workplace. Children surf the internet before they even have two digits in their age. Since the introduction of the personal computer, modern technology has placed more electronic conveniences in the hands of every member of society. Cell phones, PDAs, instant messengers, email, Global Positioning navigation devices, and MP3 players are but a few of these devices that promise a more convenient society. With the promise of convenience, however, comes an undisclosed guarantee of stress. Modern technology allows people to be instantly connected to anyone else through any number of forms of media and numerous forms of communication. People walk around with timepieces on their wrist, one or more cell phones hanging from their belt or in their purse, a contraption on their ear that closely resembles assimilation by the Borg, and carry a host of electronic gizmos to keep them informed of what is not only happening all around them, but halfway across the world too. Something must be happening all the time, the television is blasting away, a headset is pumping music into our ears, messages are being sent back and forth, and a conversation over the cell phone is occurring at once. In essence, any connection to the rest of the world is attained through some electronic means, and everyone is becoming assimilated into this electronic network whether they realize it or not. As a result, real connections with real people are greatly diminished or completely absent.

All these electronic connections are nothing more than a sophisticated form of an escape from society. What we, as a society, have attained are not connections with others, but, instead, an inner sense of loneliness. In escaping from society, we have also escaped from ourselves. By escaping, we have placed ourselves in disunity with both ourselves and those around us. With human connections replaced by wires, normal societal relationships, as defined by the traditional social structure, cannot be formed. When these normal societal relationships cannot be formed, certain natural inborn mechanisms of the mind remain intact and are able to develop naturally. When the mind develops in a more natural manner, particularly at a young age, it may often be mistaken as some type of mental disorder.

Society teaches us to behave in specific ways. From the time we are born, our behavior is regulated, modified, and controlled in every imaginable way. Multiple rules of order must be adhered to. Some rules are reasonable and necessary, and others are frankly ridiculous. A rule of order and conduct exists at home, another rule of order and conduct at work, school, church, with friends, on the internet, in social settings, and everywhere else imaginable. Natural personality traits are continually being suppressed by conforming to all these separate and distinct rules of order. In addition, unnatural personality traits are instilled in conforming with the rules of order. Over time, the mind is molded to conform to this modern disaster we call civilization. The mind is, therefore, not allowed to develop in the natural manner. Not surprisingly, anyone not conforming to the societal rules of order is often diagnosed with some mental disorder. Quite interestingly, however, those closely conforming with the rules of society generally are found to suffer from some chronic disease later in life. Specifically, artificially induced rules result in unnatural development of the mind. Since the mind and body are strongly connected, the effects of this unnatural development eventually will affect the body as well. A person having to conform meticulously to the rules of order is placed under enormous stress. This stress ultimately leads to the latent phases of the General Adaption Syndrome, eventually resulting in disease.

In certain cases, multiplicity, a normal variant of the mind, does not get suppressed. Multiplicity, one natural method of handling stress, somehow remains intact in certain individuals. In order for the mechanism responsible for multiplicity to remain intact, certain criteria must be met. This can be done by one of two possible ways, either of which must occur at an early age. These two ways, however, are not exclusive; other methods of preservation certainly can exist. Methods of acquiring multiplicity at a later age also exist, but the basic mechanism involving multiplicity is the same. The mechanisms associated with the preservation of multiplicity are quite well documented by the researchers of multiplicity. Preservation of the inborn mechanism responsible for multiplicity is not necessarily a problem, however, the mechanism may not be considered compatible with what society considers normal. Unfortunately, when multiplicity is termed Multiple Personality Disorder or Dissociative Identity Disorder, the research is directed to studying a disorder rather than a natural state of the mind. Should the researchers examine multiplicity from the aspect of that of a natural stress response, the research may actually make some sense.

The first method to preserve multiplicity is avoidance of stress and the consequences of stress at an early age. In other words, allow the child to do what the child wants to do, without any consequences for what would normally be termed misbehavior. This can easily be accomplished by not exposing an individual to the societal rules of order, and therefore allowing the mind to develop in a more natural manner. By not being required to conform to any rules, any consequences associated with breaking the rules or order cannot possibly exist. This subsequently allows the mind to develop in such a way to handle any stressor in a natural manner. Without any learning process involving any so-called civilized method of handling stress and conflict, the natural mechanism involved in the handling of stress is able to develop unhindered. Multiplicity, a natural stress response, therefore, remains intact.

The individual who has not been exposed to the stress associated with conforming to societal rules of order, thus escaping the consequences of nonconformity with the protocol of rules, is actually in a much healthier state than those individuals who have been highly trained in the system. As a result, persons who have preserved the mechanism of multiplicity are far more capable of avoiding the consequences of stress in modern day society. A counselor, whether a psychologist or psychiatrist, examining such a person would be at a loss to find any childhood trauma, whether physical, emotional, or chemical, contributing to multiplicity. The counselor, however, is searching for a cause for a condition that they would consider to be a disorder. Since multiplicity is the normal condition for this patient, and not a disorder, no cause will be found.

Early exposure to stress is the second method to preserve the mechanism of multiplicity. In this case, some form of stress, either chemical, emotional, or physical stress, is presented to the individual, but no learned or conditioned response to stress has yet developed. When this is the situation, the only response available to a stressor is any number of natural responses. Some type of naturally occurring inborn mechanism, therefore, takes over and in order to handle the stress. If the mechanism available is multiplicity, a personality switch will occur. Once a personality switch occurs, the mechanism is firmly in place, and subsequent personality switching becomes more readily available to the individual as a response to stress. Again, a counselor examining such a person would be unlikely to discover any childhood trauma as the cause of multiplicity. In this case, the personality that was present at the time of the stress may have been switched out of, perhaps permanently. With the personality switched out, the associated memory set is unavailable for recall.

The individual capable of multiplicity who has been exposed to any form of stress associated with the early experiences of life is most likely to have the cause of multiplicity identified being directly attributed to the trauma associated with the stress. The diagnosis of the disorder is most often put forth by a psychologist or psychiatrist many years later. Substantial evidence is often found in the patient history supporting the diagnosis. Conversely, in this situation, much information is also absent from the patient's chart. Omission of this information is not necessarily intentional, but is often unknown to the patient. Early childhood trauma, sexual abuse, or mental abuse generally falls into the category of omitted information. This failure to uncover either a stressor or trauma leading to multiplicity is because a personality switch occurred, and the memory associated with the incident has been switched out of the current personality, and therefore unavailable for recall. This inability to recall events is often termed *repressed memory*, and, in the case of multiplicity, is an integral part of the switching mechanism. A person with multiplicity of this origin is often subject to extensive counseling. Counseling, in this case, would be best applied to understanding multiplicity rather than attempting to reverse a condition that is firmly ingrained in the neurology. In gaining an understanding of multiplicity, the patient is better equipped to understand him or herself, and able to adapt more easily to the stressful modern lifestyle.

Since multiplicity primarily originates early in life, the neurology associated with the mechanisms of personality switching is well developed long before the individual ever sees a counselor. As a result, counseling efforts to reverse multiplicity invariably fail. This failure is because the condition is not actually a disorder, but, instead, is a normal neurological state of the mind allowed to develop in a natural way. Neurons cannot simply be rewired in such a way to eliminate the mechanisms associated with multiplicity. Developing a medication to target the mechanisms of multiplicity is impossible, and is about as feasible as developing a medication to cause someone to forget their name. As a result, medical treatment is not only impossible, but is also not indicated.

Multiplicity can also be acquired, and this deserves special mention. Acquired multiplicity has its origin in a forced personality change, and is usually, but not always, accompanied with very stressful situations. When a distinctly different personality has been instilled in the individual, the potential for multiplicity then exists. As classical example, a soldier, who lived a completely different life before entering military service, is placed in a position where a personalty change is mandatory and sudden following enlistment. This change involves the adopting disciplinary characteristics markedly different from the every day life the person was previously accustomed. In other words, a personality change was mandatory and forced. The newly installed personality is trained to follow orders, handle the stress of the battlefield better, and to respond in specific ways to certain events. The battlefield is clearly a severe form of stress, which can be handled reasonable well by the trained soldier. When the tour of duty is complete, enlistment is up, and the soldier returns to his or her previous way of life, the old personality again surfaces. The ex-soldier, perhaps years after being in the battlefield, is walking down the street and hears an automobile engine backfire. The similar sound of the engine backfire to a gun or other sound heard on the battlefield, causes the person to relive the stress of the battlefield. Under the proper circumstances, an immediate personality switch occurs. As a result of this switch, the ex-soldier may run for cover, attack an innocent bystander mistaken to be the enemy, or react in a way consistent with battlefield behavior. The medical profession incorrectly calls this post traumatic stress syndrome, which is a meaningless diagnosis that does not even begin to explain how or why this behavior occurs. Recognizing this as acquired multiplicity, however, would serve to explain completely why the events occurred as they did.

Multiplicity, then, is a natural response of the mind to some form of stress. The personality switch associated with multiplicity is not limited to only the mind, but manifests in the body and in the spirit as well. The type of stress is of either chemical, physical, or emotional origin. No matter the type of stressor, the personality switch occurs when no method to escape from the stress is possible, or no available means to deal with the stress. When presented with this type of stress, the person capable of multiplicity can deal with the stressor, or switch to a different personality set which is more able to handle the stress. In switching personalities, the consequences of stress are successfully avoided by, or handled differently by, the newly presented personality.

When a personality switch does occur, the person is sometimes aware of the switch, and at other times completely unaware of the switch. If one is aware of their multiplicity nature, any switch will most likely be evident. For those who are unaware that they are capable of multiplicity, any personality switch would be somewhat of a bizarre experience, with no explanation at all to account for what they have experienced. Once the concept of multiplicity is understood, however, the circumstances around the experience of switching makes perfect sense. The experience of a personality switch varies from person to person, and is almost always accompanied by some type of subtle neurological sign or symptom.

The medical profession defines multiplicity as a disorder. In the usual context of medicine, a great show is put on, backed by poorly conducted research, meaningless diagnostic criteria, and practitioners who have no true knowledge of what they are trying to understand and treat. The medical profession would be frightened to consider the possibility that multiplicity is not a disorder at all, but, instead, a normal condition of the mind. To give any consideration to multiplicity as a normal condition would completely shatter a profession so deeply involved in inventing and defining disorders involving any behavior that they consider as not being normal. Beating a normal condition of the mind into submission is not necessary. To beat multiplicity into submission, whether through behavior modification or drugs, is an act of hostility, therefore inducing further stress to the individual. Furthermore, to assign multiplicity into to a category of a normal variant would require many other diagnoses of psychological origin to also be termed a normal variant. Since the medical profession is often unwilling to learn any form of alternative healing methods, any true understanding of multiplicity is far beyond their reach.

The medical profession will undoubtably dislike the definition of multiplicity contained in this chapter. The primary reason is that the medical profession has not discovered the explanation presented here first. The definition of Multiple Personality Disorder, as put forth by the medical profession, leads to nothing but a maze of dead-end streets. With poorly formed theories, defective research protocols, and the unwillingness to accept the principles of alternative diagnostic and healing methods, no plausible explanation has ever been offered by the medical profession for the involved switching mechanism. As a result, their questions will remain eternally unanswered within the framework of the medical paradigm. To change their position on multiplicity would require discarding decades worth of research, something that should, but most likely will not, be done.

Just what, then, is going on during the personality switch of multiplicity? In the field of Applied Kinesiology, an elementary concept exists known as neurological switching that fully explains what transpires during a personalty switch. One basic type of switching familiar to all kinesiologists is called K-27 switching, which, by the way, is not the switching mechanism involved in multiplicity. The switching mechanism of multiplicity is more complex, requiring diagnostic testing by a kinesiologist to uncover. In some cases, multiple switching mechanisms may be involved, explaining the overlap in certain memory sets and some behaviors. Neurological switching occurs as a natural response to some form of stress, and has its origin in the mind. When a neurological switch occurs, not only is the possibility of a personality change likely, but changes are evident in the chakras and meridians as well. Any changes that manifest in the spirit subsequently will affect the physical body and mind. When neurological switching occurs, various changes are readily apparent in the musculoskeletal system to the Applied Kinesiologist. The casual observer may even notice gait and postural changes that classically follow neurological switching. Often, a change in accent or inflection may also be noticed in the voice. Using specialized kinesiology, the practitioner can neurologically switch the subject from one personality to another, therefore effectually working on each personality to restore harmony of the body, mind, and spirit. With an understanding of multiplicity and the switching mechanisms involved, the person can learn to recognize neurological switching when it does occur or learn to neurologically switch at will, therefore ultimately adapting better to the stress present in modern day society.

Multiplicity is, then, a highly sophisticated normal variant of the mind that has its origin in the mind, which affects the physical body and spirit as well. It is not known to what degree every individual is capable of multiplicity, but if the capacity is to be preserved, it apparently must be done at an early age. The ability to switch at will, or to handle any personality switches properly that may occur, has been termed a *non-disordered multiplicity* by those who have experienced this ability. Individuals who are capable of multiplicity, in a sense, have a distinct advantage in any society in which the members of that society must follow multiple rules of order, are under constant stress, or when each day is filled with highly unpredictable events. Modern Western civilization is representative of such a society.

A better way to treat multiplicity is to teach the person how to identify particular stressors associated with a personalty switch. By identifying potential stressors, better management of the associated stress can be learned. This will subsequently reduce the need for a personality switch to occur as a stress management response. For the person capable of multiplicity, a personality switch invariably will occur. When the switch does occur, great value will be found in having options available to handle the switch. Multiplicity, then, can be best addressed by a psychologist working in conjunction with a kinesiologist who is familiar with neurological switching mechanisms. An understanding of what has happened and why it has happened is invaluable to not only those capable of multiplicity, but to others around them as well.

If it isn't broken, then don't fix it.

Chapter 14
Environmental Toxins

In our environment, numerous substances and organisms can potentially have a detrimental effect on health. These are termed environmental toxins or environmental pathogens. When we think of environmental toxins, pesticides, landfills, air pollution, and water pollution come to mind. While these are certainly sources of environmental toxins, they are just the tip of the iceberg and hardly representative of the scope of the toxicity of our environment. The term environmental pathogen, while not as commonly used, refers to bacteria, molds, fungi, or any other microbial organism that can cause harm to the body. Fecal coliform bacteria, cyanobacteria, and black mold are a few examples of environmental pathogens. Environmental toxins therefore encompass inorganic toxins, organic toxins, and pathogenic organisms.

One cause of disease we previously identified was:

Something enters into the body that should not be in the body.

All environmental toxins fall into this category. Ingestion of any toxin has absolutely no role in health. While the body can effectively eliminate certain toxins found in the environment, other toxins either cannot be readily eliminated from the body or are eliminated from the body very slowly. When this happens, damage to the body results. Since this damage often occurs at the cellular and sub-cellular level, it often goes undetected until considerable damage has accumulated. By the time damage is detected at the system level, the disease process initiated by the toxin has been in progress for quite some time. Obviously, removing ourselves from the exposure to the toxin is the appropriate countermeasure. In addition, methods can be used to hasten the elimination of certain toxins from the body. Fortunately, in most cases, the body is able to repair the damage cause by these toxins.

Toxins are a unique form of stress encountered by the body in the sense that they not only invoke the body's natural stress response as chemical stressors, but also have a mechanism of toxicity that subsequently causes tissue damage. This tissue damage further invokes the body's stress response. In essence, the natural stress response of the body is invoked by both by the toxic chemical stressor and the tissue damage caused by the toxin.

For every controversy regarding any toxin presented in the discussion, two opposing positions can be found. One position is that the substance is known to be toxic and therefore can cause harm to the body. This position is substantiated by biochemists, professors, and other independent researchers. The other position maintains that the toxin is safe. This is the position that will calm the public, and is often financed by those having a vested financial interest involving that toxin in one way or another. One cannot legislate away the detrimental effects of a toxic compound. In addition, propaganda cannot be used to reduce the toxicity of a toxin.

Governments have issued documents defining safe exposure levels to various toxins, such as Mercury and other heavy metals, pesticides, and various organic and inorganic compounds. The safe exposure level is determined through extensive research, and the safe exposure limit is typically set at a level where symptoms are not evident. This research is performed by men and women who have PhDs and specialize in biochemistry and human disease. Various factors are taken into consideration and, based upon the findings, a number is generated representing the upper limit of safe exposure. The fundamental problem with this methodology is that we talking about a toxin. The safe exposure level of the toxin is therefore zero. If the PhD performing the research arrived at a safe exposure level of zero, they would be fired from their job, plain and simple. The truth is that, since these toxins are present and eliminating them is impossible, something must be done to make the public feel safe. Exposure limits, therefore, are set, published, and adhered to, giving the illusion of safety. This amounts to nothing more than a game of "how much can we get away with and not get caught." In other words, a game is being played in setting limits to how much damage that can be done to the body, and, at the same time, keeping the damage undetected as far as physical or mental symptoms are concerned. The stated intent of setting these limits is always related to, in one way or another, the protection of the health of the public. The real reason, however, is to avert any legal liability as a result to exposure to these toxins. Obviously, not being a participant in such a game would be in the best interest of health.

The same nonsense of setting safe limits is also applied to human laboratory tests designed to measure exposure to toxins. In this case, however, the nonsense is carried quite a bit further. Limits of the presence of heavy metals, various organic and inorganic compounds, or other toxic compounds are set for the urine, blood, or hair by various organizations. Several quantitative methods are available for determining whether a toxic level exists. Different organizations publish different limits of these toxins, and no agreement can be found as to what constitutes a safe level. To complicate matters further, occupational limits in exposed workers are also defined, and safe exposure levels to the toxins used in industry are different from the limits for the general population. For example, for the general population, the upper limit of Lead found in the blood should not exceed 19 µg/dl. For industrial exposure, the limit defined by the Occupational Safety and Health Administration (OSHA) is 40 µg/dl. If the level exceeds 60 µg/dl, according to OSHA, the employer must remove the employee from exposure to the hazard. While it appears that these limits are as a result of careful and extensive research, they represent nothing but pure nonsense. The question arises as to why 39 µg/dl is safe and 41 µg/dl is not safe. Another question arises as to why employment in industry warrants a higher safe exposure level as opposed to someone who does not work. The cynical observer would question why all these figures published by the government all mysteriously ends in a zero. Why is 40 µg/dl the accepted limit, and not 37.5 µg/dl? For any test designed to measure the level of a known toxin in the body, regardless of whether the toxin is being measured in the blood, urine, hair, or other tissue, the only safe level of that toxin is zero. Furthermore, determining safe levels of exposure based upon the factor of employment is, at best, absurd.

Biochemistry is a very well defined and well understood scientific field. Biochemistry does not lie. If the biochemist can clearly demonstrate the disruption to the biochemical processes of the body caused by a particular toxin, and can clearly show exactly how the toxin is toxic, no further discussion or argument is necessary. If a particular compound is shown to disrupt a particular chemical reaction through a specific mechanism of action, no guidelines or legislation issued by any governmental organization is going to affect the biochemical reaction. When something is defined as a toxin, in most cases the mechanism of actions is clearly understood and demonstrable. In other cases, the mechanism of action of the toxin is unknown, which, in a way, is indicative of a potentially more dangerous toxin. If the mechanism of action is not known or not fully understood, no one really knows exactly how that toxin is poisoning the body. A toxin in which the mechanism of action is unknown is analogous to Pandora's Box.

Just what are the sources of these environmental toxins? When one is found, what courses of action do we take? The answer to these questions depends greatly on what the toxin is. We will look at a few of the toxins present in today's society, and how it affects the body. For each toxin presented in the discussion, substantial evidence is known to exist regarding its toxicity, with the mechanism of action, also called the mechanism of toxicity, clearly defined in most cases. Many papers and writings list symptoms of toxicity associated with various toxins. While the symptoms associated with toxicity are an important part of diagnosis, the symptoms have little, if anything, to do in defining why the toxin is harmful to the body. The proof lies in the biochemical mechanism of toxicity. The mechanism of toxicity of a substance is the biochemical proof required to classify a chemical compound as a toxin. The mechanism of toxicity, if known, is presented.

Fluoride

One common toxin present in today's society is fluoride. Marketed as a preventive of tooth decay, fluoride is present in drinking water and toothpaste. Fluoride can cause a myriad of health issues and can contribute significantly in the development of various chronic disease processes.

Once ingested, fluoride initially acts locally on the intestinal lining, causing irritation. Once absorbed into the body, fluoride binds Calcium ions and can lead to hypocalcemia (decreased serum levels of Calcium). Low blood levels of Calcium can cause cardiac arrhythmias, altered sensation, tingling or numbness in hands and feet, muscle spasms, depressed deep tendon reflexes, and a host of other disorders. Fluoride also causes hyperkalemia (increased serum Potassium) resulting from the release of Potassium by cells. Fluoride inhibits acetylcholinesterase, causing signs of cholinesterase inhibitor poisoning such as hypersalivation, vomiting, and diarrhea, to name a few. Fluoride also interferes with the coagulation mechanisms of blood. Other effects are hypomagnesemia (decreased serum Magnesium), and hypoglycemia. All these, however, are just symptoms of the ingestion of fluoride.

Although fluoride causes a variety of symptoms in the body, the mechanism of toxicity of fluoride reveals the true nature of the toxin. Fluoride has a direct toxic effect on cells, and interferes with many biochemical reactions. Fluoride disrupts the Krebs cycle by interfering with oxidative phosphorylation and glycolysis, and this interference is its primary biochemical mechanism of toxicity. Oxidative phosphorylation and glycolysis are biochemical reactions involved in energy production that occur in every cell of the body. When the term *energy production* comes to mind, one might be inclined to think of the energy needed to carry out the activities of daily living, but this is only part of the picture. If the affected cell is an immune system cell, immune system function will be compromised. If the cell is a brain cell, thought patterns can be affected. If the cell is a liver cell, the body's metabolism can be affected in many ways. If the cell is a peripheral nerve, transmission of nerve impulses through that nerve will be impeded. In other words, every cell of the body is a target of the toxic effects of fluoride. This should clarify the scope of the mechanism of toxicity of fluoride. Nearly every biological effect of fluoride occurs as a result of this disruption. Ultimately, damage to multiple organs and systems results, leading to a variety of chronic diseases.

The only preventive and corrective measure is to avoid fluoride completely. Any nutritional requirement of fluoride by the body is suppled through the diet, and no supplementation, either through drinking water or toothpaste, is necessary. Purchasing fluoride free toothpaste and drinking fluoride free water is the best approach. Well water does not contain fluoride, except for certain isolated areas of the world. If well water is not available, consider drinking

Why Am I Sick? And What To Do About It

bottled water or purchase a water filter that can eliminate the fluoride from publically supplied water.

Mercury

Mercury is another environmental toxin of great concern. Exposure to Mercury occurs from breathing contaminated air, ingesting contaminated water, consumption of contaminated food (particularly fish), and from dental filings. A high level of Mercury in the body causes damage to the brain, kidneys, and the developing fetus. The central nervous system is very sensitive to all forms of Mercury, and repeated exposure can cause permanent neurological damage. Acute effects of high levels of Mercury vapors include lung damage, various gastrointestinal effects (nausea, vomiting, and diarrhea), various cardiovascular effects (high blood pressure, palpitations), skin rashes, irritation of the mucosa, and eye irritation.

Rather than enumerate and explain symptoms of Mercury toxicity, examining the mechanism of Mercury toxicity would be more valuable. By doing so, we gain a better understanding of the scope of problems associated with Mercury toxicity. Mercury compounds have a strong affinity for thiol chemical groups, which are found in certain amino acids, which make up proteins. Mercury strongly binds to these thiol groups. This is the mechanism of action that renders Mercury toxic. Proteins and enzymes contain these thiol groups, and are found in all tissues of the body. This explains the broad scope of Mercury toxicity, and the extensive biological effects that result from exposure to the toxin. Mercury compounds fall into the class of toxins called nonspecific enzyme inhibitors. Other heavy metals, such as Lead and Arsenic are also in the class of nonspecific enzyme inhibitors, causing similar biological effects. An enzyme inhibitor essentially prevents a biochemical reaction involving that enzyme from occurring. It does not take a genius to figure out that if a particular enzyme or biochemical reaction exists in the body, it is probably there for a good reason. Furthermore, if the enzyme is damaged, it does not take a biochemist to realize that the biochemical reactions dependent on that enzyme have now been compromised.

Mercury, or amalgam, fillings should be removed by a holistic dentist and replaced with a less toxic alternative. Certain procedures must be followed when removing Mercury fillings to reduce the exposure of the patient to further Mercury exposure. A holistic dentist will take extreme care in the removal of these filings to prevent any Mercury from entering the body. If a patient has a Mercury filling removed and spits out a mouth full of ground up metal, chances are very good the fillings were not removed properly. Not surprisingly, dentists, their professional organizations, and anyone else who holds potential financial liability, are the only groups who steadfastly deny the toxic effects of Mercury amalgam filings. In consideration of the fact that removed Mercury filings must be disposed of as toxic waste, the position that regards Mercury as nontoxic probably warrants some reconsideration.

What is of concern, however, is how a compound with clearly known and toxic characteristics can somehow be deemed to be safe when installed in a tooth.

If the Occupational Safety and Health Administration sets limits for Mercury exposure, even the cynical observer might come to the conclusion that the metal might be toxic to some degree. If a biochemist can demonstrate that Mercury binds to thiol groups, the mechanism of toxicity is clearly understood and well documented. What is difficult to understand, however, is what has been deemed so special about these Mercury amalgam dental filings. This special dental Mercury almost appears to have been imparted some divine characteristic in the sense that it is claimed not to have the same toxicity that other Mercury has. Mercury is Mercury, and, no matter the source, it carries the same mechanism of toxicity. To admit that Mercury amalgam filings are toxic will undoubtably expose the dental profession to class action law suits by patients who have suffered health consequences resulting from the effects of Mercury toxicity.

Mercury has appeared in many products intended to be introduced into the human body, and is known under different names. One such chemical compound containing Mercury is thiomersal, known in the United States as thimerosal. Thiomersal is used as a preservative for vaccines, contact lens solutions, and certain types of cosmetics. Thiomersal, used as a preservative in certain vaccines, has been blamed for the development of autism in babies. The thiomersal issue is yet another controversy that will never end. In the body, thiomersal is metabolized to ethyl Mercury and thiosalicylate. Ethyl Mercury is an organic Mercury compound. An organically bound heavy metal can move throughout the body more easily than if it was not organically bound. This is because an organically bound heavy metal looks more as if it is supposed to be in the body than a heavy metal that is not organically bound. Little research can be found regarding the toxicity of thiomersal, and for clear and obvious reasons. If thiomersal, used as a preservative by pharmaceutical companies, is found to be toxic by medical researchers, numerous class action law suits will undoubtably be filed. Pharmaceutical companies fund much of the medical research. If a pharmaceutical company funds research to explore the toxicity of Mercury, and discovers that their own products can cause harm, they will be submitting direct evidence to the plaintiff's attorney to be used against them in a class action lawsuit. Biochemistry, however, does not lie. The mechanism of toxicity of Mercury in the body is clear. Thiomersal is not yet another divinely created form of Mercury that is magically nontoxic.

Mercury toxicity has become a highly publicized and political issue. We can either choose to believe independent biochemists who have clearly demonstrated the mechanism of toxicity of Mercury, or choose to believe what lobby-influenced government organizations and the manufacturers of the Mercury-based products in question are telling us. Biochemistry clearly shows the mechanism of toxicity of Mercury. The lack of credible research on the subject of Mercury tells us that no one involved in medical research wants to undertake the task, and for obvious reasons. Any effort to prove that Mercury is nontoxic will ultimately draw the opposite conclusion. Biochemistry simply does not lie, the mechanism of toxicity is clear, and nothing more needs to be said regarding its toxicity.

Mercury may be removed from the body by chelation therapy. The chelation process involves the use of chelating agents designed to remove specific classes of toxins from the body. The type of toxin present in the body determines the specific chelation agent used. Chelation agents can be administered orally or intravenously, depending on the type of chelation agent used. The best chelating agents for Mercury are (Dimercaptosuccinic acid (DMSA), 2,3–Dimercapto–1–propanesulfonic acid (DMPS), and alpha lipoic acid (ALA). Chelation therapy can potentially deplete the body of certain trace minerals; therefore, supplementing the diet with trace minerals during the chelation therapy may be necessary. It is suggested that chelation therapy be supervised by a qualified natural health practitioner or holistic medical doctor. Chelation agents can be purchased at better health food and independent vitamin stores.

Stachybotrys chartarum (Black Mold)

Black mold, or *Stachybotrys chartarum*, is a greenish–black mold. It can grow on material with a high cellulose and low nitrogen content, such as fiberboard, gypsum board, paper, dust, and lint. Mold growth occurs in areas of high moisture, and is most typically seen in areas of water damage, excessive humidity, water leaks, condensation, water infiltration, or flooding. Constant moisture is required to support growth of *Stachybotrys chartarum*. Mold spores travel through the air, and may enter the home through open doorways and windows. Mold is often hidden from plain view, growing under bathroom vanities, in crawl spaces, behind walls, and in heating and air–conditioning duct work. Any damp area found in the home is a potential breeding ground for mold.

Stachybotrys chartarum can produce extremely potent trichothecene poisons. All molds produce other secondary metabolites such as antibiotics and mycotoxins. Many people are familiar with penicillin, an antibiotic produced by the mold *Penicillium notatum*, discovered in the early twentieth century. Mycotoxins are also products of the secondary metabolism of molds, and are not so friendly. Mycotoxins are nearly all cytotoxic, meaning that they disrupt biochemistry and other biological processes at the cellular level. Mycotoxins can disrupt cellular structures such as the cell membrane, and interfere with protein synthesis, and interfere with DNA transcription. Mold spores, which often contain high concentrations of mycotoxins, can be inhaled directly into the respiratory tract, causing severe irritation.

Exposure to *Stachybotrys chartarum* can irritate mucous membranes, causing allergic rhinitis and a host of other respiratory problems. Central nervous system effects may include headaches, dizziness, a decreased attention span, or difficulty in concentration. Since the mold contains mycotoxins, which can enter the bloodstream, every cell in the body is potentially affected.

Anyone who lives in an environment in which *Stachybotrys chartarum* is present, or any mold for that matter, must take steps to remove the mold. Once the mold is removed, preventing the reestablishment of the mold is very important. It is suggested that an expert in mold removal be consulted, rather than attempting the removal yourself. Remember, when buying a home, if visual evidence of mold exists, it is a dead giveaway that more mold is also lurking in unseen places, such as in air conditioning ducts, within walls and under carpets. Do not use the presence of mold as a negotiation point with the seller. Your health is not something to negotiate. Homes built on crawlspaces are particularly vulnerable to mold growth, since ventilation is often poor and, in some areas, dampness prevails. If a damp crawlspace that breeds mold is found, a foundation contractor can lay a membrane barrier over the dirt, and pump several inches of concrete over it, eliminating the dampness.

Water Contamination

The causes of water contamination are ever expanding and range from industrial and agricultural runoff to improper use and disposal of household chemicals and everything between. The poor management of industrial waste and chemicals has become extreme, as evidenced by traces of contaminants found in nearly every public water supply. Contaminants from agricultural run off into rivers and streams are particularly a problem because these contaminants disrupt the delicate ecosystem of rivers, lakes and streams before they eventually make their way into the public water supply. Industrial and agricultural sources are not the only contributors to water contamination. The use of consumer pesticides, herbicides, fertilizers, and household chemicals are also largely to blame. Everything disposed of, whether in the trash or down the drain, has potential to contaminate the water supply.

The public water supply is a source of many types of environmental contaminates. These contaminants vary greatly, depending on the area of the world, properly working sewage systems, the presence of certain industries, and many other factors. Some contaminants, such as Arsenic, occur naturally in water in certain areas, whereas in other areas the water is Arsenic free. Many contaminants found in water, however, are from industrial sources. Water contaminants fall into three categories, inorganic toxins, organic toxins and biological contaminants. Biological contaminants are living organisms that can cause disease by being ingested and causing harm, or secreting toxins that harm the body.

Inorganic toxins include the heavy metals Arsenic, Lead, Mercury, and Cadmium. Heavy metals bind to thiol or sulfhydryl groups found in proteins, thus causing damage to the protein. If the protein happens to be an enzyme, the enzyme is then rendered useless by the heavy metal. An enzyme damaged to the extent that it has been rendered useless is called a *denatured enzyme*. Heavy metals, by denaturing an enzyme, are therefore, as a group, classified as nonspecific enzyme inhibitors. Heavy metal toxins can potentially affect every cell in the body. Symptoms associated with heavy metal toxins are not readily apparent until the person is exposed to a particular level, which varies somewhat from person to person. Despite whether symptoms are apparent, damage to the body from these toxins occurs nevertheless.

Other inorganic toxins include nitrates and nitrites. Nitrates are converted to nitrites by nitrogen reducing bacteria in the intestinal tract. Nitrites are particularly a serious problem for infants under the age of six months. Nitrites, upon entering the blood stream, will bind to the hemoglobin found in erythrocytes (red blood cells). Oxygen cannot be carried by hemoglobin bound with nitrite, resulting in Blue Baby Syndrome. Lack of oxygen can cause shortness of breath, brain damage, asphyxiation, and possibly death to the infant. Adults can tolerate higher levels of nitrites than infants, but this does not imply that nitrites are safe for adults to consume. Nitrates can react with amines or amides in the body, forming nitrosamine, a chemical known to cause cancer. Well water should be tested periodically for the presence of nitrates and nitrites.

Organic toxins have their source primarily from industry, agriculture, and the home. Examples of organic toxins include benzene, chloroform, polybrominated biphenyls (PBBs), polycyclic aromatic hydrocarbons (PAHs), and vinyl chloride. Pesticides and herbicides also fall into the category of organic toxins. Trihalomethane, a by-product of the chlorination process, is also an organic toxin and is found in most public water systems, and has been implicated in cancer. While organic toxins are typically found in trace amounts, it only takes a small amount of these toxins to inflict damage to the body. In addition, many organic toxins accumulate in the body's tissues, and cannot be easily broken down or eliminated. Dichloro-Diphenyl-Trichloroethane, commonly known as DDT, is one example of an organic toxin that can accumulate in the tissues. The half-life of DDT in the environment is approximately 15 years. This means that if one pound of DDT was sprayed on a particular property, 15 years later one-half pound would remain. Thirty years later, one-quarter pound of DDT would still exist in the environment, clearly demonstrating the scope of the problem.

Biological contaminants commonly found in the water include coliform bacteria, the *Giardia lamblia* organism or its cysts, Cryptosporidium, several types of protozoa, and various types of anaerobic and aerobic bacteria. The severity of any illness resulting from exposure to biological contaminants largely depends on the health of an individual's immune system and the type of biological contaminant. In the person with a healthy and balanced immune system, exposure to most biological contaminants would result in mild to moderate discomfort for a short period. In the immunosuppressed individual, exposure to a biological pathogen may result in hospitalization or death.

A newly emerging biological contaminant of water, cyanobacteria, also known as blue-green algae, is found in just about every type of water environment and have made its way into water distribution plants. While cyanobacteria have been always present in the environment, the increase in its appearance can largely be attributed to the contamination of water with other nutrients, such as nitrates and phosphates. The increased variation in global atmospheric temperature in recent years may also play a role. Anomalies in surface sea temperatures have also been noted in recent years, undoubtably a contributing factor in the recent rise in cyanobacteria. Cyanobacteria release toxins, and are broadly termed cyanotoxins. Cyanotoxins are cytotoxins, which can cause damage to any cell or tissue found in the body. Not only are cyanotoxins toxic to humans, but are also toxic to both fish and other wildlife as well. Cyanotoxins can accumulate in fish and other organisms, which eventually make its way to the dinner table.

The rate of cancer has increased to the point that one in three persons can expect to get cancer sometime in their lifetime. The increase in cancer is, in part due, to the presence of trihalomethanes, which is a carcinogen created when chlorine reacts with organic matter found in the water. Trihalomethanes are also known as chloroform, bromoform and dichlorobromomethane. Ingesting known carcinogens cannot possibly be compatible with good health. Wild animals, for the most part, do not get cancer. Wild animals also do not drink chlorinated water from the public water supply. They get their water from streams, ponds and lakes. Household pets, particularly dogs, have been shown to get cancer at a rate that closely tracts that of humans, clearly linking cancer to something in or around the modern home. Even the casual observer can see the link between chlorinated water and cancer.

A drastic increase in degenerative diseases has been observed during the twentieth century, and has no signs of stopping. The presence of fluoride, heavy metals, and organic toxins in water are all contributors to the modern day chronic disease plague. The indications are that the water supply worldwide is becoming more contaminated, making the situation even worse. In China, for example, pure, fresh water is becoming a very scarce commodity. The decreased availability of fresh water worldwide will undoubtably contribute to future diseases, yet unknown, to society.

The problem of contaminated water, however, is not entirely caused by the presence of industrial toxins in the water supply. Federal and local regulatory agencies involved in delivering drinking water to the population through the public water supply constitute a significant part of the problem. This is perhaps best exemplified by the 2007 drought in the Southeastern United States affecting Lake Sidney Lanier, a lake maintained by the U.S. Army Corps of Engineers. Lake Lanier supplies drinking water to a significant part of North Georgia. The political fight between the states of Georgia, Alabama, and Florida with the Corps of Engineers has endangered the public water supply at the expense of preserving two species of mussels, the Fat Threeridge Mussel (*Amblema neislerii*) and the Purple Bankclimber Mussel (*Elliptoideusslo ltianus*) and a fish, the Gulf Sturgeon (*Acipenser oxyrinchusdesotoi*), which reside in a Florida river. This argument between Georgia, Alabama, Florida, and the Federal Government has persisted for decades. As the level of Lake Lanier drops due to federally mandated water releases to protect the various endangered species, any contaminants in the lake become more concentrated. Contaminants present on the surface of the water are physically closer to the supply pipes of the water pumping equipment. Both the increased concentration of contaminants and the closer proximity of surface contaminants to the numerous supply pipes poses a serious threat to the public water supply. As the lake drops to record levels, the political bout continues, the water supply is in even greater danger, and the unsurpassed stupidity of the governing officials responsible for decision making cannot be more evident. In yet another case involving gross governmental incompetence, the problem can easily be solved by constructing a facility to house and propagate the endangered species. When the drought is over, the species can then be restored to their natural habitat. It appears, however, that the government is more interested in fabricating a crisis than in the well-being of its citizens.

Why Am I Sick? And What To Do About It

Persons who live in areas with an endangered water supply should make contingency plans to protect their health. Any plans made should take into consideration the potential of both natural disasters and man-made disasters. Appropriate measures may include drilling a private well, storing an adequate supply of drinking water, installing appropriate water filtering systems, or moving away from the affected area altogether.

For anyone who is connected to the public water supply, toxins can be eliminated by installing a whole house water filter. Unfiltered water from a public water supply is not compatible with good health. For any home connected to a private well, a filtering system is generally mandatory. The type of filtering system installed is dependent on the toxins present in the water. Often, multi stage filters are required to address the wide variety of toxins present. A typical installation may include a carbon-based filter followed by a submicron membrane filter. For well water, a sediment pre-filter is usually added to the array of filters to filter out large particles. Installation of a water filtering system will cause a decrease in water pressure to some degree. If this is a concern, two identical filtering systems can be installed in parallel, thus restoring the water pressure to a more acceptable level. The other advantage of the parallel installation of filter cartridges is that the filters do not have to be changed as often.

The ideal water filter system would be a three-stage filter followed by an ultraviolet sterilization unit. In this configuration, the first stage would be a sediment filter to eliminate any large particles found in the water supply. The second stage would consist of an activated carbon filter to eliminate any organic chemicals, including chlorine, which may be present. The third stage would consist of a thin film composite membrane, also known as a reverse osmosis filter. An option to this configuration would also include a second activated carbon filter to trap any chemicals missed by the first filter. If the second activated carbon filter is used, it should be installed before the reverse osmosis filter. Some organic chemicals can damage the reverse osmosis membrane, therefore, in any filtering system, the reverse osmosis filter should be the final filtering step. If an ultraviolet sterilization unit is used, it should always be the last step in the filter apparatus.

Quality water testing equipment and test strips can be purchased from the Hach Company. Test strips are available to evaluate the levels of Arsenic, chlorine, ammonia, Iron, Copper, nitrates, nitrites, phosphates, and many other contaminants found in water. These test strips are easy to use, and are inexpensive. The address and website of the Hach Company may be found in Appendix I. Water test kits are also available for the consumer market, which are designed to test tap water. Many of these kits contain test strips from the Hach company.

Bisphenol-A

Bisphenol-A was first synthesized in the nineteenth century, and was considered in the 1930s for possible use as a synthetic form of estrogen. Bisphenol-A is used by modern polymer chemists in the synthesis of polycarbonate plastics, epoxy resins, and polyvinyl chloride (PVC). Polycarbonates are used in many consumer products such as water bottles, food containers and plastic sunglass lenses, to name a few. Bisphenol-A is a dangerous environmental toxin.

Bisphenol-A is known to be a xenoestrogen. A xenoestrogen is either a natural or synthetic substance that has the same biological effect as estrogen in the human body. In other words, a xenoestrogen is an estrogen mimicking compound. Specifically, bisphenol-A is an estrogen receptor agonist, which means it can activate estrogen receptors in the body, causing physiological effects similar to estrogen. For that reason, bisphenol-A is classified as an endocrine system disruptor. The effects of endocrine system disruptors cannot be confined to just one part of the endocrine system. Endocrine system disruptors affect the entire endocrine system and subsequently the whole body.

Xenoestrogens have been known to decrease sperm counts and testosterone levels in males, and are implicated in breast cancer in females. Long term exposure will eventually cause other endocrine system problems, as with all endocrine system disruptors.

Some polymers used in composite dental fillings and sealants also contain bisphenol-A. This hardly gives us, as a society, any good choices, neurotoxic Mercury amalgam or endocrine disrupting bisphenol-A. Glass ionomers, which is a mixture of glass powder and acrylic, is possibly a better alternative, and is best suited for non-chewing surfaces of the teeth. Glass ionomers, however, can release small amounts of fluoride. For chewing surfaces of teeth, either porcelain inlays or crowns are a much better alternative than a known endocrine system disruptor.

Not surprisingly, the same controversy that surrounds the use of Mercury in dentistry also surrounds the use of bisphenol-A. Any biochemist can clearly demonstrate that bisphenol-A is a xenoestrogen compound, and show its effect as an estrogen receptor agonist. Dentists and their professional trade organizations deny that the bisphenol-A present in dental filings and dental sealants causes any harm. Understanding the logic behind this position is difficult, since the bisphenol-A contained in dental fillings is the identical bisphenol-A examined in research. In claiming that the bisphenol-A found in composite filings and sealants acts differently than the bisphenol-A used elsewhere is again to believe that this special dental bisphenol-A has some miraculous properties imparted to it. Bisphenol-A, along with Mercury, appears to be granted some divine pardon of its toxicity when installed in a tooth. As with Mercury, admission that bisphenol-A is toxic will expose the dental profession to even more class action law suits.

The toxic effects of bisphenol-A exposure can be eliminated by not using products made from the compound. Avoidance of bisphenol-A is mandatory for anyone suffering an endocrine system problem. No level of exposure to an endocrine system disruptor is safe.

Power Lines

Power lines emit electromagnetic radiation. This characteristic, however, is not unique to power lines. Microwave ovens, television and radio transmitters, and cellular phone transmitters all emit electromagnetic radiation. The electromagnetic radiation associated with power lines is a broad-spectrum emission, meaning the radiation comprises many different frequencies of electromagnetic energy.

Electromagnetic radiation exposure clearly has effects in the human body. X-ray technicians employed in hospitals must wear a radiation sensitive badge to monitor their exposure to radiation. Likewise, when the medical professional takes an X-ray, precautions are taken to prevent unnecessary exposure to any region of the patient's body. This is accomplished through collimating the X-ray beam and using Lead shields to protect radiation sensitive areas of the body. Casual examination of a microwave oven reveals a radiation screen behind or embedded in the front glass panel. This is to prevent any radiation from escaping from the cooking area. If the radiation were not harmful, no precautions would be necessary to protect the user of the oven from radiation leaks. The Federal Communications Commission publishes radiation exposure limits based upon the recommendations of several national and international organizations. Standards have been published regarding radiation exposure, for example the IEEE C95.1 standard that defines radiation limits for most of the electromagnetic spectrum from 3 kHz to 300 GHz. Contributing organizations to these standards are the National Council on Radiation Protection and Measurements, the International Commission on Non-Ionizing Radiation Protection, and the United Kingdom's National Radiation Protection Board. If electromagnetic radiation were not harmful, no logical reason to impose limits of radiation exposure would be found.

Various organizations and studies attempt to dispel the dangers of electromagnetic radiation exposure. These studies are usually funded by organizations who have a financial or other interest in the outcome of the research. The groups of scientists involved in these studies undoubtably have extensive knowledge in radiation physics and molecular biology. Unfortunately, these scientists have less than adequate knowledge of meridians and the nervous system. While the standards regarding radiation exposure primarily address potential DNA mutation, this is only a part of the picture of the dangers of electromagnetic radiation. The effects of electromagnetic radiation on the nervous system and meridians are ignored by these studies.

We have learned from our study on meridians that whenever electrical current flows down a pathway, a resultant electromagnetic field results. If the meridian is placed into an electromagnetic field, the flow of energy through the meridian will be disrupted. Various cells, including neurons, are sensitive to electromagnetic fields. Introducing an external electromagnetic energy disrupts the energy flow in meridians and nerves in an unpredictable manner. This, in itself, should be sufficient reason to avoid living in the presence of strong electromagnetic radiation.

The best protection from the electromagnetic radiation emitted by power lines is simply not to purchase a home where these high voltage lines are installed. Health is never something to negotiate with the seller.

Antibacterial Soap

Antibacterial soap is marketed as a product intended to kill pathogenic bacteria on the skin. Certain types of bacteria found on the skin are beneficial, and some can be problematic. Antibacterial soap kills both the beneficial and problematic bacteria.

Normal, non-antibacterial soap is also quite effective in killing bacteria that may be present on the skin. Bacterial cell membranes are formed by congruently placed lipid chains, just like the cell membranes of a human cell. Washing with soap disrupts the cell membrane of the bacteria, therefore killing the bacteria. The outer layer of human skin is composed of dead epithelial cells, and is not easily disrupted by soap as the delicate membrane of the bacteria. Although both antibacterial and normal soap are efficient in killing bacteria, antibacterial soap contains chemicals that are potentially harmful to the body, and should therefore be avoided.

Many antibacterial soaps contain a chemical called triclosan. The formal chemical name of triclosan is 2,4,4'-Trichloro-2'-hydroxydiphenyl ether. Current research indicates that even a minute amount of triclosan causes disruption of the endocrine system. Triclosan, therefore, is classified as an endocrine system disruptor. Triclosan is also found in certain toothpastes, deodorants, mouthwashes, and in some cleaning products. By causing disruption to the endocrine system, serious health consequences can result. The specific targets of triclosan are the thyroid hormone receptor sites. The mechanism of action of triclosan is found in the ability of this chemical to bind with thyroid hormone receptor sites. The normally circulating thyroid hormones subsequently, as a result of triclosan binding these sites, cannot be properly utilized. The feedback mechanism to the Hypothalamus and Pituitary is subsequently disrupted. This creates a form of HPA (Hypothalamus Pituitary Axis) dysfunction, which can subsequently affect all other hormones as well. Thyroid hormone associated gene expression can also result from exposure to Triclosan. This characteristic is particularly a problem in younger children, causing abnormal development rates and patterns. Products that contain triclosan should therefore not be used.

Endocrine system disruptors are, in themselves, a special class of toxin. This is due to the characteristic that, by disrupting one segment of the endocrine system, the entire endocrine system will eventually be disrupted. The endocrine system is delicately balanced, and any disruption to this balance has extensive effects on every system of the body. The entire endocrine system is regulated by the Hypothalamus and Pituitary; disruption to any part of the endocrine system subsequently disrupts the Hypothalamus and Pituitary as well. In essence, if one endocrine system failure is found, another endocrine system failure is almost certain in the future. For example, Thyroid failure, specifically hypothyroidism, is often followed by adrenal exhaustion a short time later, usually on the order of several months.

As a side note, since any soap can disrupt cell membranes, it should not be used to wash out a child's mouth. The mucous membrane lining of the digestive system is much more sensitive than the outer epithelial layer of the skin. Another method is therefore advisable to correct the child's colorful vocabulary.

Aluminum

Aluminum is a risk factor in several neurodegenerative disorders. Alzheimer's disease is the one most commonly linked to Aluminum. Evidence for the Aluminum implication in Alzheimer's disease is supported by the presence of Aluminum in neurofibrillary tangles in brain tissue. Other dementia disorders appear to be linked to Aluminum as well. Aluminum is clearly a neurotoxic agent and its toxicity is clearly demonstrable in experimental animals. The relationship between Aluminum and organic brain disease is more than casual. Despite the fact that sufficient biochemical proof exists that Aluminum is a neurotoxic agent, the controversy surrounding Aluminum will seemingly never end.

Antiperspirants often contain Aluminum compounds. Aluminum chlorohydrate is one of the most common Aluminum-based compounds used in these products. The pores in the axillary region are very permeable. Systemic absorption of Aluminum can take place when placed on the skin in this area. While the absorption rate may not be great, the continuous presence of Aluminum in the axillary region over periods of years can cause significant absorption. Natural deodorants, manufactured without Aluminum-based chemicals, are safer alternatives. Natural deodorant products are typically available in better health food stores.

Aluminum present in cookware presents yet another potential source of Aluminum entering the body. Aluminum is readily absorbed by foods cooked in Aluminum cookware. This is particularly true for acidic foods. Any Aluminum cookware should be discarded. Cookware marketed as Aluminum, but is coated with non-stick surfaces, does not pose the same risks.

Certain brands of antacid tablets also contain Aluminum. Aluminum hydroxide is the form of Aluminum commonly found in these preparations. The digestive tract is much more permeable than the axillary region, permitting greater absorption of Aluminum through the intestinal tract. Antacids that contain any form of Aluminum should therefore be avoided. If an antacid is needed for some reason, a product using Calcium or Magnesium is a much better alternative since Calcium and Magnesium both have at least some nutritional value and are not toxic to the body.

Some brands of baking powder also contain Aluminum. Aluminum free baking powder is also available, and is the preferred product. When purchasing products from a bakery, making sure their products are made with baking powder free of Aluminum is advisable. It is interesting, now that the public is becoming more aware of the toxicity of the environment, that certain companies manufacturing these baking products are advertising on the label that they are aluminum free. If Aluminum was not toxic, the manufacturer would not bother to make an Aluminum-free alternative.

Arsenic

Everyone knows Arsenic is toxic, but since there is none laying around the house, everyone feels safe. Sources of Arsenic, however, are more common than one might think.

The mechanism of toxicity of Arsenic is very clear. Arsenic inhibits the enzyme *pyruvate dehydrogenase*, which is an auxiliary enzyme of the citric acid cycle, also known as the Krebs Cycle. By inhibiting *pyruvate dehydrogenase* the conversion of pyruvate to acetyl coenzyme A is decreased. This produces an overall decrease in the activity of specific pathways of the citric acid cycle. As a result, the production of adenosine triphosphate (ATP) is decreased. Adenosine triphosphate is important because it is the primary usable energy source found in all living cells. If energy decreases enough, cell death results. Enough cell death leads to body death.

Interestingly, the toxicity of Arsenic is downplayed by several regulatory and public health agencies. This position is in direct contradiction to the mechanism of toxicity of Arsenic found within the citric acid cycle. Believing any of the downplayed statements regarding the toxicity of Arsenic made by public health organizations would not be wise. These statements contradict the proof of toxicity clearly demonstrated by biochemistry.

For approximately twenty years, Arsenic was the most common preservative applied to wood. This process is called pressure treating, where the preservative is forced into the wood under pressure. The preservative is an aqueous solution of Copper, chromate and Arsenic. These chemicals, which are used in pressure treating wood, make the wood less susceptible to insect and fungal attacks. Pressure treated wood is used to build playground equipment, outdoor decks, and various other outdoor wooden structures. The Arsenic in pressure treated wood can be released from sawing or sanding the wood, by direct contact with the wood, or when the wood is burned. If the wood is wet, direct contact with the wood can cause the Arsenic to be absorbed into the body directly through the skin.

On January 1, 2004, a law went into effect in the United States banning the use of Arsenic in the pressure treatment of wood. If Arsenic were safe, this legislation would be unnecessary. Unless it is certain that the deck or structure in question was built with wood manufactured after that date, it is advisable never to walk on the pressure treated deck barefoot, especially when the wood is wet. Playground equipment manufactured with wood built before that date also poses a serious problem. If children routinely come into direct contact with wood, the equipment should be discarded. Sealing the wood with spar urethane is another option, however, the surface may become quite slippery when wet, increasing the potential for a child to slip and fall.

Well water is another source of Arsenic. In some regions of the world, ground water has a very high Arsenic content. This is particularly true in the Western United States. In other areas, ground water is relatively Arsenic free. Well water should be tested periodically for Arsenic content. If Arsenic is found to be present in the well water, an appropriate filter should be installed to remove it.

Arsenic can be removed from the body by a process called chelation. Meso 2,3-dimercaptosuccinic acid, also known as DMSA, is commonly used as the chelation agent. DMSA binds to a heavy metal, such as Arsenic, Lead and Mercury. This sequesters, or binds to, the metal, and allows it to be carried away and eventually excreted. 2,3-Dimercapto-1-propanesulfonic acid (DMPS) is also a commonly used chelation agent for Arsenic. Chelation therapy can potentially deplete the body of certain trace minerals, therefore, supplementing the diet with trace minerals during the chelation therapy may be necessary. Chelation therapy should be supervised by a holistic health provider who will monitor for the potential depletion of trace minerals.

Aspartame and Other Artificial Sweeteners

Artificial sweeteners are just that – artificial. It does not matter what they are called, who tested them, who claims they are safe, artificial sweeteners are still artificial, have no place in the body, and are not safe. The reasons why they are not safe vary from product to product. One issue, however, remains constant. With artificial sweeteners, a chemical is being ingested into the body that has no business being there. That, in itself, should be convincing enough.

For an artificial sweetener to mimic the taste of sugar, it must first be soluble in water. In addition, the molecule must be able to bind to a specific receptor molecule that is located on the surface of the tongue. This receptor, known as a G-protein coupled receptor, triggers a sequence of events resulting in nerve signals carried to the brain. The presence of these signals is interpreted as sweetness by the brain. G-protein coupled receptors, however, are not limited to the tongue. These receptors are also found in the intestinal tract, and also present signals to the brain. These nerves do not go to the brain for no reason at all. The nerve signals from the intestinal G-protein coupled receptors instruct the brain that a certain type of food is in the intestinal tract. Specifically, the presence of these signals originating from the intestinal tract is telling the brain that sugar has been consumed, and will be absorbed shortly. Expecting a rise in blood sugar levels, the biochemistry of the body reacts accordingly. When an artificial sweetener is consumed, the brain receives false signals, but the cascade of neurological and biochemical events occurs nevertheless. In faking out the body's neurological and biochemical mechanisms, the body has been prepared itself to receive nutrients, specifically carbohydrates, but the nutrients never show up in the bloodstream.

No evidence can be found indicating that sugar substitutes help people lose weight. In reality, the opposite is true. Hunger is triggered by the hypothalamus, a gland in the brain. When a person gets hungry, the hypothalamus is what initiates the hunger, causing the person to eat. If the person eats food containing an artificial sweetener, the body's hunger mechanism is not satisfied. As a result, the appetite is continuously stimulated until the nutritional demands of the body are finally satisfied. If other calories are found in the product containing the artificial sweetener, these additional calories are most likely contributing to the body's fat reserves. Sugar free cakes and cookies are a perfect example. Sugar-free products often have a very high fat content. Sugar free does not necessarily mean calorie free.

Aspartame is one artificial sweetener. Two isolated amino acids, aspartic acid and phenylalanine, are bonded, or fused, by a third chemical, methanol. Aspartame is metabolized in the body back into its three components, aspartic acid, phenylalanine, and methanol. Methanol is toxic to the body. Methanol is broken down in the liver, forming formic acid and formaldehyde. Methanol is known to cause retinal damage in the eye, and interfere with DNA replication, and is a known carcinogen. Proponents of aspartame admit methanol is release during the chemical breakdown, but state the amount is very little, therefore acceptable. This is quite an odd viewpoint since methanol should not be found in the body at all. This is analogous to claiming a small amount of cyanide is not dangerous.

The body also must deal with the excess phenylalanine and aspartic acid. Excess amounts of these amino acids must be broken down in the liver. With an understanding of proper nutrition, no one would ever consider continuously flooding their body with the same amino acid supplement several times a day. Using amino acids in that way would entail purchasing free-form phenylalanine amino acid capsules, and taking a few every time some food is consumed. Taking an amino acid supplement in this manner is ridiculous, and frankly stupid. If this person entered a doctor's office with some chronic disease, the first thing the doctor would do is suggest the patient stop taking such a supplement, especially in such an excessive amount. Routinely using aspartame as a sweetener is no different. However, aspartame metabolism is not understood by the typical medical doctor, so no advice is ever offered regarding the cessation of products that contain it.

A particular problem arises with aspartame because the transport of phenylalanine into the brain is mediated by a carrier mechanism shared with other amino acids in the same class. Among these other amino acids are tyrosine and tryptophan. Tyrosine is the precursor amino acid to both the neurotransmitters dopamine and norepinephrine. Tryptophan is the precursor to the neurotransmitter serotonin. Limiting the transport of tyrosine and tryptophan into the brain limits the conversion to the aforementioned neurotransmitters. This results in the associated enzymes that perform the conversion to become relatively unsaturated. When tyrosine and tryptophan are again able to be transported by the carrier mechanism, the cascade of biochemical reactions involved in neurotransmitter synthesis will occur quite rapidly by the unsaturated enzymes and hung biochemical reactions. This can cause mood swings, seizures, hyperactivity, emotional instability, depression, and a host of other neurological and psychological issues.

Sucralose, a relatively new artificial sweetener, is somehow always being advertised as "natural" or "safe." One would have to ask why this is so. Perhaps it could be because no other previous artificial sweetener has come on the market without a controversy. What has in effect happened is that the industry has learned to combat any negative publicity before it begins. By advertising the product as safe, the manufacturer gets a head start on any controversy. By advertising the product as natural, it sounds like an acceptable product. Sucralose, incidently, is not a natural product. If sucralose were natural, it would be found in nature, which it is not. Sucralose is prepared in the laboratory from sucrose, by a chemical reaction that substitutes three chloride groups for three hydroxyl groups. This cannot be construed as natural. Sucralose, being advertised as a safe sugar substitute, carries the implication that other sugar substitutes are unsafe. It is interesting how the manufacturer of one product can often inadvertently tell the truth regarding the safety of a competitor's product.

The IUPAC chemical name for the chemical sucralose is 1,6-dichloro-1,6-dideoxy-ßß-D-fructofuranosyl-4-chloro-4-deoxy-ßß-D-galactopyranoside. Sucralose contains chlorine, as the formula clearly indicates, evidenced by the terms *dichloro* and *chloro*. Sucralose can be absorbed into the body; therefore, the associated chlorine has the potential to be absorbed into the body. The Material Safety Data Sheet for sucralose states that "Hazardous Decomposition" of sucralose can occur, decomposing into "carbon dioxide, carbon monoxide, and minor amounts of hydrogen chloride." Hydrogen chloride is the proper chemical name of hydrochloric acid. Chlorine is toxic to the body, and is known to cause cancer. When found to cause cancer, chlorine is always found to be bonded to an organic compound. Information can be found stating the chlorine found in sucralose is in the form of chloride, and is therefore safe. A chloride ion is defined as a covalently bonded chlorine atom bound to an inorganic or organic molecule. This does not imply safety. Chlordane, an insecticide, also contains chlorine atoms bonded in the same way. Organochlorides, as a general rule, are not considered safe. The chemical sucralose, being synthetically chlorinated and unnatural in every respect, has no business whatever being in the body. This fact alone should be sufficient to end of the discussion regarding the safety of sucralose.

Saccharin is the artificial sweetener with which the controversy will seemingly never end. In the 1960s, Saccharin was proven to cause cancer by many research groups. In 1977, the Food and Drug Administration proposed a ban on Saccharin, but since Saccharin was the only artificial sweetener in that era, the ban was met with great public opposition by many groups, including diabetics. The U.S. Congress placed a moratorium on the ban, but required the product to display a warning label saying that the use of Saccharin may be carcinogenic. While all the controversy was transpiring, research has indicated that Saccharin was not carcinogenic after all. As a result, in 1991, the Food and Drug Administration withdrew its proposed ban on Saccharin. In 2000, the U.S. Congress repealed the law requiring Saccharin products to carry a health warning label. Saccharin, however, is another synthetic chemical intended to fool the body into thinking it is consuming something that it has not.

The research efforts into the carcinogenic properties of Saccharin were, however, not a wasted effort. One very valuable and important lesson has been learned from this research, which is not readily obvious, cannot be overlooked. Examination of the extensive research surrounding Saccharin has clearly proven that Albert Einstein was correct in his assessment of research as evidenced by his statement "If we knew what it was we were doing, it would not be called research, would it?" So, in 1965, Saccharin caused cancer, and, in 2000, Saccharin did not cause cancer. Interestingly, the chemical formula of Saccharin did not change at all between 1965 and 2000. This same methodology of research and the associated protocols are used today to determine the safety of newly proposed artificial sweeteners. The lesson learned is research into the safety of chemicals ingested into the body, no matter how carefully conducted, cannot be trusted. This is becoming more obvious, as evidenced by the large number of drugs allowed on the market that are later proven to have serious detrimental side effects.

Stevia is another sweetener, and is rapidly becoming popular. Stevia, unlike artificial sweeteners, has a natural source. This source is plants in the steraceae (sunflower) family. Extracts from the plant are reported to be 300 times the sweetness of sugar. Stevia, as with the other artificial sweeteners, has been the target of many controversies. Since Stevia occurs naturally, it does not require any patent or license to produce it. This causes a political controversy in addition to the standard controversies surrounding health issues. Nevertheless, the continuous use of any highly refined extract in concentrations far beyond what is found in nature is unadvisable.

To this date, natural forms of carbohydrates, whether fruit, vegetable, starch, or grain, have yet to be proven to cause cancer.

DEET

DEET, chemically known as N,N-diethyl-m-toluamide, is a commonly used insect repellent. It is typically applied to the skin or clothing. DEET is also used as an insect repellent to protect pets. DEET is classified as a pesticide.

DEET can enter the body through several ways. These include absorption directly through the skin, inhalation, and accidental ingestion. As an insecticide that is applied to the skin, transdermal absorption, that is, absorption through the skin, is the greatest concern. A major concern of DEET is it has been reported to accelerate the dermal penetration of other pesticides.

DEET's primary toxic effect is in the central nervous system. Central nervous system effects due to acute exposure of DEET are confusion, jerking of muscles, muscular hypertonicity (tight muscles), and various gastrointestinal effects. More serious effects include seizures and coma. The mechanism of action of DEET is unknown, which should raise several concerns. When the mechanism of a chemical is unknown, it means literally no known reason how and why the chemical is toxic. DEET and its metabolites can remain in the skin for several weeks following application. Repeated application of products containing DEET over a period of days causes an increase the accumulation of DEET in the skin. This subsequently increases the probability of an acute toxic reaction.

Many natural alternatives to DEET are available. Many essential oils have insect repelling properties. In fact, the essential oils found in plant's are part of the plant's immune system. The purpose of the plant's immune system is to keep the plant from being consumed by insects and other pests. Commercially available products labeled "DEET Free," or marketed as natural insect repellents are made from these natural essential oils. These products, which do not carry the same risks as DEET, are better alternatives.

Smoking

Not too many better ways can be found to introduce such a wide variety of toxins into the body than smoking. Cigarette smoke is reported to contain more than 4,000 chemical compounds, many of which are known carcinogens. It is doubtful that even one of these chemicals is of any benefit to the body. Inhaling toxic chemicals, which subsequently must be eliminated from the body, is not conducive to good health. The dangers of smoking have been well documented. The smoker who desires good health should therefore quit.

Some toxins familiar to many people contained in cigarette smoke are carbon monoxide, nicotine, benzene, benzopyrene, nitrogen oxides, hydrogen cyanide, formaldehyde, urethane, acetaldehyde, ammonia, vinyl chloride, quinoline, and hydrazine. Hydrazine, incidently is a component of rocket fuel. Toxic heavy metals contained in cigarette smoke include Arsenic and Cadmium. Nickel is also a component of cigarette smoke, and is capable of evoking various types of immune hypersensitivity reactions. Nicotine, the addictive chemical in tobacco, is technically part of the immune system of the tobacco plant. Insects consuming the leaves of the tobacco plant die. This places nicotine in the category of an insecticide.

As a result of the wide variety of toxins entering the body through smoking, the body is in a constant state of chemical toxicity. These toxins are chemical irritants to the various tissues of the body. The long term presence of chemical irritants will most likely place the smoker in the exhaustion phase of the General Adaption Syndrome described by Hans Selye. The exhaustion phase of this syndrome is not conducive to health. The patient in the exhaustion phase of the General Adaption Syndrome will ultimately develop any number of chronic diseases.

People often smoke to keep their weight down. While this approach may appear to work for a person in their early twenties, continuing to smoke invariably will lead to the advanced stages of the General Adaption Syndrome. In these advanced stages, elevated cortisol levels will always be found in the body. Elevated cortisol levels have been shown to be associated with excess abdominal fat. The young person who continues to smoke to keep a trim figure will eventually find large accumulation of abdominal fat that predictably shows up their thirties or forties. Fat deposits of this type are next to impossible to lose when cortisol levels are high. Losing abdominal fat, therefore, requires that a person not be in the advanced stages of the General Adaption Syndrome, which, subsequently, requires the person to stop smoking.

Perfumes and Cosmetics

The cosmetic industry appears to be unregulated in the sense that any chemicals used in the manufacture of the associated products are proprietary and therefore undisclosed on any packaging. Any attempt to discover the ingredients in any particular cosmetic is a futile effort. Any successful independent analysis of the ingredients of cosmetics will require expensive equipment and a team of organic chemists. By not being required to disclose the ingredients appears to be treated as free license to include potentially toxic chemicals.

Certain people have sensitivities to perfumes and other body scents. Nearly everyone, at one time or another, has suffered a headache following exposure to some perfume or body scent. This sensitivity is often as a result of inhaling the chemicals found in these products. Two primary ways exist by which these chemicals can enter the body. The first method of entry is absorption directly through the skin. The technical term for this is *transdermal*, and is the same method by which certain medications, such as birth control and pain medications, are administered. The second method by which absorption of chemicals can occur is through the lungs. The lungs exchange carbon dioxide and oxygen with the environment. Other chemicals can inadvertently be absorbed through the lungs as well, many of which are toxic to the body.

It is amazing how many people who complain of fibromyalgia, chronic fatigue, autoimmune diseases, migraine headaches and other chronic ailments continue to use these products. Worse yet is the practice of using the same scent or product repeatedly. Repeated exposure to nearly any chemical product can induce hypersensitivity or, in some cases, an allergy. When the immune system gets involved, one can be certain that the problem of an allergy is not going to go away spontaneously.

The inclusion of toxic chemicals in cosmetics can most readily be demonstrated by the October 2007 discovery of Lead in various brands of lipstick. The fact that Lead can make its way into the final product by intent is sufficient evidence that the entire cosmetic industry is not to be trusted. Furthermore, believing that the manufacturer was unaware that Lead was present in the products is naive. Another alarm sounded in December 2007, when mascara, eyeliner and skin creams preserved with Mercury were banned for sale by the state of Minnesota, in the United States. Thiomersal, the Mercury compound used in these cosmetics, is also found in the solutions used to disinfect and sterilize contact lenses. If these well known toxic chemicals are intentionally included into various products, the question arises as to what other undisclosed toxic chemicals are included in other products.

The best advice regarding the use of these products for persons with chronic ailments is simply to stop using synthetic body scents altogether. If a scent must be used, essential oils are a better alternative. Essential oils also have been long known to have therapeutic benefits associated with them. Lavender, for example, is known to help induce relaxation and help with muscle spasms. Lemon grass essential oil is reported to have uplifting properties. Essential oils can be found at bath shops, on the internet, and through massage therapy supply stores. When purchasing essential oils, it is best to select products that are purified, and not mixed with other oils.

Insecticides and Herbicides

Insecticides kill insects; herbicides kill plants. Some of these products are selective in nature, which means they act on a specific organism or class of organisms. Others are broad-spectrum, meaning they kill just about everything. These chemicals are, by definition, toxic. They are intended to kill. Reading the label of the product should be convincing enough. Pesticides and herbicides are also toxic to humans, birds and other wildlife. These toxic chemicals can be inhaled or absorbed through the skin. The chemicals eventually make their way into ground water, lakes, streams, and in many cases, the public water supply. Little controversy exists regarding the dangers and toxicity of pesticides and herbicides. The mechanisms of toxicity of any of these products are well documented, and surprisingly, not denied. The manufacturers of these chemicals must be applauded for their honesty regarding disclosure of the toxic effects of the chemicals contained in the products.

The use of pesticides and herbicides should obviously be kept to an absolute minimum. Walking barefoot on areas where pesticides and herbicides have been applied almost guarantees absorption to some degree through the skin. Using these products near a well should be always avoided. The chemicals can make their way into the well through ground water and runoff from rain, eventually making their way into drinking water.

Rather than itemize each herbicide or pesticide and reiterate what each product label already admits, it might be more beneficial to demonstrate how nature provides a much safer and natural alternative.

Perhaps the best insecticide ever discovered is d-limonene, a chemical found in the skin of all citrus fruit. The mechanism of action of d-limonene is to disrupt the protective lipid coating of the exoskeletons of insects. This disruption causes them to die. The presence of d-limonene in the skin of citrus fruit provides an impervious barrier to attack by insects. Additionally, physical contact with d-limonene is essentially nontoxic to humans as compared to commercially available pesticides. Products containing d-limonene are commercially available for use as insecticides.

Subterranean termites have posed a particular problem for homes constructed with wood for years. Chlordane, a highly toxic insecticide, was the standard termiticide used for many years to control subterranean termites. The use of

Chlordane was discontinued in the United States in 1988, but is still manufactured for export. Chlordane is one of the most toxic insecticides ever developed. Termites, however, having a very fragile exoskeleton, are the perfect targets for any chemical that has a mechanism of action of exoskeleton disruption. The citrus extract d-limonene kills termites on contact. It is interesting how nature often provides a simple solution to even the most complicated problem.

A door to door water filter salesman came by the office and wanted to show the effectiveness of the products he was selling. Since it was lunchtime, I gave him his ten minutes. The water that came through the portable filter apparatus actually tasted good. He then began a dissertation of how effectively toxic chemicals are removed by this filter, and nothing toxic will pass through the filter into the water I would drink. I told him I would buy two of the filters right now if he drank the water that came out of the filter from the X-ray chemicals from the film processor in the darkroom. I explained to him that the chemicals were more than 95% water. He quickly reconsidered his position about how good his water filters were. He left without making the sale.

Chapter 15
Modern Medical Mistakes

Certain medical problems are typically not treated correctly by the medical profession. In some cases, the treatment offered actually makes the condition worse. This is the case when the treatment is focused on eliminating symptoms associated with the problem rather than correcting the actual cause of the disease. When this happens, the disease process continues unabated, and the patient is given a false sense of security because the pain is gone or the symptoms have subsided.

When the patient enters the medical facility, they are primarily concerned with a symptom that has arisen, and that something may be wrong. The doctor, on the other hand, has a waiting room full of people and often does not have time for a one hour dissertation of the cause and prevention of disease. Treatment, then, is focused on symptom reduction. So, if the patient is constipated, they get a 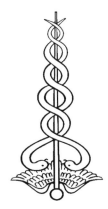 laxative, if the patient is congested, they get a decongestant, if the patient has green mucus, they get an antibiotic. If the patient cannot sleep, they get a sleeping pill, if they are depressed, they get an antidepressant, and so on. If blood work was performed, it is much the same story with a different twist. If T3 levels are low, they get a thyroid medication. If cholesterol levels are high, they get a cholesterol lowering medication. If they are anemic, they get a shot of B-12 or an iron pill. This type of medical care focused on symptomatic relief is dangerous, for it allows the underlying condition to progress to a more advanced stage while remaining undetected, systematically destroying the person's health. One would have to question whether it ever occurred to anyone why the symptom appeared to begin with, or why the blood test results were out of range.

Proper ways exist to treat certain disorders. Treating a disorder properly requires extensive time on the part of both the health practitioner and patient, and often extensive education and participation of the patient. In today's health care system, insurance will pay for the drug for palliative relief, but often will not pay for the proper care leading to resolution of the patient's condition. Proper treatment very often requires certain lifestyle changes, which contributed to the condition to begin with, on the part of the patient. As a result, many points of resistance to treatment develop. The health care practitioner does not have the time, the patient does not have a full understanding of the problem, insurance will not pay for the care, and the patient is unwilling to make certain changes. The patient dedicated to getting well will break through these barriers and ultimately obtain health and wellness.

Examples cited in this chapter are representative of disorders and issues that are often improperly addressed by modern medicine. The disorders discussed are by no means to be considered a complete list of disorders that fall into this category.

Acid Reflux Disease

Acid reflux disease, heartburn, or Gastroesophageal reflux disease (GERD) occurs when hydrochloric acid that is supposed to be contained within the stomach enters the esophagus. The hydrochloric acid enters the esophagus because the cardiac sphincter, also known as the gastroesophageal sphincter, remains open and allows the acid to flow back up instead of being contained within the stomach. The medical doctor would typically prescribe a drug to decrease or stop the production of stomach acid or an antacid to neutralize the stomach acid. By eliminating or neutralizing the stomach acid, the burning in the esophagus is stopped. Unfortunately, because the hydrochloric acid has been neutralized and rendered ineffective, the digestion of protein has been severely impaired.

The amino acids that result from the digestion of protein are needed in order to rebuild the esophageal, stomach, and intestinal linings. Hydrochloric acid is necessary for protein digestion, without it protein digestion cannot occur. If protein is not digested, no amino acids are present for assimilation into the bloodstream. Without amino acids, repairing the erosion is difficult, if not impossible, for the body. The result is, over time, the condition only gets worse.

The proper approach would be to rebuild the intestinal lining, and making dietary changes to prevent the acid reflux disease of recurring. Initially, supplementing the diet with free-form amino acids, which are predigested proteins, would give the body the building blocks necessary to rebuild the lining. Free-form amino acids are easily absorbed and do not require further digestion as do natural proteins found in food. The use of free-form amino acids during the regeneration of the digestive tract lining will allow the patient to still use an antacid to suppress the uncomfortable symptoms of the reflux disease for the short term. An appropriate free-form amino acid supplement will contain all of the essential amino acids. Once the esophageal lining is repaired, the use of digestive enzymes, as discussed in the chapter on nutrition, should prevent the problem from recurring. Free-form amino acids are available in most health food and vitamin stores.

Acid reflux disease was in progress months or years before the symptom of pain or burning was present. As the body ages, the production of hydrochloric acid diminishes. At the age of 65, the body produces only about 25 percent of the hydrochloric acid it did at the age of 18. Acid in the stomach is required to close the cardiac sphincter. If less that adequate amounts of acid in the stomach exist, the cardiac sphincter does not close properly, allowing acid to reflux into the esophagus. The long term solution to this problem is to supplement each meal with broad-spectrum digestive enzymes, which include hydrochloric acid in the form of Betaine HCl to increase the acidity of the stomach. These enzymes will close the sphincter preventing the reflux of acid, and aid in the efficient digestion of food. So, acid reflux disease results because of too little acid in the stomach, not too much acid as commonly believed.

While hydrochloric acid is necessary to digest protein, any acid, if in the proper concentration, will cause the cardiac sphincter to close. This is partly why ginger ale is often used as a remedy for an upset stomach. The ginger has a calming effect on the stomach, and the acid in the soft drink helps close the sphincter. To the generation who lived in the early twentieth century, soft drinks were touted as a cure-all for digestive tract disorders. With the arrival of modern technology, digestive enzymes, which include hydrochloric acid, produce superior results in closing the sphincter.

Sleep Disorders

Sleep disorders fall into many categories. One common complaint is the inability to fall asleep easily. Another complaint is ineffectual sleep, where the patient wakes up often during the night and does not feel rested. Most sleep disorders are as a result of a combination of neurotransmitter imbalances and stress. These two factors result in disrupted circadian rhythms. The question, then, is what is causing neurotransmitter imbalances and stress.

If a person were taken up into an airplane, strapped into a parachute, and jumps out, norepinephrine levels would most likely spike to enormously high levels. When the person lands, should they lay down an hour later and try to sleep, chances are that they will lay wide awake for several hours. The rise in certain neurotransmitters, such as norepinephrine, will keep the person awake for a time far longer than normal. A day later, norepinephrine levels will crash, and the person will most likely sleep longer that average. In this example, the body has been placed under stress, resulting in elevated neurotransmitter levels, subsequently disrupting the person's circadian rhythm. In a day or two, in the normal healthy person, the circadian rhythm will return to normal.

Circadian rhythms, also known as the sleep-wake cycle, are highly dependent on melatonin timing. Disruption of melatonin secretion is often evidenced by early morning awakenings in predisposed individuals. In order for melatonin timing to follow an appropriate pattern, an individual must wake up in the morning and go to sleep at night. While this sounds ridiculously simple, it is amazing how many people violate such a simple rule and expect to sleep well. Evidence also suggests that lack of exposure to sunlight will disrupt the circadian rhythms by affecting the timing of melatonin secretion. Daily naps, waking up using an alarm clock, attempting to relax using depressants, and attempting to remain awake by using stimulants are just a few additional ways to disrupt circadian rhythms. Ophthalmic factors, such as cataracts, partial blindness, and illumination factors, such as exposure to sunlight, also have an effect on melatonin timing. In many individuals, the lack of exposure to bright sunlight allows melatonin levels to remain high during the day, often resulting in the feeling of sleepiness or feeling lethargic. In these persons, melatonin timing has been disrupted, and the person feels sleepy during the day, and wide awake at night.

To sleep properly, the body must be relatively stress free. One cannot expect to sleep well if under constant stress. If acute stress is not handled properly, norepinephrine levels remain high, resulting in disrupted circadian rhythms. If the person is under chronic stress, the stressed condition of the body is worse than if under acute stress, also resulting long-term disruption of circadian rhythms. Cortisol, produced by the adrenal glands when the body is under stress, is known to be elevated in persons with chronic sleep disturbances. Elevated cortisol levels activate a liver enzyme called *tryptophan pyrrolase*, which breaks down the amino acid tryptophan, decreasing the amount available by the body to make both serotonin and melatonin. Lack of serotonin and melatonin propagates further disruption of the circadian rhythm. Unless chronic stress is eliminated, one cannot simply expect to attain normal sleep patterns. Acute stress must be handled properly to minimize disruption to the circadian rhythms. Anyone unable to sleep well has most likely has entered the latent phase of the General Adaption Syndrome as described by Hans Selye. The chapter on stress has an in-depth discussion of this syndrome and how it subsequently affects health.

Sleep disorders, then, is a symptom of another underlying disorder. Whatever the underlying disorder is, it affects neurotransmitter levels and most likely involves a significant degree of stress. When the medical doctor prescribes a sleeping pill, he or she is actually treating a symptom of another disorder. In most cases, this other disorder is chronic stress. When the underlying disorder is corrected, sleep patterns will ultimately return to normal, provided, of course, that nothing is done to disrupt the natural cycle intentionally. The body knows how much sleep it needs and when to sleep.

Antibiotics

Antibiotics are over prescribed by the medical profession today, and little argument can be found against that fact. Antibiotics are prescribed when any hint whatever of a bacterial infection is found, never mind the fact that the body has an immune system that, in most cases, is perfectly capable of handling the infection on its own. Antibiotics are also prescribed when a patient has the common cold, which is caused by a virus, not bacteria. This makes no sense at all, since the antibiotic does not act to eradicate a virus. Bacteria mutate rapidly, and antibiotic resistant strains survive and are spread across society. Following a course of antibiotics, any antibiotic resistant strains of bacteria have not been killed, and still pose a threat for an even more serious infection. New, more powerful antibiotics are developed to conquer these new super bugs, but the bacteria are always one step ahead. As a result of this endless antibiotic treatment of infections, the immune system does not develop in a normal manner, being less capable to fight off any similar future infection that may occur. A few cases, however, can be found where antibiotic treatment is indicated. When this is the case, a method is known of how to take the antibiotic to minimize the unintended effects of disrupting the normal bacterial flora of the intestinal tract. In addition, subsequent to antibiotic administration, a way fortunately exists to correct any of these unintended effects that remain in the wake of treatment.

Specifically, what are these unintended effects associated with antibiotic administration? A person who has absorbed antibiotics, whether by a prescription drug or through antibiotic laden food, is not quite the same kind of organism that he or she was initially. Significant alterations in the presence and balance of the bacterial flora have occurred, therefore altering to a great extent the biochemical processes that are occurring within that person. Because the balance of the microorganisms has been significantly altered, most of the beneficial effects these microorganisms have on health have been lost. Bacterial flora found in the intestinal tract significantly influences digestion and the immune system. The more one interferes with the delicate balance of symbiosis, the more one can expect disease to result. The value of these microorganisms and the role they play in health is only beginning to be understood.

Believing that an antibiotic can cure a bacterial infection is quite plausible, and in fact, little argument can be found against that belief. The problem is that, in curing one bacterial infection, another type of infection has arrived in its place. When an antibiotic is taken, it not only attacks the unwelcome foreign invader that caused the infection, but it also attacks the beneficial bacteria in the digestive tract. This is not surprising, after all, an antibiotic is designed to kill bacteria, both the good and bad. Interestingly, the immune system has a tendency to leave the beneficial bacteria in the intestines alone. This symbiotic relationship between the beneficial bacterial flora of the intestines and the human immune system cannot occur simply by accident. When the beneficial bacteria of the intestines die off as a result of the antibiotic, a yeast overgrowth then occurs. This yeast is called *Candida albicans* and *Candida krusei*. With the proliferation of yeast, the bacteria stand little, if any, chance of reestablishing themselves. This invariably results in a chronic yeast infection leading to chronic digestive problems, immune system imbalance, and a host of other disorders.

Antibiotic use and its direct correlation with intestinal yeast overgrowth and damaged balance to the intestinal bacterial flora balance are a serious problem found in today's society. Because a properly working digestive system is important in overall health, an entire chapter has been devoted to restoring the natural balance of the intestinal flora and correction of other digestive issues. One question, however, is if an antibiotic is really necessary, what can be done, if anything, to prevent a yeast overgrowth?

Taking an oral antibiotic will always destroy the great majority of the beneficial bacteria that reside in the intestinal tract. A *Candida albicans* and *Candida krusei* yeast infection will subsequently follow. Candida is a yeast that is undesirable in the digestive tract. Candida damages the intestinal lining, ferments sugar, and excretes toxins into the digestive tract. A beneficial type of yeast exists, however, that normally inhabits the intestinal tract. Since all intestinal microorganisms compete for space, if the beneficial yeast can be introduced into the intestine, it will, to a considerable degree, inhibit the growth of the highly undesirable *Candida albicans* and *Candida krusei*. This beneficial yeast is *Saccharomyces boulardii*. If taken concurrently with the antibiotic, *Saccharomyces boulardii* will proliferate throughout the intestines, thus taking up space left by the bacterial flora killed by the antibiotic. The presence of *Saccharomyces boulardii* will leave little space for an undesirable *Candida albicans* and *Candida krusei* infection to take hold. *Saccharomyces boulardii* is available in supplement form and can be found in better health food and vitamin stores and through the company Original Medicine®. The address and website of Original Medicine® can be found in Appendix I.

The development of a *Clostridium difficile* infection following antibiotic administration is one of the greatest dangers of antibiotic use. *Clostridium difficile* is a spore forming bacteria that are found in the intestinal tract of children. *Clostridium difficile* is the major cause of colitis and antibiotic associated diarrhea in children. Concurrent administration of *Saccharomyces boulardii* with the prescribed antibiotic preparation will minimize the probability of contracting a *Clostridium difficile* infection. The mechanism by which *Saccharomyces boulardii* offers this protection is through the production of a protease enzyme, which prevents a specific toxin, *Clostridium difficile toxin A,* from binding to intestinal receptors. Specifically, the protease enzyme destroys Clostridium difficile toxin A.

Following the course of antibiotics, enzymatic reduction of the levels of the *Saccharomyces boulardii* yeast and replenishment of the normal bacterial flora of the intestinal tract by using probiotic supplements would be the course of action. Reduction of the subsequent yeast overgrowth by taking the supplement is accomplished by using a supplement that contains enzymes specifically designed to break down the yeast. Common products used to break down the yeast contain the specific enzymes called cellulase and hemicellulase, and other enzymes specific to destruction of any yeast. Products containing these enzymes also contain specific proprietary blends to aid in the elimination of the yeast overgrowth. Concurrently performed with the destruction of the yeast is restoration of the normal bacterial flora of the intestines. This is accomplished with probiotic supplements. Effective anti-yeast and probiotic products are listed in Appendix I. Further discussion of this topic can be found in the chapter entitled *Digestive System Restoration*.

Body Piercing

Ear piercing has been around for centuries. In recent times, various forms of body piercing have also become popular, particularly with the younger generation. Disposable piercing instruments have made this a safer practice as compared with the use of reusable instruments decades ago. Using disposable instruments along with modern hygiene standards has dramatically reduced the transmission of blood-borne infections.

Even if the aftercare instructions are followed meticulously, a piercing will occasionally get infected. When this occurs, it is generally observed to occur shortly following the procedure. The typical medical approach is to remove the jewelry, and prescribe oral antibiotics. Removal of the jewelry from a person who has looked forward to this personal adornment causes emotional grief, and, in most cases, removal is not really necessary. In addition, in the great majority of cases, oral antibiotics prescribed to treat the infection also are not necessary. Oral antibiotics, as previously mentioned, cause disruption of the intestinal flora, leading to yet another problem that must then be treated. Antibiotic ointments, available without a prescription, are often used, and is a very poor choice in the treatment of a piercing that has gotten infected. Applying petroleum-based products within the pierced body part is difficult, which is where the infection actually is. Furthermore, the label on the antibiotic ointment states that the product is for external use only. Since the infection is an internal infection, not an external infection, the use of such preparations is inappropriate.

If a piercing has become infected, the infection must be treated as soon as possible. Waiting too long may cause the infection to spread throughout the body, therefore complicating matters. The best antibiotic preparations for treating an infected piercing are ophthalmic antibiotic preparations. Ophthalmic antibiotic preparations are in liquid form, allowing the antibiotic to enter the pierced body part easily, delivering the antibiotic directly to the site of the infection. Since ophthalmic antibiotics are prescription drugs, they will have to be prescribed by a medical doctor.

Following the aftercare instructions provided by the piercing shop should minimize the chance of any infection. Most infections are caused by playing with the jewelry, so keeping the hands off the jewelry is important until the piercing has healed.

A Pharmaceutical Research Failure

The purpose of a drug is, in one way or another, modification the biochemistry of the body. In modifying the course of a biochemical reaction, a certain effect can be realized, therefore changing the course of events of the biochemical reactions that sustain life. Pharmaceutical companies perform research leading to the manufacture of drugs intended to affect human biochemistry. The specific method by which the drug modifies the biochemistry of the body is termed the *mechanism of action* of that drug. It is the mechanism of action that defines specifically what the drug does.

One such well-known mechanism of action of is that of aspirin, a drug familiar to everyone, in which non-selective inhibition of the enzyme *cyclooxygenase*, a COX-2 enzyme, occurs. Other anti-inflammatory medications have a similar mechanism of action. Many drugs have a mechanism of action that is unknown or poorly understood. Thalidomide is a drug prescribed in the late 1950s to early 1960s to combat the morning sickness commonly experienced by pregnant women. During that time, the mechanism of action of thalidomide was very poorly understood. Later research proved that thalidomide has an antiangiogenic effect (inhibit the formation of new blood vessels) and, in addition, is an immune system modulator. As a result of poor research methodology, limited knowledge of biochemistry, and the goal of corporate profit, a drug was released to the market that caused serious birth defects. Many other drugs are approved for medical use without sufficient research. Diethylstilbestrol, commonly known as DES, is another drug in which insufficient research has been conducted before being released to the public. With one controversy after another, not a day goes by that some drug is implicated in having serious side effects.

The human intestinal system is populated with many types of microbes. These microbes, which include both beneficial bacteria and yeast, are found in enormous numbers. These beneficial organisms have their own biochemical processes that occur, many of which have been proven to interact in various ways with human biochemistry. No research, however, is performed to discover how the mechanism of action of a drug affects the biochemical processes of these microbes. By ignoring the action of a drug on these beneficial organisms, any disruption of the associated biochemistry goes undetected. These undetected changes may, in fact, be causing subsequent detrimental effects to human biochemical processes. In a normal healthy person, a greater number of beneficial microbial organisms exist in and on the body than cells can be found in the human body. When one considers this fact, research should clearly take into consideration the action of any drug on these microbes.

Metabolic Syndrome

Another syndrome that has recently arisen and is gaining popularity is called metabolic syndrome. Metabolic syndrome is a combination of several cardiovascular risk factors, including high blood pressure, high triglyceride levels, high cholesterol, abdominal obesity, glucose intolerance, and a

Why Am I Sick? And What To Do About It

nonspecific pro-inflammatory state of the body. Metabolic syndrome is also called insulin resistance syndrome. Metabolic syndrome is often blamed on consumption of refined sugar, particularly soft drinks. While these products may be contributing factors in metabolic syndrome, they have nothing at all to do with the real issues surrounding the overall decline of health seen with the syndrome.

Metabolic syndrome is a warning. The warning to the patient diagnosed with metabolic syndrome is to make a major change in their lifestyle now, or diabetes, heart disease, and a plethora of chronic disease issues are nearly certain in the future. A patient diagnosed with metabolic syndrome is most certainly under chronic stress, and has most likely been for several years. Metabolic syndrome illustrates quite effectively what happens to the body as a result of chronic stress. Specifically, stress results in both tissue and organ damage resulting from the prolonged exhaustion phase of the General Adaption Syndrome, discussed in the chapter on stress. In the case of metabolic syndrome, the body is quickly losing its ability to regulate various critical physiological components of metabolism.

The medical doctor will typically treat metabolic syndrome by treating the individual key components of the syndrome. Blood pressure medication would typically be prescribed for the elevated blood pressure. The medical doctor might also advise the patient to lose weight, but typically not offer any suggestions on how to lose it. If the patient is significantly obese, surgery may be offered as an option. A cholesterol lowering medication would likely be prescribed, and a goal of 160 mg/dl might be suggested. To address glucose intolerance, another pill would most likely be prescribed, along with the suggestion that the patient change their diet. The pro-inflammatory state would most likely be ignored, unless a specific cause can be identified. Any treatment protocols focused on treating the individual symptoms that are present essentially ignores the true underlying disorder. Treatment will often bring blood pressure, cholesterol, and blood glucose levels to within normal levels. Predictably, a few years later, increased dosages of medications will be prescribed, along with a few new ones for yet another problem that has arisen. This will give the illusion that the disease is now under control, but the underlying disorder is left untreated and none of the factors originally causing the disease have been addressed.

Metabolic syndrome is just another name for the exhaustion phase of the General Adaption Syndrome. We could name the disorder sedentary chronic stress syndrome, but naming a disorder in such a fashion is along the lines of being socially unacceptable. Specifically, metabolic syndrome is a perfect illustration of what happens in the exhaustion phase of the General Adaption Syndrome. Metabolic syndrome has a strong correlation with a long-standing history of lack of physical activity, as shown by the long term Oslo Study. A myriad of cardiovascular risk factors results from lack of exercise and poor diet. Unfortunately, in the case of metabolic syndrome, no one in the medical profession wants to confront the patient with the truth. The truth is that the patient does not exercise, is overweight, has a disrupted digestive system contributing to both the pro-inflammatory state and elevated cholesterol. Often, the patient has had a high fat diet of fast food and refined sugar for quite some time. Other digestive system disorders likely exist as well, such as acid reflux disease or ulcerations of the intestinal lining. Examination will usually reveal an unacceptably high resting heart rate. The truth is that the patient is headed for a heart attack, stroke, or other cardiovascular incident. While these may not be imminent, the probability increases with each passing year. The truth is that diabetes is just around the corner, and lifestyle changes must be made now in order to avert it.

The alternative practitioner, or holistic medical doctor would take a different approach in treating the patient diagnosed with metabolic syndrome. This would initially include restoring the digestive system, giving particular attention to eliminating candidiasis and restoration of the intestinal flora. A permanent change in diet would be required if the patient is to regain health. In addition, the patient would be instructed to lose any extra weight. This would be done through exercise and a change in diet. Supervised weight loss programs are ideal for this type patient. Abdominal obesity occurs as a result of prolonged elevation of cortisol levels, which is a good indicator of chronic stress. Exercise is mandatory for the person diagnosed with metabolic syndrome, and should be supervised by a qualified health care practitioner. Treatment should also be focused on eliminating stress regardless of the source, therefore eliminating the accumulated effects of stress. The natural health practitioner may also suggest certain dietary supplements to address any other issues on an individual basis. These dietary supplements are prescribed in such a way that specifically speeds the path to healing and health, and may be adjusted from time to time based upon patient progress. Any program used to reverse metabolic syndrome will represent a significant change in the patient's lifestyle. Unfortunately, no other choice can be found.

Metabolic syndrome is the equivalent of a four-alarm fire. Action is required now. Otherwise, further damage to the systems of the body will result. Do not think that this condition will be resolved with a pill. No pill will come along to cure metabolic syndrome. Serious lifestyle changes are required, and the faster they are initiated, the greater the chances of restoring health.

Fungal Infections

Fungal infections of the skin are quite common in today's society. The signs and symptoms of a fungal skin infection depend largely on the type of fungus and the part of the body affected. The infection may appear as red, scaly, darkened of splotchy colored skin. In many cases, the affected area is itchy. Fungal rashes can sometimes be confused with other skin conditions, such as eczema or psoriasis.

Fungal infections are classified based upon what type of fungal organism is involved, and the location of the fungal infection on the body. Most fungal infections have a common name associated with it. Tinea pedis, also known as Athlete's Foot, is caused by a variety of fungi and sometimes bacteria. Tinea cruris, commonly known as "jock itch," typically will cause an itchy, red rash in the groin area. It is commonly seen in athletes who sweat a lot. Often in the person who has athletes foot, scratching the feet followed by scratching or touching the groin may spread the infection from one place to another. Tinea versicolor, sometimes known as Pityriasis versicolor, is a fungal infection that can occur anywhere on the body. Tinea versicolor appears like dark areas on pale skin and light areas on tanned or darker skin, and usually becomes more apparent when a person has a suntan.

Fungi can be spread by sharing towels, combs, and other personal care items with an infected person. Walking barefoot on wet gym carpet is a sure way to get Athlete's Foot. Polyester clothing does not breathe well, and sets up a perfect environment for a fungal infection to occur. Occasionally, fungus will grow under the nail bed. This is commonly contracted from nail shops using improper sterilization procedures.

Over the counter fungal medications are available, and usually have to be applied for several weeks to eliminate the fungus completely. Stronger forms of topical ointments and oral antifungal agents are available by prescription. Once a fungal infection becomes systemic, it is very difficult to eliminate. Systemic fungal infections usually only occur in those persons who are immunosuppressed.

Most fungi have the ability to sense light with light-sensing proteins. Some fungi, such as *Saccharomyces cerevisiae*, commonly known as baker's yeast, cannot sense light. Ultraviolet light is known to kill fungus and other pathogens. A common use of ultraviolet sterilization is in fish tanks and air-conditioning units to kill bacteria, viruses and fungus. Ultraviolet sterilization units are also available to kill pathogens in the water supply to the home, and are usually inserted right into the water line.

The same ultraviolet light that kills fungus in the environment can kill fungal infections found on the skin. Exposure of the skin to ultraviolet light can therefore eradicate a fungal infection. Persons who frequently visit the beach and tanning beds rarely, if ever, have fungal infections. A few trips to the tanning bed or a little time in the sun each day are about all it takes to eliminate fungal infections of minor to moderate severity. Today, everyone is warned about the dangers of ultraviolet light, and how being in the sun is going to age the skin prematurely, and increase the risk for developing skin cancer. Because of medical and media hype, everyone stays out of the sun, which is equally, if not more unhealthy. The key, as with most issues, is moderation.

Nail fungus is particularly a problem, which requires special attention. If a fungal infection is found under the nail beds, using nail polish is the worst thing someone can do. This is because the nail polish blocks any sunlight exposure to the nail bed, including ultraviolet light that would ordinarily kill the fungus. But, because the fungal infection does not look pretty, the person attempts to hide the infection. The first mistake made is to cover it up with nail polish, which gives the fungus the perfect environment to thrive. Obviously, nail polish should not be used when fungus is found in the nail bed. When the toes are involved, the second mistake made is to refrain from wearing open toe shoes or sandals. Socks, shoes, and sneakers block light and help to retain moisture on the skin, making the perfect breeding ground for more fungus.

Heat and Ice for Sprain and Strains

Following trauma, the patient is usually given care instructions by their medical doctor or the attending staff at the emergency room. The patient who is diagnosed with either a sprain or a strain may be given a prescription for an anti-inflammatory or muscle relaxant. If the pain is significant, a pain killer may be prescribed as well. Often, these instructions outline the use of either heat or ice for the injury.

Emergency rooms and medical doctors, in many cases, seem to offer the wrong or conflicting advice on using heat and ice for traumatic injuries. The improper use of heat and ice can actually make the symptoms worse and delay the healing process. Furthermore, additional conflicting advice is often given by some family member or friend, thus complicating matters. At times, better advice is seen coming from friends and family as compared with that given by the emergency room. Understanding the use of heat and ice is simple, and follows some basic rules. A good understanding of the inflammatory process is beneficial to understand these basic rules. Once an understanding of the inflammatory process is gained, the basic rules can be applied with confidence, therefore reducing healing time.

A sprain refers to a ligament, and means the ligament has been stretched, partially torn, or ruptured. A strain refers to a muscle, and means that the muscle has been stretched beyond its elastic limit, and, as a result, muscle fibers have been torn to some degree. When a muscle is torn, blood escapes from the vessels supplying the muscle, and this can often be visualized under the skin. When a ligament is sprained, little, if any, blood escapes into the surrounding tissue.

Whenever a sprain or strain injury occurs, inflammation of the tissue will immediately follow. The four cardinal signs of inflammation are rubor (redness), calor (elevated temperature), dolar (pain), and tumor (swelling). The result of these four inflammatory responses is a specific loss of function of the affected area. One example of loss of function is decreased range of motion of a joint. Another example of loss of function is impaired nervous system function due to inflammation exerting direct pressure on the surrounding nerves. Direct pressure on a nerve impedes nerve transmission, and can result in numbness, tingling, pain, altered sensation, or muscular weakness. The inflammatory response of the body resulting from tissue injury is often quite exaggerated. Excessive inflammation can actually inhibit healing. Steps taken to reduce inflammation can subsequently speed healing of the affected area.

The rate of healing of a specific type of tissue is proportional to its blood supply. The tongue has one of the best blood supplies of any organ of the body, and, if injured, it heals very quickly. Anyone who has bitten their tongue and caused a minor bleed knows that it is healed the very next day. The skin and muscle tissue have a reasonably good blood supply, and any injury to these tissues is quick to heal, although not as fast as the tongue. As compared to the skin and muscle tissue, bone has somewhat less of a blood supply. As a result, a fractured bone requires a much longer time to heal than a strained muscle or an abrasion of the skin. Ligaments have a very poor blood supply, increasing healing time dramatically compared to muscle tissue or bones. The blood supply to ligaments is so poor in comparison, that a torn ligament often requires surgical intervention to correct. A sprained ligament can take several months to heal fully. Intervertebral discs have no blood supply to them. Intervertebral discs obtain their nutrients by a process called imbibition, where nutrients move from the end plate of the vertebra into the disc at night time when the disc is mechanically decompressed during sleep. Metabolic waste products diffuse out of the disc during the day when the nucleus is at a relative positive pressure. This slow rate of nutrients into and out of the disc explains why disc degeneration is prevalent, the injured disc degenerates faster than the body can effectively heal it.

The rate at which inflammation occurs in a particular tissue is also proportional to the blood supply of that tissue. Muscle tissue, skin, and fat become inflamed much quicker following an injury than does a ligament or spinal disc. This explains why, following an automobile accident or other trauma, certain injuries are not apparent until several days later. A whiplash injury is a sprain of the ligaments and strain of the muscles of the neck. While not part of the classical whiplash definition, injuries to the joints of the spine and the intervertebral discs occur quite often. The full scope of a whiplash injury is typically not apparent until approximately five days following the automobile accident. This is because the inflammation of the muscles, ligaments, joints, and disc occurs at different rates. Likewise, the healing rates of the tissues involved is different. Muscle strains will heal much faster than the sprained ligaments. The disc, with no blood supply at all, is often the slowest to heal, and is also the slowest to inflame following an injury. An inflamed disc does not respond to oral anti-inflammatory medications. Oral anti-inflammatory medications are delivered to the structures of the body through the blood. With no blood supply, anti-inflammatory medication cannot be delivered to the disc. A steroidal anti-inflammatory injection directly into an injured disc is often done in severe cases of disc inflammation.

During the acute phase of an injury, the primary goal is to reduce the body's inflammatory response to injury. This is when ice is used. Ice will reduce bleeding of the damaged tissue, and reduce swelling. The application of ice will also prevent the area from becoming stiff, minimizing loss of function. Excessive swelling can significantly inhibit healing by altering the blood supply to the affected area. Swelling can exert pressure on the blood vessels, altering the flow of blood in both arteries and veins in undesirable ways. Pressure on a vein, for example, will cause the decreased return of blood from the area, and swelling will subsequently increase.

Ice should be applied as quickly as possible following the injury to the affected area. Ice is typically applied for 10 to 30 minutes at a time, followed by 45 to 60 minutes off. The usual recommendation is to repeat this procedure for 24 to 48 hours. This is a reasonable time for a muscle strain. When sprains that involves a joint or the spine is involved, ice therapy may be required for longer than two days, since in these cases the swelling is often slow to subside. The length of time for each application of ice varies, and is dependent on several factors. First, the body part thickness is taken into consideration. For example, the bones of the wrist are very close to the surface of the body, so ice would be applied to the wrist for a duration shorter than say, for example, the lumbar spine, where the spinal joints lie deep beneath the surface of the skin. Another factor taken into consideration is the person's body type. A person of an endomorphic build, who has a large amount of body fat, will require ice being applied for a longer time, since fat acts like an insulator. The person of an ectomorphic build, who is very thin, would not need the ice applied for as long of a time, since little fat exists to act as insulation. When these factors are taken into consideration, it explains the wide time frame of 10 to 30 minutes suggested by most authorities for ice application. When using ice, care must be used to avoid frostbite, wrapping the ice pack in paper towels will usually suffice. The icing phase should continue as long as inflammation is present.

After the icing phase is complete, typically a few days, tissue mobilization should begin. This is accomplished by light exercise and stretching to mobilize the joint. This does not mean going back to the gym and setting power lifting records or back to power yoga class just yet. Gently moving the affected body part through its range of motion is sufficient at this point. The intensity of the mobilization efforts should increase gradually each day. Physical therapy, under the supervision of a licenced physical therapist, is, by far, the most appropriate treatment during the tissue mobilization phase of an injury. Following the protocol prescribed by the physical therapist will result in a greatly decreased likelihood of a permanent injury. The physical therapist will also prescribe exercises to be done at home. The worst thing to do once the inflammation has subsided is to lie in bed all day. Laying around in bed all day will prolong the healing time of most musculoskeletal injuries.

Never use heat on a new injury. Heat will increase inflammation, increase bleeding, subsequently making the condition worse. This is because heat causes the blood vessels to dilate, increasing the blood flow to the affected area. As a result of using heat on an acute muscle tear or other injury involving broken blood vessels, an increased probability exists of an adhesion forming. Since adhesions are extremely difficult to treat, often requiring surgery to remove, preventing their formation is very important.

When the acute inflammation phase has ended, heat can then be applied. Therapeutic sources of heat are heating pads, microwaveable heat packs, heat creams, hot water bottles, warm baths, or infrared lamps. Heat helps to relieve muscle spasms, which invariably follow trauma. The typical duration for heat application is thirty minutes to two hours. When heat is applied, great care must be taken to avoid burning the skin. The heat should be warm, not too hot. If the heat feels too hot, it most likely is too hot.

Moist heat therapy is often used with chronic injuries, rheumatoid arthritis, and chronic pain. Moist heat is also effective for the acute muscle spasms found following trauma. Unlike dry heat, moist heat provides a water medium that aids conducting the heat to the affected body part. As a result, moist heat generally provides deeper penetration than dry heat at the same temperature and application time. Moist heat also offers better pain relief than does dry heat. The purpose of moist heat is reduction of acute muscle spasms and chronic pain relief.

Dry heat, such as electric heating pads and infrared light, draw out moisture and toxins through the skin. The purpose of dry heat, therefore, is detoxification of the body. Dry heat is beneficial following a strenuous workout to help eliminate the accumulation of toxins that accumulate in the muscle tissue, thus reducing soreness. Excessive use of dry heat may cause dehydration, so replacing fluids and electrolytes is important while undergoing dry heat therapy. Laying in the sun is actually a form of dry heat, and has other benefits as well. While dry heat has many benefits, dry heat is less effective than moist heat in the treatment of traumatic injuries.

Alternating heat and ice is often prescribed for concurrent treatment of inflammation and muscle spasms. A much better solution is to obtain massage therapy from a professional massage therapist following a soft tissue injury. Ice will reduce inflammation, and the proper type of massage will both reduce muscle spasms and help to reduce inflammation. Cross-tissue massage will also help prevent the formation of adhesions, which are a common result of tissue injury. Cross-tissue massage, incidently, is the most reliable method to prevent adhesion formation. A professional massage therapist, therefore, can accomplish much more than alternating ice and heat. Massage, in conjunction with the icing phase of an acute injury, is a superior to alternating heat with ice.

The use of heat and ice are contraindicated on persons with heart disease, hypertension, diabetes, deep vein thrombosis, dermatitis, arterial blockages and other conditions in which blood supply regulation is impaired. If heat or ice is prescribed to patients with these conditions, following the prescribing doctor's advice carefully is imperative.

TENS Units

TENS stands for Transcutaneous Electrical Nerve Stimulator. A TENS unit is often prescribed for patients who are in either acute or chronic pain. A TENS unit is a small electronic device that delivers a controlled electrical signal through electrodes placed on the skin. If used properly, the device can be quite effective in the control of both acute and chronic pain. TENS units are often prescribed by medical doctors, chiropractors, or physical therapists. While a TENS unit can be purchased from many online sources, it is a prescription device, a prescription must therefore be obtained prior to its use. The units are typically packaged with operational instructions only. Additional instructions regarding proper calibration and electrode placement are determined on an individual basis by the prescribing physician.

Some people claim great benefit from using the TENS unit, while others experience no pain relief at all. Whenever a TENS unit is found to be ineffective in relieving pain, the most likely reason is that the dials and switches on the unit have not been set correctly. Improper electrode placement is also commonly observed when poor results are obtained. If operated with Incorrect settings or improper electrode placement, the TENS unit does nothing more than drains the 9-volt battery inside the unit. If the correct settings are used in conjunction with proper electrode placement, the TENS unit will most likely provide pain relief as advertised and intended.

Only two pain relief protocols are possible with a TENS unit. These are known as the Gate Control Protocol, and the Acupuncture Protocol. The Acupuncture protocol is also known as the Descending Pathway Inhibition protocol. Either protocol requires the device settings to be set in a very specific manner. The Gate Control Protocol is often prescribed for acute pain, and causes inhibition of the ascending pain pathways, effectively decreasing the intensity of pain signals reaching the brain. The Acupuncture protocol is often prescribed for either acute or chronic pain, and induces endorphin release through stimulation of specific spinal cord tracts. Endorphins are the natural, opiate-like, painkillers of the body, therefore pain relief afforded through the Acupuncture protocol continues for several hours after the TENS unit has been turned off.

The use of a TENS unit for other purposes, such as to relieve muscle spasms, reduction of edema, trigger point stimulation, or to build muscle is an inappropriate application of the device. Relief of muscle spasms, the reduction of edema, and trigger point stimulation, are all, however, appropriate applications for more powerful interferential units. Interferential units cost several thousands of dollars and the associated applications are generally limited to in-office use by qualified practitioners. Some interferential units are also capable of a protocol called *Russian Stimulation*. Russian Stimulation is the protocol used to build muscle tissue through electrical contraction of muscle tissue.

The purpose of a TENS unit is to stimulate the nerves located in lamina II and lamina V of the posterior horn of the spinal cord. These are the nerves that are responsible for pain transmission. These nerves operate on a principle which increases the efficiency of pain transmission if the cause of the pain continually remains present. This increase of pain transmission efficiency is called *wind-up*, where the neurological synapses in the spinal cord become more efficient at conducting nerve impulses, essentially increasing the body's sensitivity to pain. The terms *neuroplasticity* and *synaptogenesis* have come into popular usage recently, and refer to this condition of wind-up of the neurological synapses. This increased pain perception is the body's way of getting a stronger message through to the brain to alarm the person that something is wrong. Once the cause of pain is removed, the neurological synapses will then *wind-down* and return to normal, becoming less efficient at pain transmission. If the nerves, however, are allowed to attain a chronic wound-up state, the wind-down process is exceedingly prolonged. In some cases of chronic pain, wind-down has not occurred as it should. The TENS unit is very valuable in preventing the wind-up of the synaptic connections. In preventing any wind-up of the neurological connections, the probability of chronic pain is decreased.

Older TENS units have a variety of switches and dials to allow the user to configure the unit for the appropriate protocol. The newer digital TENS units also have various controls on them; the unique feature with these modern units is the digital LCD readout and buttons instead of dials. On both the newer and older units, some switches and dials are located inside the unit, often inside the battery compartment. These hidden switches and dials are the ones that must be set in a precise manner to obtain optimal results. One switch, which may or may not be present, is the *Mode* switch. The mode switch should always be set to the **continuous** position, unless specifically instructed otherwise by the prescribing physician. Two dials will be found inside the compartment of the older models. One dial will be labeled either *Frequency* or *Pulse Rate*, and will be calibrated in Hz. The other dial will be labeled either *Pulse Width* or *Pulse Duration*, and will be calibrated in microseconds (µsec). On the digital models, these settings are usually modified by first selecting either the frequency or duration from the configuration menu, and then, using the buttons labeled ▲ or ▼, entering the appropriate setting. These settings are of the utmost importance, the appropriate settings for either protocol are shown in Table 15.1. Outside the unit the intensity controls can be found. These must also be set correctly for optimal results. The appropriate intensity settings for either protocol are also found in Table 15.1.

Electrode placement is another issue that arises when poor results have been obtained with a TENS unit. The entire purpose of a TENS unit is to stimulate the nerves located in lamina II and lamina V of the posterior horn of the spinal cord. Electrodes must be placed in such a way to stimulate the nerves that are found in a wound up state. Optimal electrode placement, therefore, would require that the electrodes are placed adjacent to the spinal cord to stimulate the required nerves properly. Electrodes placed on the hands, arms, leg, or other remote place in the body, will do little to stimulate structures located within the spinal cord itself directly, but does offer some degree of pain relief. When electrodes are placed along an area of the body away from the spine, they must be placed along the nerve distribution directly related to the pain. Another common error often seen is to place the electrodes too far apart, for example, one electrode placed on the neck and the other electrode on the low back. Electrodes placed this far apart do not allow sufficient current to flow through the target structures. Without any current flowing through the target structure, no meaningful stimulation to the neurological structures involved occurs. Consequently, any error in electrode placement will result in little or no pain relief.

Electrodes should be placed no closer than one centimeter, or farther than ten centimeters apart. The effectiveness of the treatment decreases when the electrodes are placed farther than ten centimeters apart. A good rule of thumb is to leave the distance equivalent of one to two electrodes between the electrodes placed on the skin. Closely placed electrodes will provide a more superficial and concentrated stimulus. When placed farther apart, a deeper, but less concentrated, stimulus is realized. The electrodes should be placed to the left or to the right side of the spine, never directly over the center of the spine. Electrodes, however, may be placed on either side of the spine if the pain is related to the nerves on both sides of the spine.

Proper placement protocol, therefore, requires that the electrodes are placed in such a way to stimulate the precise neurological level associated with the area of pain. For example, if the pain is of neurological origin is due to disc compression of the sixth cervical right nerve root, the pain is often felt in the thumb and index finger of the right hand. The proper electrode placement would be overlying the mid cervical and the upper thoracic (T2) region on the right side of the spine, thus delivering the majority of the electrical current between the electrodes to the affected nerves. If the pain, however, is due to trauma to the C6-C7 facet joint at the base of the neck, the pain is often felt as referred pain in the right scapular region. Optimal electrode placement in this case would be similar to that of the example cited regarding disc compression. In this case, electrodes inappropriately placed over the shoulder region or mid back would be relatively ineffective, since no true neurological relationship exists between the region of pain and the structure responsible for causing the pain. The appropriate neurological levels to be stimulated, therefore, are best determined by a qualified practitioner. The practitioner will take into consideration the type of pain, such as local pain, referred pain, radicular pain, or any combination these, and determine the cord level(s) which are best stimulated to address reduction of the pain.

The use of a TENS unit is contraindicated in patients with a pacemaker, electronic insulin pump, any other electronic implant, in the presence of any malignancy or infection, and over the uterus during pregnancy. The evaluation of other conditions that may constitute a contraindication will be performed by the prescribing physician.

Protocol	Frequency (Hz)	Pulse Duration (µsec)	Intensity	Duration of Treatment
Gate Control	High 80-120	Narrow 50-100	To sensory perception	20 to 30 minutes or longer, as instructed by the prescribing physician.
Acupuncture	Low 1-10	Wide 200	To patient tolerance	20 to 30 minutes each session

Table 15.1   TENS Protocols and Settings

Ear Tones

Many people report hearing periodic annoying tones in their ears. One type of tone is that of a very pure pitch, and usually occurs only in one ear at a time. The pitch of the tone heard can be very low to very high, and lasts for several seconds. When this tone occurs, the intensity remains relatively constant for five to thirty seconds, then suddenly decreases over a period of a two or three seconds. This is termed an *eartone*. An eartone is not to be confused with tinnitus. People whom experience eartones also may experience momentary blocks in hearing which may last several seconds. These momentary blocks in hearing sound as if someone pressed the mute button for a few seconds. This is termed an ear block.

These momentary eartones and ear blocks are typically of no medical concern and do not require extensive medical tests to diagnose. In most cases, examination of the ear will be found to be unremarkable.

The structures involved in hearing during the formation of each ear are a result of both genetic and developmental factors. As a result of these factors, in some persons, the structure of the inner ear is tuned to resonate at certain frequencies. Specifically, electrolyte levels in the chambers of the cochlea, in conjunction with the bony structure of the ear, create a tuned resonant system. If the electrolyte levels are at some predetermined level, which varies from person to person, under the correct conditions a resonant state of the structures involved can be entered.

Since we have clearly identified a resonant structure, any electromagnetic signal with the appropriate characteristics can cause the system to resonate. Since the resonant structure in question is found in the inner ear, resonance will be translated by the associated neurology into a tone or other variation in hearing. The question, then, is what can cause this system to go into resonance. Solar flares generate electromagnetic energy, and subsequently this can cause the eartone or ear block. The shifting tectonic plates of the Earth momentarily disrupt the planet's magnetic field, another cause of the eartone or ear block. In the case of shifting tectonic plates, the eartone or ear block is often a precursor to earthquakes. Seismologists have detected subtle electromagnetic changes in the Earth's magnetic field prior to a seismic event. In stands to reason that, since the body is affected by these electromagnetic fields, sensory perception of changes in the magnetic field can be perceived by certain individuals under the appropriate conditions. Persons who experience these phenomena are termed *earthquake sensitives*.

Treatment of Psychological Disorders

A psychological illness is an illness in which clinically significant aberrations in cognitive thought patterns occur in an individual, subsequently leading to partial or full disability of the individual, or the inability to function as part of society. Psychological disorders are often termed a mental illness. What is considered a psychological disorder encompasses a wide scope of primarily symptom-related conditions. Schizophrenia, bipolar disorder, depression, obsessive-compulsive disorder, delusional disorder, attention deficit disorder, various personality disorders, post traumatic stress syndrome, and stress itself are just a few of these psychological disorders. These disorders, regardless of the name, are all linked to the balance and action of neurotransmitters and their associated receptor sites in the brain. These disorders also have significant environmental factors associated with them. In some cases, neurotransmitter aberration is caused by a history of unusual or repeated thought patterns.

Modern medicine has developed many highly specific medications for treating disorders termed as psychological disorders or psychological illness. Medications of this type generally target specific neurotransmitter sites, either by blocking the action of that neurotransmitter or by prolonging the action of that neurotransmitter in one way or another. Some medications selectively target specific neurotransmitter binding sites, and others, being more general in nature, target an entire neurotransmitter system, such as the serotonin system. Other medications affect multiple neurotransmitter systems, such as the group known as the monoamine neurotransmitters, which includes norepinephrine, dopamine and serotonin. Monoamine oxidase inhibitors (MAOIs) are one class of drugs that targets multiple neurotransmitter systems. By various mechanisms of action, the activity of these neurotransmitters can be enhanced or suppressed, causing a predictable change in behavior of the individual. The medical doctor, then, examines the list of patient complaints, and prescribes a medication that adjusts the neurotransmitter most likely to eliminate the symptoms associated with the patients complaints or observed behavior.

Neurotransmitters and other substances involved in neurotransmission include dopamine, serotonin, norepinephrine, acetylcholine, Gamma-aminobutyric acid (GABA), glycine, Substance P, endorphins, enkephalins, dynorphin, histamine, glutamic acid, Aspartic acid, purine, in addition to more than fifty neuroactive peptides. Both electrolyte levels and blood sugar levels influence neurotransmission within the nerve itself. Hormone levels can affect the mood, and therefore affect thought patterns. Thought patterns also influence both neurotransmission and the formation of synaptic connections. Alcohol, can also affect neurotransmission in very well known ways. In addition, for any given neurotransmitter, many variations of receptor sites are known to exist. Receptor sites are not permanent static structures; they are created and removed by the body over time. In addition, synaptogenesis can occur, creating either new or more efficient neurological pathways.

To believe that any psychological disorder hinges on the effect of a single neurotransmitter and its associated receptor sites is not sound medicine or sound science. Medications that target specific neurotransmitter mechanisms are used because they appear to some degree alleviate the symptomatic complaints of the patient. Unfortunately, by alleviating the symptoms of one disorder through the use of a medication, new disorders are subsequently created. Medications used to treat depression, for example, are well known to produce "sexual side effects," in other words, some degree of sexual impotence. Logic dictates that if the correct receptor site was identified and subsequently targeted by an appropriate antidepressant medication, the depression would be cured with no side effects. The mere fact that a sexual side effect, or any other side effect for that matter, occurs, is evidence that the wrong receptor site or neurotransmitter was targeted. Neurological side effects are also suggestive of the fact that other neurotransmitter sites outside those that are specifically intended to be targeted by the medication are also involved. The medication, while appearing to work, is most likely causing further neurologically related problems, the effects of which may not be known until years later.

By blocking receptor sites, the body either creates more receptor sites, develops a new neurological disorder, incurs some form of neurological damage, or plain and simply just dies. This is best documented with commonly prescribed antipsychotic dopamine blocking agents. Lethal catatonia and neuroleptic malignant syndrome have been clearly implicated in the blockade of dopamine receptors. Other diseases, such as tardive dyskinesia, are evidence of irreversible brain damage that occurs as a result of dopamine blocking action of these antipsychotic medications. If the drug were actually targeting the correct neurotransmitter sites, the patient would be cured. The schizophrenic or psychotic patient is never cured by these medications although symptoms are alleviated, which is strong evidence that the medication is not even an appropriate treatment for the disease in question. Again, as with antidepressant medication, long term use of antipsychotic medications eventually will lead to diseases and disorders that were not originally present. This is evidence that the selected drug is targeting the wrong neurotransmitter and receptor sites, and is therefore an inappropriate treatment that appears only on the surface to work. In the case of the schizophrenic or psychotic patient, neurology suggests that glutamate receptors in the prefrontal cortex of the brain are also involved to a significant degree. Gamma-aminobutyric acid, the primary inhibitory neurotransmitter of the brain, is most likely involved as well. A problem arises, however, because the action of Gamma-aminobutyric acid and glutamate cannot be affected with the degree of specificity as can be done with other neurotransmitters, such as dopamine and serotonin. This causes a significant problem for pharmaceutical manufacturers in the sense that a problem cannot be specifically addressed by a manufactured chemical.

The modern medical mistake in this case, then, is that most all disorders involving thought processes are not as a result of aberrant activity of one neurotransmitter. With more than sixty known substances involved in neurotransmission, it is naive to believe that only one of many neurotransmitters somehow got out of balance, and, as a result, caused some clearly defined specific condition. Worse yet is the belief that a manufactured chemical can actually cure the disorder. Whenever a psychological disorder is present, much more than a chemical is needed to restore the health of the individual.

Invented Psychological Disorders

Certain psychological disorders are literally invented, and should not even be classified as a disorder. The reasons that they are often defined as disorders are either to classify the condition thus justifying treatment for the condition medically, to force an insurance company to pay for the treatment, or to make someone feel better by simply giving a name to whatever they might be perceive as wrong. The treatment of an invented disorder is just as invented as the disorder itself. These invented disorders often simply rename the symptom that is present. The symptom of the invented disorder is actually a symptom of another underlying disorder that needs to be identified. This places the invented disorder into a class called a diagnosis of absurdity. A few of these disorders, and what the diagnosis is supposed to mean, are listed in Table 15.2. This list of disorders is by no means to be considered complete.

Invented disorders carry another problem with them. While they seem ridiculous when originally defined, time well ingrains them into medicine, and they become generally accepted as a disease or disorder. Eventually, the disorder becomes a common household word, and no one gives a second thought to what the disorder really is. If any thought were given to what is actually being described as a disorder, reconsideration of the diagnosis and search for a more meaningful explanation for the symptom would be demanded by the patient.

Name of the Disorder	Meaning or Explanation
Body Dysmorphic Disorder	The patient does not like the way their body looks
Depersonalization Disorder	A feeling a disconnection from one's body
Impulse Control Disorder NOS	Patient has a pattern of doing something on impulse
Hallucinogen Intoxication	Intoxication due to a hallucinogen. Duh ... that's why someone took the drug in the first place
Mathematics Disorder	The inability to perform or understand math
Conduct Disorder	The person has bad conduct
Personality Change Disorder	The personality of the patient has changed for some known or unknown reason
Mental Disorder NOS	Unspecified or unknown mental disorder
Attention Deficit Disorder	Person has difficulty paying attention and concentrating
Intermittent Explosive Disorder	Periodic severe or uncontrollable rage
Eating Disorder NOS	Any unexplained or uncategorized eating disorder

Table 15.2   Diagnoses of Absurdity

By defining these disorders, what happens is that the process of diagnosis stops prematurely because a named problem has been found. This essentially prevents the true underlying disorder or disease from being discovered. In not discovering the underlying causes, the patient's condition will never improve because, as all too common in modern medicine, the true underlying conditions are left untreated. By treating only the symptoms, the underlying cause is still present, waiting to be manifested in another manner.

In the case of Personality Change Disorder, for example, the question is why did the person's personality change? Take, for example, a female teenager whose personality suddenly changed for no apparent reason. It could be, perhaps, that the teenager is just in a bad mood because they could not understand how to do their math homework, which is clear evidence of Mathematics Disorder. The teacher calls the parents, concerned that the student has trouble concentrating and paying attention in class, and suggests to the parents that their daughter may have Attention Deficit Disorder. Repeated demands by the parents for their daughter to do her math homework lead to the teenager getting really cranky and irritable, which is another well known and documented disorder called Conduct Disorder. In fact, the parents have suspected Conduct Disorder for quite a long time. Both the parents and the teacher, however, did not recognize that the reason that the student was unable to do her math homework was because of Hallucinogen Intoxication, which clearly occurred as a result of another disorder, Impulse Control Disorder, earlier that day. In other words, the teenager impulsively smoked pot at lunchtime while at school with some of her friends. Hallucinogen Intoxication subsequently has lead to the teenager feeling a little disconnected with herself while in math class, and is clearly a case of Depersonalization Disorder. Hallucinogen Intoxication also, has at least one generally expected side effect, which has lead to the teenager accidently eating a half gallon of ice cream and a 2-liter soft drink after school. A little later, upon looking in the mirror, the teenager appeared to look a little fatter, her belly button ring looked weird, and her jeans were a little tight, and she was not at all happy with her appearance. This severe case of Eating Disorder has inevitably lead to an acute case of Body Dysmorphic Disorder, clearly evidenced by the fact that she was not happy with her appearance. The daughter, being more concerned about the appearance of her midriff than her math homework, caused the parents to get very frustrated. Finally, the parents just throw their arms up in the air and say to their daughter, "We don't know what is wrong with you anymore!" The parents, by not knowing what is wrong with their daughter, have discovered quite by accident yet another disorder afflicting their teenager, Mental Disorder NOS (Not Otherwise Specified), which clearly explains everything. Finally, the teenager screams, slams the door and runs outside. This sudden outburst by the teenager suggests that perhaps Intermittent Explosive Disorder might be another factor involved. When confronted about her Intermittent Explosive Disorder, the teenager is quick to suggest that she thinks an explosive disorder sounds more like it refers to a bomb.

With eleven ridiculous diagnoses applying to the teenager, the true cause remains a mystery to everyone involved, except the teenager. If anyone had even bothered asking, the teenager might have just said that she was having a bad day because her boyfriend dumped her earlier that day. But, since no disorder called Boyfriend Dumped Me Disorder exists, the fact that she got dumped cannot possibly be the problem. Nevertheless, getting dumped by her boyfriend was the underlying condition for everything that happened during that entire day. Obviously, getting dumped was the true underlying problem, not the activities that happened because of getting dumped.

Inventing other disorders can be done just as easily. All one has to do is to find some behavior considered undesirable, define it, and then call it a disorder. The level to which this has already been done in medicine borderlines on absurdity, and indications are that, in the future, even more ridiculous disorders are on their way. Since the medical profession appears to be able to create any disorder at will, in the above example we might as well just say that all of the adults who are involved have a severe case of Teenager Intolerance Syndrome. This would provide a clear explanation of the entire scenario described above as understood from the perspective of the teenager. Clearly then, the adults are in need treatment, and not the teenager. So, the teenager goes back to school, and tell her friends that her parents had a bad case of TIS (Teenager Intolerance Syndrome) yesterday.

By issuing and accepting a diagnosis of absurdity, we have essentially built a roadblock to proper treatment of what is actually responsible for the symptom or behavior. If the diagnosis of absurdity was never issued to begin with, finding the true cause of the problem would have been much easier. It is quite a shame that such monumental efforts are put into documenting such absurd disorders.

What, then, explains the existence of these invented disorders? Disorders of the mind that are typically diagnosed before the age of 25 are often a result of different rates of development of the various regions of the brain. The brain does not develop according to a rigid schedule; some variation in developmental rates is to be expected from one individual to another. If the rate of development of one region of the brain greatly exceeds the norm, or for some reason significantly lags the norm, the affected individual is often labeled with either a disease, disorder, or learning disability. Complicating matters even further are instances in which certain areas of the brain develop at a rate faster than the norm, while other regions of the brain in the same individual develop at a slower rate. Variations of development rates of the various areas of the brain are not, in fact, a disorder of any type at all. What these so-called disorders are, however, are normal variants that the individual will undoubtably outgrow after the age of 25 when the nervous system is fully developed. Most psychological disorders assigned to anyone under the age of 18 fall into this category. What the teenager needs is a little leeway for individual differences in development, not rigid academic performance standards or gross intolerance of temporary behavioral problems. The problem lies not in the development of the individual, but in a society that demands flawless and rigid performance in every facet of life from children, adolescents, and teenagers who are forced to conform to unreasonably rigid standards.

Ironically, another medically defined disorder, Multiple Personality Disorder, which has clearly defined and obvious mechanisms associated with it, is labeled as a controversial diagnosis. If Multiple Personality Disorder was properly understood by the medical profession, the understanding of the condition could at least be given to the patient.

Attention Deficit Disorder

In the previous section, Attention Deficit Disorder was identified as a diagnosis of absurdity. This popular diagnosis deserves special attention. This classification is because the disorder, in fact, really does not exist. Both Attention Deficit Disorder and Attention Deficit Hyperactivity Disorder (hereafter referred to as Attention Deficit Disorders) are yet other invented disorders to classify, and therefore medicate, children who do not meet either a predefined performance or behavioral standard. By prescribing a medication, the child becomes more controllable in the school environment in which he or she is forced to conform.

Much research has been funded on the subject of Attention Deficit Disorders; a cursory search of one online research repository returns more than one thousand published research papers on the subject. Examination of this research indicates that Attention Deficit Disorders have a strong genetic basis, a nutritional basis, neurotransmitter involvement, linked to child abuse, linked to organic pollutants, has a correlation with social class, linked to cigarette and alcohol consumption during pregnancy, associated with childhood Lead exposure, is a result of brain injury, or is caused by food additives. In addition, MRI studies have shown children with Attention Deficit Disorders have structural differences in cortical gray matter and cerebral volume differences, but, until recently, these claims have remained vague and nonspecific. The list of postulated causes is seemingly endless. Much of this research has been directed toward looking for an external cause that simply will not be found. Nevertheless, to keep the research money flowing and researchers employed, the search for the cause of a nonexistent disorder continues year after year.

Recent research indicates that the classical drugs used to treat Attention Deficit Disorders have no long term benefits. Short term effects of the drugs used in treatment are limited to making the student more manageable in the classroom. This new research, which employs the use of Magnetic Resonance Imaging, has revealed that certain areas of the brain develop at different rates than other areas. Those diagnosed with Attention Deficit Disorders are found to have slower development of the brain's prefrontal cortex, the area that controls attention and planned movements. Conversely, the motor cortex, which is responsible for movement, is found to develop faster in children with Attention Deficit Disorders. In other words, the area of the brain that is responsible for carrying out movement has developed faster than the area of the brain that conceives and plans the movement. Other areas of the brain are most likely involved, but are beyond the detection capability of modern instrumentation. Since the brain is fully developed at the age of 25, this explains why most people outgrow the disorder at or before that age.

Attention Deficit Disorders, therefore, are not disorders at all. If Attention Deficit Disorders are to be classified as anything, they would fall into the category of a *normal variant*. A condition is termed a normal variant when the condition is considered to be a normal condition, but occurs at a decreased frequency than is found in the general population. Expecting that everyone's brain will develop at the same rate is unreasonable. Some leeway in individual development rates must be allowed for, and prescribing dangerous drugs is certainly not the answer for anyone who is perceived as different. One must wonder what kind of damage these drugs have done to the millions unnecessarily medicated to treat a diagnosis of absurdity.

To illustrate the absurdity of prescribing medication for Attention Deficit Disorders, consider the fact that physical development and any associated athletic abilities do not develop at the same rate in every individual. Some individuals are highly gifted in sports, and this is evident in many cases at a very young age. If we were to propose that every student to perform at the physical level of these gifted individuals, and prescribe anabolic steroids to force the development of the body to bring physical performance of the less gifted individuals up to par, the proposal would be laughed at and quickly condemned as an inappropriate and unnecessary treatment. Furthermore, since the dangers of inappropriate use of anabolic steroids are well documented, the proposal will be quickly dismissed for being a risky and dangerous path to take. Why, then, would we require academic and intellectual performance to be altered by medication? Why would we endanger the proper development of a child's mind by prescribing drugs that can alter the normal course of nature? In reality, prescribing medication to treat Attention Deficit Disorders is no more logical than the ridiculous proposal of prescribing anabolic steroids to those students with inferior athletic performance.

Interestingly, those children diagnosed with Attention Deficit Disorders do not seem to have any attention deficit in either gym class or recess.

Personality Profiles and Employment

Personality profiles and psychological testing are often used in schools to help decide what type of profession is best suited for the student. Information regarding scholastic aptitude is combined with the results of any number of personality profiles, resulting in a list of professions or job classifications that may be suited for that particular individual. Personality profiles are also used by employers to determine whether a particular employee is well suited for a particular position. Personality profiles may also be used by employers for other undisclosed purposes.

Personality profiles are also used to evaluate different facets of a person's personality. Many different types of tests have been developed over the years to discover these various personality traits. It can be determined if a person is introverted or extroverted by taking a specific type of psychological test. Other tests are used to determine whether a person is more playful or more serious, or whether the person is a thinker or feeler. Left and right brain dominance can also be determined by these tests. These personality traits are readily obvious to the most casual observer.

When it comes to employment, no test can adequately determine in what profession an individual should be employed. Amid all this testing, it never occurs to anyone to anyone to ask the question "what do you really want to do for a living?" If one could imagine a hypothetical society in which the needs and desires of all the members were fully met, and, in exchange, everyone had to do some job eight hours a day, the answer to the question of an ideal employment situation becomes readily obvious. If all of a person's needs and desires were met in exchange for eight hours of work each day, what would that person be doing during those eight hours? Whatever the answer to that question is would be an optimal employment situation.

Calcium and Osteoporosis

Television commercials, doctors, and friends all have us convinced to take a Calcium supplement to prevent or reverse osteoporosis. In advanced cases, the medical doctor might prescribe some medication that promises to reverse the condition. Osteoporosis is quite a significant problem for the elderly, one traumatic fall is all it takes to shatter the pelvis or fracture a bone. The problem arises not because of the fracture itself, but, at an advanced age, healing of the fracture is very slow to occur, resulting in complications that are not seen in younger patients. Surgery is often required which is followed by several months of healing time, not to mention weeks or months of rehabilitation of the affected area.

Osteoporosis is largely preventable. The mineral portion of the bone is a mineral called hydroxyapatite. The molecular formula of hydroxyapatite is $Ca_5(PO_4)_3(OH)$. Two molecules of hydroxyapatite are required to form the crystalline unit found in bone tissue. Bone also contains other trace minerals, such as Copper, and Potassium. Osteoporosis occurs when hydroxyapatite is broken down to restore depleted Calcium levels in the blood. If the breakdown of hydroxyapatite is prevented, osteoporosis can be prevented.

Ingestion of Calcium alone is insufficient to reverse or halt osteoporosis. Attempting to prevent osteoporosis through Calcium therapy, in fact, causes other disorders. When dietary Calcium is elevated with respect to Magnesium, absorption of Magnesium is inhibited, and hypomagnesemia (decreased serum levels of Magnesium) results. Hypomagnesemia results in cardiac arrhythmias, weakness, muscle spasms, neurological complaints, loss of appetite, digestive system complaints, and certain personality changes. The intake of Calcium and Magnesium in the diet should be a 2:1 ratio; that is, for every 1000 mg. of Calcium ingested, 500 mg. of Magnesium should also be ingested. This nutritional balance is largely ignored by proponents of Calcium therapy.

Osteoporosis is often caused by excessive ingestion of carbonated beverages. From chemistry, we know that an acid is neutralized by an alkaline substance. Carbonated beverages contain phosphoric acid and carbonic acid. Phosphoric acid and carbonic acid must be neutralized by an alkaline substance in the body. Phosphoric acid is known to disrupt the Calcium / Phosphorous ratio of the blood. The Calcium ion, Ca^{++}, is the most convenient and best alkaline ion around, and is used by the body to neutralize the acid. Ingestion of carbonated beverages subsequently leads to a decrease in serum levels of Calcium. Since the physiology of the body is programmed to keep the serum Calcium level between 8.5 and 10.2 mg/dl, any deficit in serum levels is quickly restored by transferring Calcium from the bones to the blood. The elevated serum phosphate level and decreased serum Calcium level subsequently cause Calcium to be quickly removed from bones to restore homeostasis. Avoidance of carbonated beverages, then, is one of the best preventatives against osteoporosis.

Resistance training or weight bearing exercise also provides great protection against osteoporosis. Resistance training is often thought of as weightlifting, but done properly, Pilates, kayaking, swimming, and bicycling are also forms of resistance training. During resistance training, force is exerted against some resistance, which ultimately leads to greater physical strength. Resistance training not only increases the size of the muscles, but also increases the strength of the tendons and ligaments as well. The stress placed on the bone by the tendons during resistance training causes the bone to strengthen and become more dense. As a result, resistance training cannot only prevent osteoporosis, but reverse it as well.

Low Back Pain

Low back pain is defined as pain, muscle tension, or stiffness below the ribs and above the crest of the pelvis. Specifically, low back pain is along and adjacent to the region of the five lumbar vertebrae. Some authorities consider low back pain also to include the pelvic region and sacrum. Low back pain can also include sciatica, which is radicular pain felt in any combination of the posterior thigh, calf, and foot. Low back pain has several causes. The causes discussed in this section refers to biomechanically related low back pain, specifically, low back pain of a non-organic cause.

The pain associated with low back pain comes from multiple anatomical structures. Pain can be felt from any combination of the four structures affected, which include direct pressure of a disc on a nerve, the facet joint, ligaments, and the associated muscles. The first, and by far most serious of these sources of pain is the direct pressure of the disc on a nerve, causing radicular symptoms along the path of the nerve, also called sciatica. Direct pressure on the nerves can also cause muscular weakness. The facet joints, which are the pair of joints between each vertebra, are another possible source of pain. When any joint capsule is stretched, pain results, and the facet joints of the spine are no exception. Ligaments can also be a contributing source of low back pain. Ligamentous pain typically feels like a dull ache. Muscle spasms are almost always present when low back pain is present. In the case of severe low back pain, the muscle spasms can be so intense that any movement at all is excruciating.

The medical approach to low back pain is symptomatic relief through the prescription of anti-inflammatory medications and muscle relaxants. In cases of severe low back pain, a pain killer may also be prescribed. A lumbar support brace is often prescribed, and is useful at times to give the muscles found in spasm some well needed rest. Oral anti-inflammatory medications address inflammation of the facet joint and surrounding muscular tissue. Oral anti-inflammatory medications are delivered to the tissues through the blood. Since the disc has no blood supply to speak of, anti-inflammatory medications do not significantly reduce disc-related inflammation. Ligaments also have a relatively poor blood supply, however, oral anti-inflammatory medications are more appropriate for a sprain because the tissues surrounding the ligament are what is primarily inflamed rather than the ligament itself. Medical treatment is focused primarily on symptom reduction. Nothing is typically done from a medical perspective to resolve any underlying causes of low back pain.

Chiropractors approach low back pain from a different perspective. Specifically, the goal of chiropractic care is to correct the cause of skeletally related low back pain. This involves correction of a condition known as a vertebral subluxation, in addition to the use of adjunct therapies focused upon the reduction of muscle spasms and reduction of the associated edema. When a subluxation occurs, in addition to the pain felt in the low back, nerve function is also found to be impaired. If a sufficient amount of pressure is exerted on a sensory nerve, pain, numbness, tingling, or any other altered sensation, can be felt anywhere along the path of the nerve. If pressure is placed on a motor nerve controlling a muscle, the muscle will either be weak or go into spasm. Chiropractic care will restore proper alignment of the vertebra, thus addressing the root cause of low back pain. In correcting the alignment of the spine, the causes of the inflammation and muscle spasms are removed.

Most low back pain can be attributed to one of two causes. The first cause of low back pain is weak abdominal musculature in comparison to the overall muscular strength of the rest of the body. The second common cause is tight hamstring muscles, located in the back of the thigh. Tight hamstring muscles are often accompanied by tight quadriceps muscles, which are located in the front of the thigh. Regardless of the treatment rendered, the underlying issues initially causing low back pain must be identified and addressed, otherwise the low back pain will be sure to return in the future.

The abdominal muscles are a very flat and wide muscle. Whenever a flat and wide muscle is found in the body, its primary function is most likely stabilization. Another muscle with this characteristic is the Tensor fascia lata muscle, which serves as a stabilization muscle of the thigh and pelvis. The purpose of the abdominal muscles, therefore, is to stabilize the body while standing erect. If the abdominal muscles are weak, the muscles of the low back are forced to take over the stabilization function of the abdominal muscles. The lumbar erector muscles of the low back are very strong muscles. Their primary function involves lifting movements, and is not considered a primary stabilizer muscle of the spine. Being forced to act as a stabilization muscle with little or no help from the weak abdominal muscles, the low back muscles will prematurely fatigue, most notably at the end of the day. In cases of severely weakened abdominal muscles, finding the lumbar erector muscles to be in a state of constant fatigue is not unusual. This fatigued state of the lumbar erector muscles causes the lumbar spine to be destabilized, thus drastically increasing the probability of an injury.

Persons with weak abdominal muscles are typically unable to perform sit-ups, crunches, or other abdominal exercises very well. In addition, these people generally have significant amounts of abdominal fat, which interferes with the stabilization function of the abdominal muscles, and places even a greater strain on the muscles of the low back. In the case of weak abdominal muscles, the muscles must be strengthened. Losing any fat around the abdominal area would also be beneficial, thus decreasing the physical stress on the entire body.

The hamstring muscles are located in the posterior region of the thigh. The hamstring muscles are unique in the sense that they are the only muscles outside the spine that cross two joints, the hip joint and the knee. The hamstring muscles originate at the pelvis and insert just below the knee. If these muscles are shortened and tight, the pelvis is tilted in such a way that the natural curve of the lumbar spine becomes hypolordotic, or flattened out. Any flattening of the normal curvature of the lumbar spine causes destabilization of the vertebral column, which results in both increased and unnatural pressures on the associated intervertebral discs. This can cause the spine to subluxate, subsequently causing the intervertebral discs to bulge and become inflamed, putting pressure on the sensitive nerves where they exit the spinal column. This bulging disc is sometimes improperly referred to as a slipped disc. If a disc is allowed to bulge for a period of months to years, the disc may herniate. If the disc further progresses to being severely herniated, it may eventually rupture, and will make a root canal look like quite a bit of fun in comparison. A disc rupture should be avoided at all costs.

In some instances of low back pain, the quadriceps, located in the front of the thigh, are found to be tight in addition to the tight hamstring muscles. When both muscle groups are tight, the mobility of the pelvis is severely restricted. Because the hamstring and quadriceps are very strong muscles, they exert a great restrictive force on pelvic movement during certain activities. Because of the decreased mobility of the pelvis, any stress placed on the pelvic region will most likely result in an injury to the muscles themselves, or injury to the lumbar spine. The low back, particularly the lower lumbar vertebrae at the base of the spine, must compensate for the lack of mobility of the pelvis. This compensation involves the lumbar vertebrae consistently being forced to its limits of motion; therefore, the susceptibility to injury increases. The spine and pelvis are held together by very strong ligaments. In comparison, the somewhat weaker ligaments and muscles of the low back, particularly at L4-L5, are therefore more vulnerable to injury. In any case, the weak link is the one most likely to suffer injury. The type of injury depends on the mechanics involved. The injury can be a muscular strain, ligamentous sprain, subluxated pelvis or lumbar vertebra, or any combination.

It must be pointed out that approximately 50 percent of the body's weight is above the L5 - sacral disc, located at the base of the spine. Weakening of the muscular structures in the abdominal area can place an inordinate amount of stress on the discs of the lower lumbar spine. This stress explains why the lumbar spine is the most probable location in the body to find a disc that has herniated.

Repetitive injuries to the same area of the body are an indication of an underlying structural weakness or imbalance. Once the acute phase of treatment is rendered and completed, and the pain removed, the second phase of treatment can begin. In this phase, which is not optional, properly identifying and correcting any underlying issues of musculoskeletal origin is the goal. Correction of these issues will involve exercise and stretching. The exercise prescribed depends on the underlying conditions present. Exercises must be individually tailored, taking biomechanical individuality into consideration, and must specifically address any strengths and weaknesses that may have developed over the years. Exercises that are beneficial for one person are often found to worsen a similar problem in another person. Since exercise prescription should be done on an individual basis, consulting a chiropractor, physical therapist, or skilled personal trainer who can deal with any issues at the appropriate level will result in the best possible outcome. Correcting these underlying conditions will take considerable time.

When low back pain has subsided, do not think that the actual problem has been corrected. Removal of the pain is only the first step. Prevention of future injuries requires that the underlying conditions be addressed.

Donating Blood

Blood is needed for emergencies, certain surgical procedures, and certain diseases such as sickle cell anemia. In rare cases, regular blood transfusions are needed by some people in order to sustain life. Donating blood is considered a noble thing to do, and it helps your fellow citizens in need.

Donating blood, however, does have its disadvantages. During a typical donation, approximately one pint is drawn. One pint is approximately 450 milliliters. The average adult has approximately five liters of blood. Therefore, during the donation process, about one tenth of the donors blood supply is removed. This includes one tenth of the circulating immune system as well. If one tenth of a person's bank account suddenly disappeared, they would certainly notice. If one tenth of the circulating immune system suddenly disappears, the body will similarly notice. The circulating immune system is not only consisting of leukocytes (white blood cells), but various antibodies, complement proteins, and other immune system components as well. Removal of this amount of the circulating immune system will result in a temporary state of immunodeficiency. Since the immune system is the primary defense against disease, careful consideration must be taken when donating blood, specifically in how the blood is donated.

Incidentally, five liters is about how much oil is in the average automobile. If the oil level in the automobile drops by one-half a liter, or approximately one-half a quart, most prudent people are quick to replenish the lost amount. In doing so, engine failure and any resultant repairs are avoided. How much more precious, then, is the blood that circulates in the body?

Guidelines regarding the frequency at which blood can be donated are often set by the organization who receives the donation, or by institutions who profit in some manner by the use or distribution of the donated blood. This is obviously a red flag and should arouse suspicion about whose interests are really at stake.

For the person who wants to donate blood, a process called apheresis can be used to return certain components, such as the leukocytes (white blood cells), to the bloodstream. This process is more time consuming than a regular donation session, and requires specialized equipment. This method is the preferred method to prevent any immunodeficiency due to the loss of white blood cells during the donation process.

Apheresis is expensive. Since any industry is focused upon lowering costs associated with operation, apheresis is not commonly offered as an option. Apheresis, specifically in the return of the white blood cells and other components to the donors blood supply, is clearly in the best interest of the donor. Lowering costs and increasing profit margins is in the best interests of the organizations receiving the donation. It does not take too much analysis to figure out the economic factors at play in the blood donation process.

While away on vacation at the beach, I contracted a case of conjunctivitis. Not wanting to go anywhere near a medical office, I looked around for any alternatives. The best alternative was right in front of me - the hotel swimming pool. The solution was simple; go under water and open my eyes a few times. The bromine in the pool should eliminate the infection. After all, bromine is used to kill any pathogens that may exist in the pool. The next day the infection was completely gone.

Why Am I Sick? And What To Do About It

Chapter 16
Zen

Many people are probably wondering why Zen has anything to do with the subject matter presented in this book. Earlier it was stated that a group of individuals can be found who rarely, if ever, get sick. This group is Zen masters. Since the Zen master rarely gets sick, studying why this is the case would be appropriate. While we are not suggesting everyone adopt the lifestyle of a Zen master, examining and incorporating some lifestyle habits of the Zen master into our own lives will prove beneficial. For any Christians reading this book, Jesus was the supreme Zen master of all time. Interestingly, Jesus never got sick, nor are there any recordings in the Scriptures of the apostles being laden with illness. Jesus and the Apostles lived a lifestyle quite different from that of modern day society. Interestingly, this lifestyle was similar to that of the Zen master.

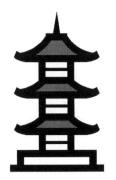

Just what does the Zen master do all day long that promotes the freedom from illness? This again, is asking the question in the wrong way. Answering the question directly will result in a daily list of activities, and will hardly do justice in obtaining true understanding of what we are seeking. So then, to answer the question, we will examine some basic Zen principles that will lead us to the answer, and then look at what the overall lifestyle of a Zen master is like. To do this though, we must have a basic understanding of Zen. With this understanding, the foundation is laid for the lifestyle of the Zen master.

The age-old saying that "if it can be explained in words, then it is not Zen" holds true even to this day. Nirvana, Zen enlightenment, the answers to Zen koans or "riddles" all cannot be truly expressed with the use of words, language or symbols. It does not stop here though. The understanding of such ideas can be grasped and understood, but the understanding cannot simply be transferred to another person using traditional methods of communication. This presents a dilemma in the sense that something is claimed to exist but cannot be readily explained or proven to another individual by using either analytical or other traditional methods. Understanding is granted to some, but seemingly denied to others. When the roadblocks to understanding are removed, understanding that was seemingly denied will become instantly clear, not only conceptually, but in experientially as well. Likewise, with health and healing, understanding is granted to some, but seemingly denied to others. The understanding of healing, similarly, is granted only when the roadblocks to true understanding are removed.

To gain understanding, comprehending a concept without the use of words is often necessary. This is because words distort the original meaning of the concept to be understood, thus opening the door to misunderstanding, misinterpretation, or something taken out of context. In Zen, understanding is most often transmitted in methods other than paragraphs composed of words and sentences. While many Zen writings exist, none can replace the understanding they are intended to impart.

One common method of transmitting understanding is the koan, which is a Zen riddle, used most notably in the Rinzai school as a method for transmitting understanding. To say that the answer to a koan can be expressed in words is simply wrong, because the only true answer is the experience of understanding. An example of a koan is:

> When you came into this world, did you fall into it as a star falling from the sky, or did you fall out of if, as a leaf falling from a tree?

Another example of a popular Zen koan is:

> Nan-in, a Japanese Zen master during the Meiji era (1868-1912), received a university professor who came to inquire about Zen. Nan-in served his guest tea. He poured his visitor's cup full, and then kept on pouring. The professor watched the overflow until he no longer could restrain himself. "It is overfull! No more will go in!" "Like this cup," Nan-in said, "you are full of your own opinions and speculations. How can I show you Zen unless you first empty your cup?"

The koan is not a question to be answered, but a concept to be grasped and understood in a method that defies traditional communication methods. The koan is intended to be meditated upon, using reflection, without the use of logical analysis and without the use of cumbersome words. Once the concept is grasped, the understanding of the concept is granted. Once words are used to express the concept, the concept is no longer pure, but tainted by the interpretation of one individual. If allowed to be expressed in words, the answer to the koan has as many interpretations as people attempting to interpret it. The purpose of the koan is to transmit understanding without the use of words.

The above Zen koan can be rewritten to help us gain understanding about the path to true healing. Our new version of the koan is:

> Dr. John, a local Chiropractor, received a patient who came to inquire about healing. Dr. John served his guest tea. He poured the patient's cup full, and then kept on pouring. The patient watched the overflow until he no longer could restrain himself. "It is overfull! No more will go in!" "Like this cup," Dr. John said, "you are full of your own opinions and beliefs. How can I show you the path to healing unless you first empty your cup?"

Our new version would lead us down the path of emptying our cup. What is in the cup are knowledge and preprogrammed notions regarding health care and the treatment of illness and disorders. In emptying our cup, we become as a child, and able to accept and understand new wisdom, leading us to the true path to health and wellness. In our koan, this is what both Nan-in and Dr. John were attempting to communicate. In other words, if we are attempting to understand an alternative healing method within the framework of modern medicine, we have entered the study in a position of distinct disadvantage. We must first rid ourselves of preconceived ideas of healing, and study the alternative form of healing within its own framework of philosophy and methodology. Once preconceived notions of health and disease are discarded, we start with the proverbial clean slate, and are better equipped to find the true answers.

We can also write our own koan. Another koan applicable to our discussion of healing, specifically regarding the toxic environment we live in, is:

> Is it the poison in a man's environment that causing his body to be sick, or is it the thoughts of a man's mind that resulted in the environment becoming sick?

That, now, is certainly something to contemplate.

Children also involve themselves in contemplation of koans, often without the knowledge that they are doing so. Consider for a moment the age-old question posed to every grade school student at one time or another, which is:

> If a tree falls in the wilderness and there is no one around to hear it, does it make a sound?

The argument of whether the tree will make a sound will go on forever. Left-brained young scientists vs. right-brained philosophers in training continue to argue this question and the next generations will continue to debate the issue with just as much success. If a student comes along and ponders the question outside the traditional sense of argument and debate, the question can convey wisdom beyond the simple yes or no answer it demands. The question, when looked at in this way, raises other questions, such as a how can a person explain to a blind man what sight is, and how can a person describe the music of a symphony to a deaf person. More applicable to healing, we can contemplate how it can be explained to a chronically sick man what health really is, or to a healthy man what it is like to be sick? Words have little place in such contemplation.

Zen enlightenment, or a state in which one is aware of one's true nature is yet another example of a concept that cannot be expressed in words. This enlightenment is not necessarily a state of complete awareness. Complete awareness would be termed Nirvana, or the ultimate state of awareness, and the penultimate state of harmony. This enlightenment is more like the complete harmony of the body, mind and spirit. A Zen master is one who has gained the understanding of this concept through experience. To tell someone "do this and you will become a Zen master" or "read this and you will become enlightened" simply does not happen. No amount of logical thought, study, classes, questioning, reasoning or rationalization is the path to Zen enlightenment or Nirvana.   Nor will the answer come through thinking. Remember from the koan that its answer cannot truly be expressed in words. Zen enlightenment or Nirvana likewise cannot be expressed in words.

Occasionally someone would ask "what is it like to be a Zen master?" The only answer is "become one and find out," which on the surface, appears to be an evasive and annoyingly sarcastic answer but no answer can be closer to the truth. That, by the way, is the kind of answer one will usually get from a Zen master. Consider for a moment trying to explain to someone the experience of skydiving. Unless one has skydived, no written or verbal explanation can come close to satisfying communication of the experience. The answer would be "skydive and find out." Likewise, with experience of enlightenment obtained by the Zen master, many analogies exist, none can replace the experience. No writing can explain or describe Nirvana. No one who has experienced Nirvana can deny its existence, and no one who has not experienced Nirvana can understand the experience.

So what is this enlightenment like? How can we understand it? This is asking the wrong question, as many, by now, have probably guessed. Perhaps, though, the best way to begin contemplation of the experience is through analogies rather than a list of descriptive items. Yet, as with the koan, interpreting and understanding the analogy cannot be adequately expressed using words. The understanding offered by the analogy is best used as a contrast between the enlightened and unenlightened, or perhaps by the experience of the transition to enlightenment, and not taken literally. At best, the analogy offers a small glimpse into a world unknown.

Consider a stadium full of spectators watching a football game. Both observers and participants of the game are found in the stadium where the game is played. The observers have an eagle eye view of what is happening from the stands yet can offer no contribution to the outcome of the event.   The participants have a limited view, and with this limited view, are expected to perform in moving the ball toward the goal. Imagine now what it would be like to be a participant on the field with the view of the observer in the stands. That person would have a clear view of what is happening and can use this to an advantage in many ways to accomplish the goal. It does not stop here. Taking it one step further, imagine if this person can foresee, to some degree, the outcome of a particular play before it occurs therefore choosing the path correctly in each instance. This is the clear view of life experienced only by those who are enlightened.

Most people see the physical world, that is, the Earth, from a three-dimensional viewpoint. Length, height, and width are observed in everything we see from the ground. While technically three dimensions exist, there exists a stumbling block to see that which is much greater. Imagine now that someone is in an airplane or helicopter and sees for the first time a view of their city from the air. This is, no doubt, a different perspective than most people are accustomed. Places, roads, buildings suddenly are in perspective with each other. The view, as seen from the sky, appears to take on a whole new dimension. What is odd is that from the air, the view more resembles a two-dimensional view, rather than the three-dimensional view seen from the ground. By removing one dimension, we see much more, gain a greater perspective, and create a paradox in the process. Again, going one step further, imagine if someone can see this view from the ground somehow. The ability to understand both perspectives simultaneously versus only one or the other illustrates the difference between the enlightened and unenlightened.

Nirvana can be described as fully accepting all that comprises one's life. Every situation and its outcome is viewed in the sense "whatever will be, will be." No attempt is made to force an experience into what it is not. No attempt is made to force the future into something that cannot be, for such an action is futile anyway and may be likened to chiseling a 50-foot granite statue using a mere stick of wood. Consider, for example, if the computer used in writing this manuscript were suddenly destroyed and no backup copy of the text existed. One choice would be to lament and toil over the fact that the work was lost forever and will take years to replace. The other would be to fully accept the disaster and to be of the attitude that, since it is lost, there is no reason to be concerned about it any longer.

Many writings exist that attempts to point one toward enlightenment or Nirvana. Once the line is crossed into enlightenment, the writings which once served as the roadmap diminish in value to the point that they are no longer of any use. This is similar to a roadmap being no longer useful once a person has gotten to their destination. Similarly, the instructions for assembling a bicycle are no longer of much value once the assembly is complete. This is exactly what is true of Dharma, or the law associated with Zen Buddhism. Once enlightened, the Dharma may be discarded by the newly enlightened master, for the destination has been reached.

Zazen, or the "sitting practice" the Zen master's meditation, is meditation in which the desired result is to cease all thinking, remaining open beyond dualistic, comparative, judgmental, and interpretive thought and is said to be enlightenment. Zazen is done without any goal or object of concentration. This is the ultimate expression of experiencing one's own existence. Again, as with the concepts previously visited, it is an experience that cannot be described in words, but, instead, the experience itself communicates all understanding.

Take a few moments and meditate without any thought process. You will probably find that your mind will drift from topic to topic, perhaps revisiting the events of the day or thinking about what you will do in the next hour. Realizing that this has occurred, you will again attempt to stop thinking. In an instant the thought process occurs again. You undoubtably will get to the point eventually when you are aware that you are not thinking. At this point you are actually thinking since you are aware that you are not thinking. This is not Zazen. In true Zazen, you are aware of the state and experience it, yet unaware that you have entered it. Nevertheless, you know that you are there. Words have no part in the Zazen experience.

Zazen is difficult; however, Zazen is very simple and easy. Zazen brings up another concept, the concept of Ku. Ku, a Japanese word, is defined as "emptiness" or "void." In the context of Zazen, emptiness is not truly void in the sense that the absence of thinking is not an absence of experience. Emptiness in this regard is not truly empty. The concept of being empty without emptiness is expressed in the sense that thought has ceased, but experiences continue without the interpretation of thought processes. In other words, life is experienced without verbal, or linguistic interpretation, therefore experienced in its purest sense. Those who go off and explore this world will never see the everyday world in the same way again.

Another way in which to meditate, without any involved thought, is to focus all attention on music. Selecting the right type of music is imperative, instrumental music used for relaxation is perhaps the best type for this form of meditation. This type music is often used during a therapeutic massage session. Other selections desirable for meditation are music in which the words are in a foreign language, instrumental music, or classical music. Rock music is simply not conducive to meditation. A high quality sound reproduction system is best for this purpose, since the reproduced audio is very close to that of a live performance. In a dimly lit room, sitting in a comfortable position, the attention is simply focused on the music. Once the music is perceived without any interference from thought processes, the music will sound as if the wall has dropped, the music will sound as if is both much closer and much farther away than the speakers are, and every note of the music will sound crystal clear. The music sounds as if it takes on a three-dimensional quality. No words will do justice in describing what this experience is like.

Other activities can benefit greatly when performed without any intervening thought process. Playing a musical instrument is a perfect example of this type of activity. If a drummer plays music without any associated thought about what he or she is doing, the rhythm and timing, in a way, just happen. The beat comes out with unprecedented ease in an undescribably fluid manner. When the drummer, however, begins to introduce words and thought processes while playing, for example "at the end of the next measure I will drop the hi-hat hit and replace it with a cymbal crash-splash combo," he or she will immediately lose timing, be offbeat, and it is all over after that. If the

Why Am I Sick? And What To Do About It

drummer, however, just does what was intended as if it is second nature, whatever intended change to the beat occurs flawlessly, without any intervention of words. In this way, thought patterns and any associated words interfere with the expression of music. Words have very little use to the musician while playing a musical instrument.

By this time, many will be convinced that not everything can be expressed in words. The truth is that very little, for that matter, can be accurately or adequately expressed in words. In some cases, words become a barrier to understanding. Words and the sentences they form may be thought of as accurate and reliable way of distorting what is intended to be communicated. For example, someone may say that the grass is green. So are the leaves on a tree. So is the color of the bug that happens to be eating the tree. Many shades of green can be seen in the landscape, so when we say something is "green," we no longer have an exact concept of what color is actually being described. To more accurately describe the green color of the grass, we can depict it as a graphical spectrum displaying the wavelengths of light reflected from the blades in their proper proportions. We can hire a physicist to describe the particular color in very specific undisputable scientific terms. To look at the grass and to see its color, we understand and experience the color without any words at all. The experience of actually seeing the color renders all other methods of communicating the color useless. Once the color is visualized, communication of the color is complete and perfect. This is Zen, and we may as well call it the Zen of color.

Zen requires the understanding of a concept to be understood by experience. Verbal or written descriptions prove inadequate to transmit understanding to another individual or provide true understanding of the concept in question. Once the concept is truly understood, it becomes evident to the one who has the understanding that the true understanding cannot be communicated using traditional means anyway. This is very evident to those who have the understanding, but not to those who do not have the understanding. In other words, it is very evident to those who are enlightened but not to those who are unenlightened.

Those who are enlightened and those are not enlightened becomes very evident when examining different healing philosophies. Western healing philosophy is seemingly devoid of any type of practice that cannot be proven analytically, in the laboratory, or by today's science. Ironically, tomorrow's science will prove what we already know to be true today. In Western civilization one must prove that something works in order for it to be accepted. For example, the conceptual model of the body, mind and spirit has been known and clearly understood for thousands of years. The model has been developed independently by numerous cultures over the ages with the same template discovered and documented repeatedly. This cannot simply be a coincidence. Western philosophy demands that the body-mind-spirit relationship be proven analytically. Eastern philosophy demands that any disbeliever in the body-mind-spirit relationship prove that both the concept and relationship do not exist. Yet when the subject of the body-mind-spirit arises, many who subscribe to the Western philosophy are quick to dismiss the concept as new age, religious, unproven, unscientific, or not relevant to healing today.

Genesis, Chapter 1, Verse 26 begins by stating ""Then God said, "Let Us make man in Our image," a clear reference to the Trinity. The term "Us" refers to the Father, Son, and Holy Spirit. This verse states that man is made in the image of the Trinity, specifically the mind parallels the mind of God, the spirit parallels that of the Holy Spirit, and the body parallels the body of Jesus. By not accepting the body-mind-spirit model, we have moved out of the realm of reality, and have entered a fictional realm where true healing then becomes a fantasy. It is no wonder, then, why many modern medical methods that address only the healing of the physical body fail miserably.

Understanding the process of healing through the spirit cannot always be expressed in words, nor can every procedure be described in a "how to" manual. Healing methods that heal through the spirit, such as Acupuncture, Reiki, reflexology, and Applied Kinesiology, among others, may be difficult to understand and comprehend. The education required to learn many of these healing methods is beyond that of medical school. A different level of understanding is to be grasped, but when someone knows and comprehends the concepts, they will then know that they have the understanding. What was previously a plethora of seemingly unrelated concepts comes together in a moment of time to make perfect sense. The veil is dropped and understanding becomes crystal clear. The one who gains this enlightenment immediately knows without any doubt whatever of its reality.

Just what, then, does the Zen master do all day long that promotes longevity, health and wellness? In the beginning of our discussion on Zen, we stated that the Zen master has attained enlightenment, which is perfect harmony of the body, mind, and spirit. This perfect harmony of body, mind, and spirit was also part of our definition of true health. The Zen student is attempting to obtain this enlightenment, learning many things from the Zen master. The secret of how to remain healthy, however, is not to be found on the list of things to learn. This leads us to believe that it is the learned lifestyle that is conducive to health. When we examine the lifestyle further, we will discover that it is not only the lifestyle that is conducive to health, but the attitude toward life as well.

The Zen master lives a lifestyle quite different that most of society. Some Zen masters live in a Zendo, a place where Zen is practiced. Others commute to their daily job, do their job, and go home like any other person in today's society. No matter where the Zen master lives and works, they rarely get sick. The Zen master is exposed to the same pathogens that everyone else is, yet rarely gets sick. The Zen master is exposed to the same potential stressors as everyone else is, and rarely get sick. The difference between the Zen master and anyone else in society is that the Zen master attempts to live in perfect harmony with their surroundings without regard to what those surroundings might be.

The Zen master does not attempt to change things that they cannot change. If something cannot be changed, no waste of mental or physical energy is used to try to change it. No reason is found to play the game of mental gymnastics, thinking in circles, or constantly worrying about something that cannot be controlled. Thinking of this sort can only lead to emotional frustration, and in some cases, emotional pain. A peace that surpasses all understanding can be found in accepting things as they are. To try to change what cannot be changed is futile, and can only lead to anxiety and frustration. To accept the current circumstances, and to move forward, is the natural way of thinking of the Zen master.

The Zen master rarely, if ever, moves past the alarm phase of the General Adaption Syndrome described by Hans Selye. If the alarm phase is entered, any stressor present would most likely be a natural event followed by the appropriate response. This would result in no long term consequences, therefore not leading to any disease process. This lack of stress, as a result of the state of mind of the Zen master, is quite a different state of mind than the average person found in society today. By not allowing external circumstances to affect thought patterns and emotion negatively, the adaption phase of the General Adaption Syndrome cannot be entered. By not being subject to chronic stress, the Zen master avoids chronic disease.

Living in perfect harmony with the physical environment is one of our requirements of health. The Zen master living in a Zendo can be found eating natural foods, often grown at the Zendo whenever feasible, or purchased from the local farmer's market. Following meals, it is time to quiet the mind, a time to rest and reflect. Meditation is often done in nature or in a room specifically designed for this purpose. At the Zendo, work sessions are common, and several hours a day are spent working, both inside and outside. Opposing modern Western tradition, the newer students are assigned light duties and simple tasks, and the more senior members and advanced students perform the heavy duties and more difficult tasks. For example, the Roshi, the spiritual leader of the Zendo, is very often the one who cleans the toilet. The new student may walk around with a check list and make sure everything has been done. Contrast that with modern day business where the Chairman of the Board of a major corporation often cannot even lift a finger to place a phone call, but, instead, instructs an administrative assistant to place the call for him or her. People at the Zendo work together toward a common goal. The work is not unlike any other work, it is just done with a different attitude, an attitude of gratefulness that there is work to do. In the Zendo, no stress, worry, or anxiety is found, only peace. In addition, no office politics, no corporate ladder, no fast food, and no rush hour traffic are found either.

Outside the Zendo, a Zen master might have a job similar to the job anyone else in society may have. The Zen master might be living around the corner, working in a local store, or repairing your home or automobile. Although the environment is quite different from that of the Zendo, the inner attitude of the Zen master is the same. It is not the environment that matters; it is the perfect harmony with that environment that is the issue. Whether the environment is the peace and tranquility of the Zendo, or at home in the big city, perfect harmony with the environment is the Zen master's way of life. This gives us concrete evidence that it is the mind set of the individual, and not the physical environment itself, that allows one to attain perfect harmony with the environment.

Living in perfect harmony within our social environment is also one of our requirements of health. This is also a characteristic of the Zen master. Everyone at the Zendo has a common goal. That goal is enlightenment, which is the perfect harmony of the body, mind, and spirit. As a result of this enlightenment, perfect harmony with the social environment also becomes a reality. This perfect harmony is not limited, however, to only the Zen master or those in the Zendo. Perfect harmony within the social environment can be obtained by anyone and anywhere in society.

A life of perfect harmony is the same type life Jesus lead. Jesus worked, meditated, prayed, taught, and lived a perfect life in perfect harmony. Jesus did not worry about anything, but, instead, trusted in his Father to provide all. By every stroke and letter, Jesus fulfilled perfectly the definition of health.

How odd, then, is it that the followers of Jesus today abandon the very ways He taught and illustrated? In some circles, a strong denial is found that health and healing can actually occur outside the medical arena. Any suggestion that faith should be placed in divine healing is treated essentially as a backup plan. Any suggestion to anoint a sick person with oil is quickly dismissed as something they did before the existence of modern medicine, whoever *they* may be. Suggestions to return to eating a natural diet are all too often dismissed as an extremist position, never mind the fact that the person offering the suggestion is quite healthy in comparison to everyone else. Anyone offering advice on living a healthy lifestyle and is often labeled as a health nut or considered to have a backward view in such a modern society. Worst of all, any prayers offered for the sick are secretly cast in doubt, and the people offering the prayers secretly place their faith in the medical system, not in God. The words "Thy will be done" are secretly meant to mean "my will be done." In reality, what we really want is for God to heal all the sick people that we are a little concerned about, offer a little praise, and then move on and forget. The notion that God does not heal someone because He perhaps wants us to learn something about the body and take better care of it seems all too foreign to accept. Anyone even suggesting such a possibility would typically be shunned or thought to have an unloving attitude. The better path would be to return to the ways instructed by God, the Creator. God is the creator. Humans are the creation. The creation does not tell the Creator what to do.

What happens quite frequently is that people live a lifestyle in complete contradiction to that which is conducive to health. They then wonder why they have contracted some disease. With this being the case, wisdom would suggest that the ways of the healthy be studied so that we can learn from them, no matter whom they are. In adopting the wisdom of their healthy lifestyle, the health they enjoy will also follow.

A mirror is interesting in the sense it presents a paradox. The paradox is that the mirror can appear to be two colors at once, both silver and the color it is reflecting.

Why Am I Sick? And What To Do About It

Chapter 17
Exercise

Exercise should be part of most people's lives. Before everyone breathes a sigh of relief and believes they are not included in *most people's lives*, read on. People generally fall into three categories, those who desperately need exercise, those who desperately need rest, and those who get the correct amount of exercise. Very few people, however, are found in the latter group.

The group of people who are getting the correct amount of exercise is already living and enjoying a healthy lifestyle. They are somewhere in the upper 5 percent of the population in terms of physical fitness. They have always been involved with athletics to some degree, and typically excel at just about any sport in which they participate. Additionally, over their lifetime, they have participated in a variety of sports, and typically have not focused on any one particular activity. After work they meet their friends with whom they 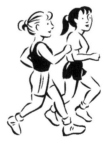 may go to the gym, play racquetball, attend a yoga class, or go for a swim or run. Exercise, however, does not dominate their life. People in this group know how to play hard, work hard, and rest well.

The group who desperately needs rest can usually be found in a job that requires physical labor on a daily basis. Construction workers, landscapers, lumberjacks, and laborers generally fall into this category. This type of employment entails constant physical activity, day after day. Persons in this group most likely do not need additional strengthening exercises. When it is time to move from one home to another, this is the person everyone wants around since he can move your washing machine all by himself. Detoxification would be more applicable to persons in this group because the muscles are working to their limit and beyond, and the by-products of metabolism accumulate within the tissue. Stretching would also be of great value to persons in this group, since overworked muscles have a tendency to tighten and shorten over time, which would be relieved by stretching.

The vast majority of the population comprises the third group, the group who desperately needs exercise. The people found in this group encompass everyone not found in the first two groups. Anyone who does not exercise or has a sedentary lifestyle can typically found in this group. Nearly all chronic disease sufferers can also be found in this group.

Physical inactivity has long been recognized as a risk factor for coronary artery disease, blood lipid abnormalities, high cholesterol, diabetes, elevated blood pressure, and obesity. Muscles that are not used become shortened and inelastic, and therefore become more prone to injury. Ligaments that are not stretched become tight and inflexible, and, like the muscles, also become more susceptible to injury. Decreased levels of physical conditioning also contribute to osteoporosis. Lack of exercise or physical activity also contributes to depression and anxiety. If this sounds like a depressing and bleak picture, it is because it is. Perhaps looking at this subject in a more positive sense is better, in order to gain a better perspective.

Physical activity has long been recognized as a significant contributor to overall health. Persons involved in regular physical activity have a significantly lower risk of all types of cardiovascular disease. In persons who exercise regularly, cholesterol is rarely an issue, and diabetes, elevated blood pressure, and obesity are of no concern since these diseases are virtually unheard of in physically fit individuals. Exercise maintains muscle mass and preserves the flexibility of ligaments. Resistance training not only strengthens the muscles, but helps maintain bone density, and helps maintain ligament and tendon strength. Increased levels of physical activity also contribute to a positive mental outlook. Exercise also promotes sound and restful sleep. Physical activity is high on the list of preventive measures one can take to ensure a life free from chronic disease. By looking at exercise in the positive sense, getting excited and motivated to begin a physical fitness program is much easier.

A widely held belief exists that physical fitness only applies to the musculoskeletal system. Nothing, however, can be further from the truth. Physical fitness not only applies to the entire body, but extends its benefits to the mind as well. This can easily be seen when that overly energetic, perpetually happy relative who is always going on some mountain climbing expedition or traveling to Boston to run in a marathon shows up at a holiday gathering. This person often bubbles out a positive attitude in every direction to the extent that others may begin to wonder whether he or she is bipolar or taking some sort of illegal pill. The truth is all this person has been doing is exercising, and a positive mental attitude is merely a side effect of the physical activity.

Why Am I Sick? And What To Do About It

Many people have been involved in physical activity and sports their entire life. In adopting a healthy lifestyle at an early age, and continuing this lifestyle into adulthood, chronic disease and illness have most likely been averted. The physically active person is often found to have a healthy diet, another characteristic contributing to overall health. John Nitti, a running back for the New York Jets in the early 1980s, has lived such a lifestyle his entire life. As of the date of this publication, Mr. Nitti still engages in running, bicycling and weightlifting, long after his football career has ended. While many people, just like Mr. Nitti, have been engaged in physical activity their whole life, others have avoided physical activity for one reason or another. It is never too late, however, to begin an exercise program.

Everyone has the ability to choose which group they belong to. Only two choices are available, the healthy and physically fit, or chronically diseased and physically unfit. The decision can be made right now to move from the physically unfit to the physically fit. Simply going for a ten or fifteen minute walk, doing a few pushups, or taking two dumbbells and exercising for a few minutes is a step in the correct direction. Some exercise is better than none at all. Five to seven hours of exercise a week is all it really takes to maintain reasonable physical fitness.

Various types of exercise exist and are categorized based upon various criteria. One categorization is done at the biochemical level, defining exercise as either aerobic exercise or anaerobic exercise. Another categorization defines the exercise based upon the goal at hand. Strength training, endurance training, flexibility training, and agility training represent goal-orientated classifications of exercise. Goal-oriented training includes both anaerobic and aerobic forms of exercise. In addition, specific training for various sports is often a combination of the various types of exercise. Any good exercise program should consist of a variety of exercise types.

Aerobic exercise refers to exercise performed in which adequate amounts of oxygen reaching the muscle cells. During aerobic exercise, the body synthesizes 38 molecules of ATP from each molecule of glucose, a very efficient biochemical pathway of energy production. This is the standard pathway of energy production for all metabolic functions in the body. Aerobic exercise utilizes this primary energy pathway. Aerobic exercise is exercise of moderate intensity, and is typically performed for an extended time without rest, generally greater than thirty minutes. Aerobic exercise increases the body's need for oxygen, and requires the heart and lungs to work harder. Distance running and bicycling are good examples of aerobic exercise.

Anaerobic exercise, on the other hand, refers to exercise which is performed without sufficient oxygen reaching the muscle cells. This involves a different pathway in the Krebs cycle than does aerobic exercise. In anaerobic exercise, two molecules of ATP are produced from each molecule of glucose, as opposed to the 38 molecules of ATP produced in the aerobic pathway. This is performed by the enzyme *lactate dehydrogenase*. This alternative pathway is much less efficient that the aerobic pathway. Anaerobic exercise is exercise of high intensity. Exercise of this type requires short bursts of very intense exertion, in which the glycogen is metabolized without sufficient amounts of oxygen reaching the cells. Weight training is the most popular form of anaerobic exercise. Sprinting is an anaerobic form of running. During anaerobic exercise, fewer calories are burned than during aerobic exercise. The goal of anaerobic exercise it to build strength and muscle mass, as a result, anaerobic exercise is somewhat less beneficial for cardiovascular fitness. The increase in muscle mass causes a person to become leaner and subsequently lose weight, because muscle tissue metabolizes a significantly greater number of calories when compared with other tissues of the body, even while at rest.

Agility training develops those skills specifically involved needed for the body to make abrupt changes in motion at will, and doing so in a precisely controlled manner. These abrupt changes in motion are generally required as a response to the actions of other competitors in a fast paced sport, such as basketball or football. Agility training also increases coordination. Other sports in themselves, such as gymnastics and springboard diving, are purely forms of agility training. Agility training is primarily a training protocol of the mind, developing those neurological pathways involved in coordination. Agility training also encompasses dance, wrestling, martial arts, and competitive diving. Earning seven Olympic gold medals and nine world championships, Shannon Miller, an American gymnast, exemplifies agility in every sense of the word.

Endurance training is a combination of aerobic and anaerobic exercise. This type of training is often associated with sports at the competitive level. Endurance training combines the goal of increasing strength with increasing aerobic capacity. The type and amount of endurance training will vary based upon the specific demands of the sport. Some competitive sports, such as bicycle racing or speed skating, require superior aerobic fitness combined with great strength and power. Eric Heiden, MD, a speed skater who won an unprecedented five Olympic gold medals and set four Olympic records in 1980, is a perfect example of a master of endurance training.

Flexibility training refers specifically increasing the range of motion of the joints. This is primarily accomplished through stretching. When stretching comes to mind, we often think of stretching muscles, but a stretching program also targets the ligaments as well, making the more elastic and pliable, therefore less susceptible to injury. Stretching is generally incorporated into any other exercise protocol. Stretching can be either active or passive. Practicing Yoga is an excellent method to increase range of motion, and decreasing muscle tension, and is an example of active stretching. Passive stretching requires another person to exert force against the muscles and joints, allowing for a more effective stretching of the muscles involved. Passive stretching requires some knowledge of biomechanics and certain specialized skills. Personal trainers, massage therapists, and chiropractors have extensive knowledge of the techniques of passive stretching. When flexibility comes to mind, one might think that a gymnast is a perfect example of one who is flexible. While this is true, Olympic wrestlers, springboard divers, world-class runners, and martial arts competitors all exemplify superior flexibility.

Strength training is often equated with anaerobic exercise. This, however, is not necessarily the case. Strength training is specifically designed to increase muscular strength. The Olympic weightlifter and power lifter are both prime examples of athletes who participate in strength training. Strength training involves performing maximal muscular contractions against some form of resistance. Weightlifting, particularly with low repetitions (1-3 repetitions per set), isometric training, and resistance training are forms of strength training. Strength training in which a single repetition is performed with very heavy weight does not raise metabolic levels sufficiently enough to be classified as a purely an anaerobic exercise. This is because, during the lift, sufficient oxygen already exists in the muscle tissue to perform the lift, and the anaerobic pathways are not activated to any further extent. Strength training utilizes both the anaerobic and aerobic pathways, but does not stress the pathway to the degree of either anaerobic or aerobic exercise. When we think of strength training, people like Arnold Schwarzenegger, Vasili Alexeyev, and Paul Anderson all come to mind. In different ways, these athletes have taken center stage as a master of strength training.

When developing an exercise program, incorporating several different types of exercise is desirable. A well-designed exercise program will include both anaerobic training and aerobic training, with a good stretching program to increase the mobility of the joints. Modifying any exercise program from time to time is also preferable. Repeating the same activities has a tendency to cause strengths and weaknesses to develop. If a muscle is constantly used in a certain way, it will become stronger in comparison to other muscles in that region of the body. When this happens, the body becomes more prone to injury. Likewise, when a muscle is not challenged by a particular exercise program, a relative weakness may develop, also increasing the risk of injury. By modifying the program, the body is challenged in new ways, therefore promoting balance by not allowing the strengths and weaknesses to develop.

When a person casually observes the activities in a typical gym, one can see people training the same muscles with the same exercises day after day, week after week. With hundreds of exercises to choose from, the amateur athletes found in the gym can be found performing the same ten or fifteen exercises during each workout session. This causes disproportionate great strength in certain muscle groups at the expense of significant weakness in other muscle groups. Since most musculoskeletal injuries are a result of muscular imbalances, limiting the types of exercises performed is inviting injury. In varying the workout program and incorporating a variety of exercises, balance of the muscle groups is promoted, therefore avoiding potential injury.

When training in the gym, unless someone is familiar with training protocols, seeking the guidance of a personal trainer is wise. When selecting a personal trainer, make sure he or she has obtained a certification in personal training from a recognized organization. Certified personal trainers are very familiar with proper exercise techniques, and are well able to identify any strengths and weakness that may be present. Subsequently, the personal trainer can custom tailor an exercise program designed on an individual basis, taking into account the many factors unique to any person. The personal trainer can also offer expert instruction in the use of the various machines that are found in the gym. The proper use of these machines is very important; if they are used incorrectly, injuries may result.

When beginning a resistance training program, gaining weight in the first few weeks is more common than to lose weight. This weight gain should not be of concern, and should not discourage anyone. The weight gain is generally attributed to the increased muscle mass, and not an increase in body fat. Deconditioned muscles adapt very quickly when subjected to resistance training. Specifically, the increase in muscle mass is attributed to both increased protein levels in the muscles and carbohydrate reserves, and not due to an increase in fat reserves. As a result of the increase in muscle mass, the body's basal metabolic rate is also increased. An increased basal metabolic rate results in the body burning more calories even while at rest. For these reasons, when beginning to exercise, measuring progress by looking in the mirror is better than measuring progress by using a scale.

Gyms are also equipped with various types of machines designed for an aerobic workout. These include treadmills, stair climbers, exercise bicycles, and elliptical trainers, to name just a few. Again, as with resistance exercise, preferred training programs will use a variety of these exercise machines to work all the muscles involved in as many ways as possible. The purpose of exercising on these machines is to raise the heart rate within the range required for aerobic activity. Table 17.1 shows the target heart rate for an individual based upon age. The theoretical maximum heart rate is also included in this table. Aerobic exercise requires that the heart rate remain in the aerobic target range, as indicated in the table. This table assumes a normal, otherwise healthy individual. If any chronic disease process exists, especially involving the cardiovascular system, it is recommended that the target heart rate, and duration of the workout be determined by your health practitioner. In addition, the table does not apply to persons taking certain medications, including, but not limited to, beta blockers and Calcium antagonists.

An individual's maximum theoretical heart rate is calculated to be 220 minus their age. The aerobic target is calculated as 60 to 80 percent of the maximum heart rate. When this target is reached during exercise, it is termed the aerobic threshold. A heart rate monitor can be used to tell when a person has reached the aerobic threshold. When a person starts breathing more deeply and the exercise becomes more difficult, it is a good indication of approaching the aerobic threshold. Aerobic exercise should, under normal conditions, be sustained for minimally 20 minutes. The American College of Sports Medicine recommends that aerobic activities should be performed for 20 to 60 minutes for maximal benefit. The duration of the aerobic session also depends on many factors, such as current physical condition or any pre-existing medical conditions. Severely deconditioned individuals, for example, may be able to engage in an aerobic workout for less than ten minutes, particularly when beginning an exercise program. The duration of the aerobic session, in this case, would be increased as progress is made. In every case, follow the health care practitioner's advice regarding exercise. He or she is familiar with any issues that may exist and will prescribe an exercise program accordingly.

Age	Theoretical Maximum Heart Rate	Aerobic Target Range
20	200	120–160
25	195	117–156
30	190	114–152
35	185	111–148
40	180	108–144
45	175	105–140
50	170	102–136
55	165	99–132
60	160	96–128
65	155	93–124
70	150	90–120

Table 17.1   Aerobic Target Heart Rate

Even while at rest, the body burns calories. The number of calories burned increases with increased physical activity. Table 17.2 shows the number of calories burned per hour for light activities.

Activity	150 Pound Person	175 Pound Person	200 Pound Person
Gardening	300	340	390
Shopping	250	295	335
Sitting	75	90	100
Sleeping	70	85	95
Standing	145	165	190
Walking – 4 mph	310	365	420

Table 17.2   Calories Burned Per Hour
Light Activities

When exercising to lose weight, how much weight lost is proportional to the number of calories burned. The number of calories burned during various activities varies greatly. In general, the greater the intensity of the activity, the more calories are burned. At the beginning of a workout session, fat and carbohydrate are burned at approximately a 50:50 ratio. As the workout session continues, the percentage of fat burned increases as carbohydrate reserves are depleted. After one hour of intense training, approximately 70 percent of the calories burned can come from fat. If the goal of exercise is to reduce fat reserves, longer workout sessions are recommended. Table 17.3 shows several types of exercises and the number of calories burned per hour. The figures stated in this table, and any similar table for that matter, will generally be plus or minus 25% from the actual amount any particular person may expend during the indicated activity. Overall, the table provides a rough guideline of the comparison of various activities.

Replacing the carbohydrates depleted during a workout session is important. How much carbohydrate that needs to be replaced is dependent on the number of calories burned during the workout. This amount is quite easy to calculate. Assuming that fat and carbohydrate were burned at a 50:50 ratio, half the calories expended were in the form of carbohydrate. This means that half the calories expended during the workout session must be replaced to restore the reserves of carbohydrate in the muscles and the liver to a normal level. The other half of the calories expended during the workout were obtained from fat, and, if the goal is to lose weight, these calories should not be replaced. From the chapter on nutrition, we learned that four calories are found in one gram of carbohydrate. Dividing half the calories expended during the workout session by four will tell us how many grams of carbohydrate must be consumed to restore the body's reserves. Another way to arrive at the grams of carbohydrate that needs to be replaced is to divide the total calories expended during the workout session by eight. When replacing the carbohydrate burned during a workout, the calories consumed must come from carbohydrate.

The importance of replenishing the carbohydrate burned during a workout cannot be understated; failure to do so will result in fatigue and irritability. In addition, failure to restore carbohydrate levels can cause the body to perceive starvation, and anything eaten will quickly contribute to the fat reserves of the body. The best sources of carbohydrate are those foods with a low glycemic index, as discussed in the chapter on nutrition. One exception to this rule, however, can be found. For a short time, generally 20 minutes, following a strenuous workout, glucose can pass through the cell membrane without the aid of insulin. Refined carbohydrates, in the form of commonly available sports drinks, can be ingested during this window and will quickly and efficiently replace the carbohydrates burned during the workout. Sports drinks are also formulated to replace electrolytes lost when sweating. The person on the treadmill who is drinking a sports drink is replacing the carbohydrate during his or her workout. This is, by far, the most efficient way to replenish the body's carbohydrate reserves.

The ideal body fat composition for a male is 12 to 20 percent. For a female, the ideal body fat composition is 15 to 25 percent. A digital body composition monitor can be purchased to monitor the progress of losing body fat. Body composition monitors are often incorporated into digital scales, and can also be purchased as a hand-held stand-alone unit. These devices provide a digital readout showing the percentage of body fat. Digital body composition monitors are more accurate and easier to use than the skin caliper method used decades ago. Tables associated with skin calipers assume that 50 percent of the body's fat reserves are stored between the muscle and the skin, and the other 50 percent is stored within the muscle. The percentage of body fat stored in either location is genetically determined, and few people fall into the 50/50 distribution ratio. Digital units have a distinct advantage in that they are accurate regardless of where the fat is stored. When using a digital body composition monitor, measuring body fat at the same time of the day is preferred. When using a digital body composition monitor, more accurate results can be obtained if a meal or water has not been consumed for two hours prior to its use.

Persons with impaired glucose tolerance should closely follow the advice of their health care practitioner regarding exercise. The person with adult onset Type II Diabetes will need to monitor their blood sugar levels closely when engaging in an exercise program. Glucose tolerance improves with increased physical activity; adjustments to medications are often required by the Type II diabetic. The person with Type I Diabetes will also need to monitor blood sugar levels, particularly around the times of increased physical activity. Adjustments in insulin levels or the type of insulin may be required, and should be discussed with the prescribing physician.

Activity	150 Pound Person	175 Pound Person	200 Pound Person
Aerobics	400	470	540
Aerobic Dancing	415	480	550
Backpacking	405	470	540
Basketball	405	470	540
Bicycling	450	515	590
Canoeing or Kayaking	405	470	540
Dancing	340	400	455
Ice Skating	415	485	550
Jogging	675	790	900
Kickboxing	700	840	960
Martial Arts	440	515	590
Racquetball	440	515	590
Skiing (Cross Country)	550	640	730
Skiing (Downhill)	440	515	590
Spinning	475	555	635
Stair Climbing	610	715	815
Swimming	600	705	805
Tai Chi	275	315	360
Tennis	550	640	730
Walking Briskly	400	460	530
Water Aerobics	290	335	385
Weightlifting	470	545	625
Yoga	360	420	480

Table 17.3   Calories Burned Per Hour
Selected Exercises

With all that said, what, then, constitutes a reasonable workout routine for the beginner? The goal of exercise is simply to improve overall health. Improved overall health includes increased strength, increased aerobic capacity, increased flexibility, improved coordination, and creating balance where an imbalance is found to exist. A properly designed exercise program will, therefore, take into consideration all these aspects of training. A workout program should be four or five days per week, with each session approximately 30 minutes in length. Table 17.4 illustrates the division of an exercise program to incorporate these different types of training. Included in this workout is what is known as *Weak Point Training*. Weak point training involves additional exercise for those areas that are known deficiencies in a person's physical abilities. For example, the individual who has sufficient physical strength and reasonable aerobic capacity, but limited flexibility, weak point training would incorporate additional flexibility training. For the person trying to lose weight, weak point training should be geared toward those activities that enhance weight loss. By spending extra time addressing any individual weaknesses, balance is created, injuries are less likely to occur, and overall fitness is improved. Weak points change periodically, requiring that activities be changed from time to time.

Day	Exercise Type
Monday	Strength Training, Stretching
Tuesday	Aerobic Training, Stretching
Wednesday	Rest
Thursday	Strength Training, Agility Training
Friday	Aerobic Training, Stretching
Saturday	Weak Point Training
Sunday	Rest

Table 17.4   Example Exercise Schedule

On days where rest is indicated, activities such as meditation, social activities, or just laying in the Sun should be scheduled. These activities are therapeutic in themselves, and should not be overlooked.

Table 17.5 shows several examples of the various types of training. In the table, several exercises appear in more than one category. This is because the activity inherently is a combination of the different forms of training. Incorporating a wide variety of activities into an exercise program is desirable, therefore averting boredom with any particular activity. A boring workout program will be quickly abandoned, so choosing activities that are enjoyable is very important. In most regions of the world, many activities, such as swimming, kayaking, and skiing, are seasonal, and many people who participate in such activities will simply substitute other forms of exercise at different times during the year. If it is too hot or too cold to jog or run, an alternative aerobic activity, such as riding a stationary bicycle, should be substituted. Running in extreme weather conditions is an injury waiting to happen. Weather conditions, therefore, must be taken into consideration when selecting any activity.

Many exercises fall into both the aerobic and anaerobic category. In most activities, both the aerobic and anaerobic pathways of metabolism are active simultaneously. The predominate pathway during any particular exercise typically determines the classification of that exercise. Weightlifting, a perfect example, is often mistaken for a purely anaerobic activity. If weightlifting is performed with light weights using a high number of repetitions with very little rest between sets, weightlifting becomes both an aerobic and anaerobic activity. Weightlifting in this manner would therefore be classified as endurance training, which is defined as a combination of aerobic and anaerobic activities. The key to aerobic weightlifting is to keep the heart rate in the target range required for aerobic activity. This principle holds true for every other exercise that classically considered as an anaerobic activity as well. Bicycling is another good example of an activity that can be either aerobic or anaerobic. Sprinting on a bicycle is an anaerobic activity, whereas distance cycling is an aerobic activity. Merrily riding a bicycle at two miles per hour, however, can hardly be considered exercise.

Category	Examples
Anaerobic	Bicycling (sprints), Isometric exercises, Kayaking, Pilates, Resistance training, Running (sprinting), Swimming, Weightlifting (moderate to high reps)
Aerobic	Bicycling (distance), Dance, Jogging, Running (distance), Basketball, Handball, Kayaking, Kickboxing, Martial arts, Racquetball, Ski machines, Soccer, Stationary bicycles, Spinning, Stair climbing, Swimming, Treadmill, Weightlifting (low weight, high reps)
Strength	Weightlifting (very high weight, low reps)
Agility	Dance, Gymnastics, Kickboxing, Martial arts, Springboard diving, Tai Chi, Twirling, Yoga
Flexibility	Dance, Gymnastics, Martial arts, Stretching, Yoga

Table 17.5   Training Examples

If the training program of a professional athlete is examined closely, all types of training are typically found to be part of the overall program. The professional athlete cannot afford to have any weak points. Any weak points will predispose the athlete to injuries, which will lead to a shortened career.

Football is a perfect example. Football training incorporates anaerobic activities and strength training (weightlifting), aerobic activities (running), agility training (agility drills), and flexibility training (stretching). In addition, during the off season, the professional athlete can often be found correcting any weak points, which improves performance on the playing field. The same can be said of Olympic athletes. Any weak points will ultimately cost them the gold medal, so the Olympic athlete is always striving to be in top physical condition.

Once an exercise program is developed, setting realistic goals is as important as exercising. Writing these goals down, and tracking progress by recording body measurements and weight, is helpful to monitor progress. Keeping track of how much weight that can be lifted or how fast it takes to walk a mile is also a valuable way to monitor progress. When progress is seen, continuing the exercise program is much easier. When a goal is met, reward yourself in a way that is meaningful. If the goal is to lose 25 or 50 lbs., reward yourself with that new outfit or a trip to the beach. Do not, however, reward yourself by eating a half gallon of ice cream. The best reward, however, is knowing that a goal has been set and then accomplished.

Having a training partner, with whom to exercise, is very valuable for many reasons. Good training partners will keep each other accountable and make sure that they do not skip workouts. Having a training partner with the same goals in mind is preferable because the exercise program used to accomplish the goals will be similar. Exercising with a partner, or with a group, will reduce the temptation to skip exercises or shorten the workout. Having the correct partner has a synergistic effect, both people will benefit in the sense that, in having the same goals, increased energy will be expended in meeting that goal. The right group of training partners will help everyone attain their goals faster.

In adopting a healthy lifestyle, exercise is a key component. The key to exercise is consistency. Try not to skip any workouts because dropping the program altogether is too easy after missing as few as two or three sessions. Some exercise is better than no exercise at all, if all that is available is 15 minutes, then use the time wisely and accomplish as much as can be done in the time available. By incorporating a variety of activities that are enjoyable, exercise becomes something that one wants to do, not something someone has to do.

A 60-year-old patient under chiropractic care was not progressing as expected. This was primarily due to some very tight muscles, so I suggested to the patient that she begin a stretching program. I recommended a Yoga video, as this will allow the patient to stretch in the comfort of her own home. After about two weeks, I asked the patient how the Yoga was coming. She replied "it's good, it is very relaxing." She stated she uses the video both morning and night, every day. Another two weeks go by and I still do not see much improvement in her flexibility. Again, I asked how the Yoga is coming. She replies that "it is very enjoyable." I then asked if any of the moves are giving her any problem. She replies "no, I enjoy them all." I then asked her to show me one or two of them, to make sure her form is correct. She replies, "Oh doctor, I was just watching the video, I didn't think I was supposed to do the moves myself." Ok, now, where did I go wrong?

Chapter 18
What Does This Mean?

In this highly automated and technical age, quick and easy access to diagnostic machines and laboratories have come to be expected, by both the patient and the doctor. Magnetic Resonance Imaging machines, Computer Aided Tomography (CAT scanners), Positron Emission Tomography scanners, (PET Scanner) and diagnostic ultrasound equipment are all found in diagnostic centers in every major city. In emergencies, laboratory tests can often be performed in minutes or hours. In non-emergency situations, results are often obtainable in a day or two, the limiting factor being transportation of the tissue sample or blood vial rather than paperwork. In the modern day medical facility, an electrocardiogram (EKG) can be performed in a general practitioner's office, the data can be sent electronically over the internet where a cardiologist reads it hundreds or thousands of miles away, and electronically sends the report back before the patient leaves the office. The even more modern computerized EKG machine can read and interpret the test itself, and provide a printed report to the attending physician immediately. In advanced research facilities, genetic mapping of the human genome is taking place. This is uncovering the cause of genetic-based disease, and, at the same time, providing the knowledge and basis for any potential cure.

Modern diagnostic equipment has not been on the scene for very long. Much of this equipment has descended from laboratory equipment used in chemistry and physics coupled with modern day computing devices. For example, the technology found in the development of the modern Magnetic Resonance Imaging (MRI) scanner has descended from the Nuclear Magnetic Resonance (NMR) technology used in organic chemistry. Nuclear Magnetic Resonance is used by chemists for identification of chemical compounds. Nuclear magnetic resonance technology was first described in 1938, but it was not until many years later that technological advances allowed the development of a viable analysis unit to be built. Modern day Nuclear Magnetic Resonance machines can easily identify chemical compounds, using computerized technology to perform most of the analysis. No machine, however, can ever take the place of a brilliant organic chemist, such as Herbert O. House, PhD. The Nuclear Magnetic Resonance machine is a tool for the chemist to make further and quicker advances, and is not a substitute for human thinking. Diagnostic equipment used in medicine should play the same role. Medical diagnostic equipment cannot replace human thinking.

This modern equipment did not, however, appear just out of the blue. Diagnostic equipment, treatment protocols, chemicals to treat disease are all a result of modern research and development. Research is done to prove the efficacy of any protocol proposed to be used in the treatment of disease. Extensive clinical trials are done to prove the efficacy of chemical compound proposed to be introduced into the human body. Research is also used to disqualify some particular treatment protocol or chemical compound should the treatment prove ineffective or dangerous to the patient. The methodologies associated with modern research have been set as the standard by Western medicine in proving the effectiveness of any treatment offered to the public.

Modern research and research protocols are in their infancy stage. Compared with acupuncture, spinal manipulation, Ayurveda, the use of herbs in the treatment disease, energy medicine and energy healing techniques, all of which have been around for thousands of years, modern medicine is clearly the newcomer on the scene. Along with modern medicine comes an integrated research and development machine with standards and protocols specifically designed to prove the efficacy of the newly developed medical techniques, pills, and protocols. Discarding all the tried and true knowledge of older healing methods, modern medicine has voted and exalted itself to the level of being the only viable method of treating illness of the body. The various arms of the modern medical research institutions demand that scholars and practitioners of these tried and true methods submit research proving the efficacy of their techniques that have been in use for thousands of years. All of a sudden, acupuncture, chiropractic, energy medicine, Ayurveda, the medicinal use of herbs, and so on, are under scrutiny and demands are made to meet standards of acceptance using research methods that have little or no application whatever in the time tested healing methods.

Acupuncture is a perfect example of a healing method that has come under scrutiny in modern times. Applying modern research methods to acupuncture is not even possible. This is primarily because the research methods and protocols employed in the modern scientific method do not apply to the spiritual entity known as the meridian, or the energy which flows through the meridian, known as ki or chi. Acupuncture, however, has been in use for thousands of years. One might wonder why an organization, such as the World

Health Organization, established on April 7, 1948, has any business at all in demanding research proving the relevance of a healing technique used successfully for many millennia. In essence, modern day society is engineering a rift between pharmaceutical based conventional medicine and well-established Eastern healing methods, such as acupuncture. Various organizations, such as the National Center for Complementary and Alternative Medicine (NCCAM) and the American Medical Association (AMA) have also studied and commented on the efficacy of acupuncture. These institutes generally regard acupuncture as safe for certain ailments, but are also in agreement that further research is warranted.

"Further research is warranted." What does this mean? Does It mean that we must look at acupuncture from a Western scientific viewpoint? Do we now perform clinical trials of the methods of acupuncture? Do we apply the scientific methods used in other types of research to prove the efficacy of acupuncture? Should the safety of acupuncture be evaluated? These are the wrong questions to ask, and also asking the questions in the wrong way, so it would be of benefit not even to address the subject from the viewpoint of Westernized medicine. Sufficient research already exists, and is found among the doctors who practice, in healing centers, and in the universities of countries that have a long history of practicing acupuncture. The problem is that organizations wishing to evaluate acupuncture cannot read Chinese, and are unwilling to review existing research performed in a manner consistent with the beliefs of the healing method. History also validates the techniques employed by acupuncture. Any method failing to deliver satisfactory results would quickly be abandoned by all but the very stupid. Any healing method that delivered reasonable results would be refined over time, evolving into a system that delivered better and better results as refinements and adjustments were incorporated into the methodology. That which is found not to work would be replaced with that which does, and the result, over time, would be a highly refined healing method. Casual observation raises the question as to why China is the most populous nation in the world. This certainly could not have come about by practicing healing techniques that are detrimental to health and kill people.

When a statement such as "Further research is warranted" appears in a document, what does this really mean? This is not the only statement of this sort to arise in medical literature and research. Similar statements often appear in research papers and publications, giving the impression that great discoveries and accomplishments are just over the horizon. When used concerning systems of healing outside modern medical research, however, these statements have a different meaning altogether. Many of these phrases completely defy logic and are quite meaningless, but often give the impression that some highly advanced mumbo jumbo is being communicated. Examining what they really mean in the many contexts they are used is advantageous to understand the modern medical system better.

Further research is warranted

Further research is warranted, when applied to any healing method, means that modern medicine recognizes the fact that the healing method works. Some acceptance of the healing method in question is granted, but full acceptance is not granted because it most likely threatens the money stream of the organizations suggesting further research be conducted. When the statement *further research is warranted* appears, no real denial of the efficacy of the healing method is usually found. Denial of the efficacy of the healing method altogether will subsequently result in embarrassment of the organization making such a claim. Since any denial of efficacy would discredit the organization making the claim, no stance is therefore taken regarding the endorsement of the method.

When the phrase *further research is warranted* is used, it often gives the impression that this further research is either planned or has already been financed. This, however, is rarely the case. Modern medicine has little to be gained in proving the efficacy of chiropractic, herbal therapies, acupuncture, or any other natural healing method in the treatment of disease, therefore does not typically fund research proving the validity of these healing methods. Since the healing methods under scrutiny are fully understood by the doctors who practice them, little or no motivation can be found to prove to the modern medical system what is already known. In addition, doctors of these other healing methods are often unwilling to donate money to support research, particularly research in which the goal is to prove what is already known. As a result, no further research is ever conducted.

Unscientific

This is a popular label affixed to anything that involves the spirit of the body–mind–spirit model. Chakras, meridians, acupuncture, Reiki, or any other methods of spiritual healing are often labeled as unscientific. Labeling something as unscientific is simply an admission that the understanding of science is inadequate or has not yet progressed to the level required to understand whatever is in question. This lack of understanding is found either on the personal level of the scientists making the claim, or in the understanding that exists in a body of knowledge as a whole. At one point, the notion of looking into the human body using a magnet, large electromagnetically energized coil, and semiconductors would have been considered unscientific. Anyone who suggested this possibility two hundred years ago would have been thought to be insane, possibly in need of trephanation. Today, the magnet, a large electromagnetic coil, and a computer manufactured with semiconductors comprise the key components of an MRI machine.

A long time ago, anatomists dissected the human body, and asked the question "What are these parts?" They began examining the parts of the body and, over time, gained an understanding of what each organ does. They then wanted to know what the fundamental substance comprising each organ is, specifically with what is each organ made. The more they asked that question, the more they realized they could not answer it, because they had no tools in order to examine the parts more closely. Then, technology brought a tool called the microscope. As crude as these early instruments were, it gave the anatomist a view into the world previously unseen. They looked through the microscope, and saw a cell. This created a new field of science, called cellular biology. Cellular biology could not exist until the cell had been discovered. These new biologists wanted to know what cells are made of, what it inside it, and what makes the cell work. The more they asked these questions, the more they again realized they cannot answer them until a much better microscope was developed. Then, the biologists, with their more powerful instruments, were able to identify smaller parts inside the cells, and again wanted to know of what these smaller parts are made. Then a chemist comes along to help the biologist, and the chemist takes the cell apart, and identifies the molecules of with which the cell is made. The biologists then take this information and, with their newly found partner, the chemist, figure out how it all fits together and how it works. Working as a team, the biologist and chemist develop the field known as biochemistry, and describe the biochemical reactions that occur in the cell. During the process of figuring out the answers, even more unanswered questions began to surface. The physicist then comes along and describes the atoms, electrons, protons, and all sorts of subatomic particles that comprise the atoms that make up the molecules found in the cell. Just when all the subatomic particles have been identified, and all of the scientists think all the basic building blocks of matter have been discovered, the quantum physicist arrives and says even smaller entities named quarks exist. The quark theories formulated by the quantum physicist form the foundation for the representation of matter and energy as a single entity. This will have a profound effect on the future understanding of the body-mind-spirit representation of the human body.

Not a single scientist, not the anatomist, biologist, chemist, physicist, or the quantum physicist, claimed that the work of the others was unscientific. Instead, the work each scientist complemented the work of the other scientists. Each used the research of the other to advance their own work. Working harmoniously with each other, the science of biology got to where it is today. When something is labeled as unscientific, such as meridian points, it is evidence that scientists do not have a sufficient understanding of the science required to understand the inner workings of the meridian system. This science, however, already exists today, and is able to prove the existence of a meridian. The problem is that the scientists who are involved in medical research lack any understanding of quarks and the advanced mathematics required to formulate the proof. The meridian system is fully understood by the practitioners who practice the methods that use them. The concept of a meridian, however, does not have to be proven to a highly skilled Chinese medical doctor who has practiced acupuncture for fifty years. Suggesting to the classical Chinese medical doctor that the concept of a meridian does not exist is the equivalent of suggesting to the Western medical doctor that the heart does not exist. Suggesting that the heart does not exist is quite absurd. To the classical Chinese medical doctor, suggesting that a meridian does not exist is equally absurd. To claim that a chakra or meridian does not exist implies that acupuncture, reflexology, Reiki, and Applied Kinesiology are all fraudulent healing arts. Conversely, to accept acupuncture as the legitimate healing art that it is, one must also accept the concepts of a chakra and meridian. One cannot believe in the efficacy of a healing art and, at the same time, dismiss the basic foundational concepts of that art as unscientific. In this way, modern medicine has entered a trap, a trap of logic from which one cannot escape.

Without an adequate understanding of quantum physics, advanced mathematics, advanced electromagnetics, and the meridian system, the researcher confined to the laboratory postulating the effects of some chemical on a neurosynaptic connection simply does not have anything close to the skills required even to begin research in the area of Eastern medicine. Dismissing a meridian as unscientific should be quite an embarrassment to any researcher. The researcher who has an understanding that Western medicine has only begun to touch the surface of meridian research, and subsequently explores this avenue of research will undoubtably offer a significant contribution to medicine.

The label of *unscientific* is not limited to Eastern healing methods. Time after time, this term is used concerning any healing art that is found to be in direct competition with modern medicine. Modern medicine, unlike any field of modern science, is quick to dismiss anything as unscientific, fraudulent, or quackery that poses any hint at all of competition with the services they offer.

Mechanism is not fully understood

This is an interesting statement made quite often, usually in reference to the biochemical processes of the body. Any chemical placed into the body will react with other chemicals in the body, or, infrequently, be inert and not react with anything. When the chemical introduced into the body reacts with some chemical, a mechanism of action is then defined. All drugs have a mechanism of action. Herbs contain chemicals that have a mechanism of action. Vitamins and minerals also have a mechanism of action. The mechanism of action refers to the specific biochemical interaction through which a substance produces an effect, whether the effect is desirable or not. In pharmacology, a mechanism of action usually targets a specific molecular target, typically an enzyme or receptor. Interestingly, toxic substances often target the same sites as the pharmaceutical or herbal remedy.

When a mechanism is not fully understood, it means that the researchers who are involved in the research either lack the required technology to discover the mechanism of action, or lack the foundational knowledge required in order to figure out what the mechanism of action is. The truth of the matter is that the mechanism of action occurs whether the researcher understands it or not. In other words, when the mechanism of action is not fully understood, the team of researchers has literally no clue why the chemical compound in question does what it does. If the mechanism of action is not understood, the question arises of what else the chemical might be doing that is not yet known about. This is a foundational deficiency of the knowledge and understanding of the biochemistry involved. The lack of knowledge on the part of the researcher, however, does not stop the chemical from participating in whatever mechanism of action with which the chemical is involved.

Lithium has been used as a treatment in bipolar disorder for many years. The mechanism of action of Lithium is unknown. This means that the action of Lithium in the neurology of the brain is not understood, but it appears to produce some desired result. Substantial amounts of research and literature use this phrase with respect to Lithium. The question arises of what other reactions this drug is participating in and what else it is doing that is also unknown.

Acupuncture has also been used to treat bipolar disorder. The mechanism of action is fully understood by the acupuncture doctor in the framework of meridian therapy. Western medicine, however, cannot understand the mechanism of action of the acupuncture treatment within the framework of allopathic medicine. In this case, the mechanism of action of a treatment is known and fully understood, but the basic foundational concepts of acupuncture have been dismissed as unscientific, therefore a roadblock has been erected preventing any understanding by the Western researcher.

The question arises of why Western medicine uses a treatment (Lithium) for a disorder (bipolar disorder) when the mechanism of action is not understood at all, and, at the same time, fails to accept the treatments of other disciplines (acupuncture) whose practitioners fully understand the mechanism of actions of their own treatments. No discernable logic can be found in the position of Western medicine regarding this, and similar, issues. In fact, this is nothing more than reductio ad absurdum.

Does not readily

The term *does not readily* is often used in circumstances where some conclusion of the research is drawn, but the researchers wanted their research to indicate a different conclusion. What was hypothesized and subsequently demonstrated is most likely not in the best interest of the organizations funding the research. The researchers initially set out to prove that something can or cannot occur, and inadvertently proved the opposite of what was originally intended. When this happens, it is often considered an undesirable outcome of the research, and terms such as *does not readily* are used to water down the conclusion. In essence, a vague conclusion appears to be drawn, leaving little or no confidence in the use of the research as a supportive reference for other researchers. On the other hand, if the research proves the original hypothesis, stronger terms such as *clearly demonstrable* are used.

The statement "Gamma-aminobutyric acid does not readily cross the blood-brain barrier" is a common example of this phrase. Gamma-aminobutyric acid will either cross or not cross the barrier. The hypothesis is that the molecule is too large to cross the blood-brain barrier. Somehow, regardless of the hypothesis, the molecule manages to cross the blood-brain barrier anyway. This is because the mechanism of action in moving Gamma-aminobutyric acid across the barrier is not fully understood (see above) by the researchers. In fact, since Gamma-aminobutyric acid does, in fact, cross the blood-brain barrier, the mechanism by which this happens must not be understood at all.

This statement has not been evaluated by the FDA. This product is not intended to diagnose, treat, cure, or prevent any disease

This statement must appear on every product, except drugs, that either blatantly or remotely make the suggestion of a health benefit or health claim. It is required by law. The following is a quotation regarding this statement from the Food and Drug Administrations documentation.

> "This statement or "disclaimer" is required by law (DSHEA) when a manufacturer makes a structure/function claim on a dietary supplement label. In general, these claims describe the role of a nutrient or dietary ingredient intended to affect the structure or function of the body. The manufacturer is responsible for ensuring the accuracy and truthfulness of these claims; they are not approved by FDA. For this reason, the law says that if a dietary supplement label includes such a claim, it must state in a "disclaimer" that FDA has not evaluated this claim. The disclaimer must also state that this product is not intended to "diagnose, treat, cure or prevent any disease," because only a drug can legally make such a claim."

The phrase "This statement has not been evaluated by the FDA" gives the impression that the FDA is in the business in evaluating health claims and the efficacy of certain dietary or other supplements. This is not the case. The label contains that phrase simply because it is required by law. Even if the claim were correct, and the supplement does, in fact, provide the cure for a particular disease, the disclaimer still must appear on the label. Scurvy, for example, occurs as a result of Vitamin C deficiency. If a Vitamin C supplement states that it can cure Scurvy if taken according to certain directions, which it in fact does, the product manufacturer still cannot legally make that claim.

But, no one really cares about the Food and Drug Administration anyway. The Food and Drug Administration is supposed to protect the public from the manufacturers of dietary supplements from making unsubstantiated claims. Let us all be reminded that the Food and Drug Administration has issued approvals for drugs such as thalidomide, diethylstilbestrol (DES), and Malathion. Malathion, an irreversible cholinesterase inhibitor, is a pesticide approved for the treatment of head lice. It is the same chemical sprayed on lawns and gardens to kill insects. With many safer alternatives available, one must wonder why such a toxic insecticide has been approved for killing head lice. The fact that drugs such as these can even enter the consumer market suggests that the public is who is in need of protection from the Food and Drug Administration.

For reasons that are not entirely understood

This is another ridiculous statement that appears quite often in literature and research. This statement implies that a conclusion has been drawn. The statement also implies little or no understanding exists regarding how or why the conclusion was drawn. Drawing a conclusion to a hypothesis requires at least a basic understanding of how and why the conclusion was drawn. If this approach were applied to mathematics, it would be immediately rejected due to obvious reasons. In fact, application of this statement, in the framework of logic, is termed *Ad ridiculum*, referring to an anomaly in logic. Statements such as *for reasons that are not entirely understood* truly defy logic when applied to research.

The phrase *for reasons that are not entirely understood* implies that little confidence in the conclusion of the research can be found, and that the conclusion drawn lies somewhere in a gray area. In other words, the research effort has failed to produce any meaningful or usable results. The task, then, is to gain a better understanding of what is actually occurring. Once whatever is being studied is fully understood, then a solid conclusion can be drawn.

The statement "for reasons that are not entirely understood, the airplane stayed in the air during the first test flight" would not give us very high confidence in either the engineering behind the plane or the engineers that developed the plane. Who, now, wants to get on the plane for the second test flight? Why, then, would we give any more confidence to medical research that uses the same term? If science and engineering embraced the same inferior standards as medical research, bridges would collapse, planes would drop out of the air, electronic equipment would fail incessantly, and automobiles would randomly explode every day.

Unproven

This buzz word is usually applied to any alternative form of treatment outside mainstream medicine. It also has been applied to the use of herbs to treat whatever condition is in question. When something is stated to be unproven by modern medicine, it simply means that medical research has not taken the initiative to prove the effectiveness of the treatment or product. The fact that the treatment or product has not even been investigated is not even considered when the term *unproven* is used.

If some treatment is labeled as unproven, no satisfactory proof satisfying the organization demanding the proof was found. Most likely, the organization has not searched for the proof. Conversely, however, no proof may even exist that indicates the treatment does not work either. An organization demands proof that the treatment works, and another organization demands proof that the treatment does not work. The hidden agenda of one organization is to deny acceptance of the treatment protocols of the other organization. Furthermore, each organization desires to be self determining, and by being independent, refuse to submit to the rules that define the other organization. What we end up with, then, is a childish game in which the healing profession can never make progress.

Risky

This is yet another commonly used buzz word is which is usually applied to any alternative form of treatment outside mainstream medicine. It is most likely used to scare the patient away from trying any alternative form of treatment. The patient often suggests alternative forms of treatment when they cannot see any progress in the current treatment of their condition. The suggestion of alternative treatment is an indication that the patient is on the verge of seeking care elsewhere, but the medical doctor does not perceive this. When the term *risky* is used in reference to any alternative healing method by the medical doctor, what is actually being stated is that the future income of the doctor is what is really at risk.

Disclaimers

Disclaimers are found in nearly every publication or website providing health information. While many reasons can be found for disclaimers, at least one good legal reason exists that any disclaimer is made. The disclaimer at the beginning of this book serves as a perfect example. It states:

> *Medical and health information is not medical advice. The content of this book provides information about health and certain health conditions. The information contained herein is presented for educational purposes only, and is not intended to be a substitute for professional medical advice, diagnosis, or treatment. We highly recommend that everyone seek the care of a natural health care provider or holistic medical doctor for proper application of this material to any specific situation. Never disregard professional medical advice or delay in seeking appropriate care because of something presented in this book, any other publication, or website.*

Most of what is contained in a disclaimer is common sense. Some of the content of a disclaimer is included for legal reasons. Specifically, the wording that states *The information contained herein is presented for educational purposes only, and is not intended to be a substitute for professional medical advice, diagnosis, or treatment* infers that anything found in this book is presented for the education of the reader. The educational material is never a substitute for the advice and guidance of a health care provider. When advice is given to the patient, a doctor-patient relationship is subsequently established. By not giving advice, no doctor-patient relationship is established; therefore, the doctor, or author cannot be indicted for practicing medicine without a license in any jurisdiction.

The information presented in any literature discussing health care may have a valid application in 99% of the population. If this is the case, the information presented in the literature will not even apply to one in every 100 persons. Statistically, if a plane had a 1 percent chance of crashing, most prudent people would not even get on the plane. One percent is a seemingly small number, but is quite large when looked at in the correct perspective. If a particular person happens to be that one in one hundred that the information does not even apply to, that person may be placing him or herself in a dangerous position without proper guidance from a qualified practitioner. Administration of health care has an enormous number of variables. No book, publication, or website can address every potential issue that may arise. For this reason, it is always strongly recommended that the advice of a qualified health care provider be obtained.

Technical factors preclude further evaluation

This and similar statements often appear on radiological reports. What this statement means is the x-ray, ultrasound, MRI scan, or other image was not of perfect quality, for one reason or another. A worse statement to appear on a radiological report is *not of diagnostic quality*. These statements are often issued in the report by the radiologist in order to avoid malpractice, and are included in the radiology report in case something serious could not be identified on the film. These statements also shift the burden of potential liability back to the party who was responsible for ordering the test. The radiologist expects a diagnostic quality film to read to formulate a diagnosis properly, and cannot be expected to see that which is obscured by poor imaging techniques. A diagnostic quality film is not an unreasonable expectation if the radiologist is expected to render a diagnosis.

When statements such as these appear on a radiological report, the imaging was not, simply by definition, of diagnostic quality. Should this occur, the imaging should be repeated. The patient paid for a diagnostic test, and the images obtained should be of diagnostic quality. In addition, the patient should not have to pay for the repeat of the test.

Some type of abnormality in the neurotransmitter system...

The use of this, and similar terms, commonly appear in research or literature concerning mental disorders. The term states that an abnormality is suspected or has been found in one of the neurotransmitter systems of the brain. Statements such as this usually read something like:

> *The majority of researchers believe that, in obsessive-compulsive disorder, there is some type of abnormality in the neurotransmitter system of the brain involving serotonin*

or

> *Research indicates that decreased levels of the neurotransmitter Gamma-aminobutyric acid is responsible for the manic phase of bipolar disorder.*

The question arises as to whether the aberrant neurotransmitter levels actually cause the disease or disorder, or occur as a result of the disorder. The first thing that must be considered is that, in research and clinical examinations, only persons with the disorder are found to have the aberrant levels of neurotransmitters. Documentation regarding the state of the neurotransmitter systems before the condition was diagnosed is essentially nonexistent. Years of unusual thought patterns can easily invoke neurotransmitter deviations from normal in any otherwise healthy subject. Imaging studies depicting brain development before the onset of the disorder are equally nonexistent. Differing rates of brain development from person to person may in fact exist, but, since these rates of development are undocumented, they are not considered as a factor in a predisposition to a disorder. As a result, genetically differing brain development patterns can predispose an individual to different thought patterns early in life. Counseling and cognitive therapy would, therefore, be most appropriate at a young age for individuals who are susceptible to the development of any disorder with a developmental basis. It is not sound logic to wait for a problem to move into the crisis phase to begin treatment. Interestingly, the medical profession attempts to detect certain illnesses before the crisis phase. Everyone is familiar with the yearly physical. Preventative dental care is recommended every six months. A colonoscopy is recommended at the age of 50. No provision, however, is made to evaluate predisposed children and teens for any early signs of issues related to the mind. Periodic evaluation of these individuals by a qualified psychologist is clearly warranted.

Any repeated activity or thought pattern can clearly result in altered neurology of the brain, involving both synaptic connections and neurotransmitter activity. For example, the neurology of a 5th level black belt martial arts master and a corporate business executive is quite different. Areas of the brain in the martial arts master which are well developed are most likely poorly developed in the business executive, and vice-versa. Placing a business executive in a martial arts contest competing against a martial arts master will most likely end in severe injuries for the businessman, providing he or she even survives the competition. Likewise, producing a business proposal for a multimillion dollar development project is not in the realm of the skill level of the martial arts expert, and will most likely end in a financial disaster. In the case of each individual, the neurology has developed in accordance with activities performed over years of activity. This neurological development is not only true for the examples cited, but applies to most everyone. We could say that the business executive has integrated physical performance deficit syndrome, or that the martial arts master has financial planning and development deficit syndrome, but this would sound somewhat stupid. Equally as stupid are some of the modern psychological disorders that are, for the lack of a better term, invented. The brain and its associated neurology are a product of what a person does over time. It is much more likely that any aberration in neurotransmitter systems occurs as a result of thought processes and lifestyle, rather than defective neurology causing the person to act in a certain way.

Neurology is not carved in stone. In order to correct disorders of a mental origin, a change in thought patterns is essential. Changing any activities that may have lead to any existing condition must also be considered. In changing activities and thought patterns, a change in the associated neurology and neurotransmission will ultimately occur. This applies to anyone, not only those who have been diagnosed with a disorder of either a developmental or neurotransmitter basis. Changing neurologically based thought patterns, however, takes considerable time and effort. In altering thought patterns and activities, anyone can be a completely different person in the years ahead, without the use of mind-altering medication.

Not everything that society does makes sense. Daylight-saving time, the ritualistic act of changing the clocks twice a year, is one such example. By changing the clocks to read one hour ahead of what the time should be during the Spring and Summer months, we, as a society, fool ourselves into thinking that an extra hour of sunlight can magically appear. Politicians, in a like way, fool themselves into thinking that changing the clocks will actually save energy. As a result of the illusion, circadian rhythms are disrupted to an extent that it takes many people weeks to adjust to the change.

We might as well propose that, for the Summer months, we change the thermometers. By changing all thermometers to read ten degrees cooler during the Summer months, we can fool ourselves into thinking that it is cooler than it really is. This, in fact, will solve the problem of global warming. Al Gore will then have to find something else to talk about.

Chapter 19
Epilog

Regardless of the disease, illness, or syndrome, a root cause existed at one time allowing the disease process to begin. The level and extent of any progression of any disease process is based upon many factors. Some of these factors are genetic, some factors originate from the patient's health history, and other factors include the diet, lifestyle, and environment. All these factors are potential contributors to any disease process. Some of these factors are under our direct control, and some are not. Genetic factors cannot be readily modified using today's science. No one can change their past, placing everything that has happened in the past essentially carved in stone. What can be modified, however, is everything that lies in the future. Since what is done today affects the health of the person in the future, positive accomplishments directed toward good health can only improve health in the future as compared to making no changes at all.

Rather than treating individual disorders and the associated symptoms that all may be present simultaneously, it is often advantageous to step back and look at the health of the individual from a different perspective. This new perspective would incorporate the philosophy that a disease is allowed to exist as a result of disharmony of the body-mind-spirit and the person's relationship with the social and physical environment. In creating harmony, we then create health. Conversely, if we create disharmony, we create disease.

The body is not a stupid organism. The intelligence to maintain health is already built into the body, and the body does not ordinarily need help in maintaining health. What the body does need, however, is freedom from anything that is detrimental to health. If some disease or illness does occur, placing the body into a position to facilitate natural healing is imperative. This not only includes changes to the diet, the use of appropriate supplements or exercise, but includes changes to the physical and social environment as well. Removal of any barriers to healing that may exist is of the utmost importance. The body is normally perfectly capable of functioning without some manufactured chemical ingested on a daily basis. If early warning signs are ignored, or, worse yet, hidden by a pill, damage is likely occurring to the body. Damaging the body beyond its ability to heal itself is entirely possible, which is a path no one wants to go down. Heart attacks, strokes, torn ligaments, and osteoarthritis are perfect examples of permanent damage that can occur.

What happens when we circumvent the natural healing process of the body is that we send the body on a detour in which it now must also recover. Not only does the body have the task of healing itself of the disease or disorder present, but also must detoxify and rid itself from a handful of ingested chemicals. All too often the ingested chemical, by suppressing symptoms, actually hinders the natural healing process or leaves the patient with a worse problem than the one that was initially treated.

The question posed in the title of this book is "Why am I sick?" The answer to this question is that some form of disharmony has been allowed to exist, leading to the illness. The second part of the title suggests that something can be done about it. What we should do, then, is to create this perfect harmony of the body, mind and spirit in whatever way possible. At the same time, making any changes possible to the physical environment to create better harmony will be advantageous in the betterment of health. Regarding the social environment, any changes that need to be made should also be undertaken to better health. In some cases, creating the life of perfect harmony may involve only a few minor changes to the diet, social situations, or daily activities. In other cases, however, it may involve selling everything a person owns, moving hundreds of miles away, and starting all over with a new mind set on life.

Create perfect harmony, and health will undoubtably follow. People will be attracted in every way to those who maintain perfect harmony. Everyone sees something in these people that they want themselves, but may not know exactly what it is. Spread the word.

The modern medical school is perhaps the only institution in which the students are less knowledgeable on graduation day than on orientation day.

Why Am I Sick? And What To Do About It

Appendix I
Where to Find Products
Referenced in the Discussion

The following agents are effective in reducing intestinal yeast overgrowths.

Fungal Forte ™
        Manufactured by:
        Original Medicine®
        5500 Village Blvd.
        Suite 102
        West Palm Beach, FL 33407

        Website: www.original-medicine.com

Candex ™
        Manufactured by:
        Pure Essence Labs™
        P.O. Box 95397
        Las Vegas, NV 89193

        Website: www.pureessencelabs.com

Quality Growth Hormone Secretagogues

Meditropin®
Symbiotropin®

Nutraceutics Corporation
2900 Brannon Ave.
St. Louis, MO 63139

Website: www.nutraceutics.com

Phone: 1.877.664.6684

The following probiotic products have demonstrated high quality.

Multi-Probiotic ™
Manufactured by:
Original Medicine®
5500 Village Blvd.
Suite 102
West Palm Beach, FL 33407

Website: www.original-medicine.com

iFlora ™
Manufactured by:
Sedona Labs®
211 Jennifer Lane
Cottonwood, AZ 86326

Website: www.sedonalabs.com

Water Testing Equipment

The following company is a superior source of water testing equipment.

Hach Company
P.O. Box 389
Loveland, CO 80539

Website: www.hach.com

Natural agents to restore Th1 / Th2 balance

The probiotics strains mentioned below have been formulated into products manufactured by Original Medicine®, a company whose product line is dedicated to restoring health using natural means.

Suppression of Th2 involves the following strains of probiotics:
1. *Lactobacillus plantarum*
2. *Lactobacillus acidophilus*
3. *Lactobacillus paracasei*
4. Fermented Arabinogalactan

These can be found in the following product:

Th2S ™

      Manufactured by:
      Original Medicine®
      5500 Village Blvd.
      Suite 102
      West Palm Beach, FL 33407

      Website: www.original-medicine.com

Suppression of Th1 involves the following strains of probiotics:
1. *Lactobacillus salivarius*
2. *Bifidobacterium lactis*
3. Fermented Arabinogalactan

These can be found in the following product:

Th1S ™

      Manufactured by:
      Original Medicine®
      5500 Village Blvd.
      Suite 102
      West Palm Beach, FL 33407

      Website: www.original-medicine.com

Therapeutic Light Boxes

When purchasing a therapeutic light box, certain factors must be considered. These factors involve not only price, but the engineering and service behind the product as well. By engineering, we must consider whether the manufacturer examines current research, and improves the products as more research becomes available. By service, we are concerned about the availability of replacement parts, specifically bulbs.

The following company was founded in 1985 and has been found to satisfy all the above criteria:

> The Sunbox Company®
> 19217 Orbit Drive
> Gaithersburg, MD 20879-4149
>
> Website: www.SunBox.com
>
> Phone:
> 1.800.548.3968 (toll-free in U.S.A. & Canada)
> 1.301.869.5980 (local suburban Maryland & international)

The following agent is effective in the prevention of Candida yeast overgrowth when taking antibiotics.

S. boulardii
> Manufactured by:
> Original Medicine®
> 5500 Village Blvd.
> Suite 102
> West Palm Beach, FL 33407
>
> Website: www.original-medicine.com

Appendix II
Finding Qualified Practitioners

Finding a qualified practitioner can be an easy task or it can be hard. Asking your friends, family, or business acquaintances who may have seen a natural health care provider is often the best place to begin your search. Referrals from people who have been helped by a particular doctor is often the best place to start. Once a practitioner has been found who can help, a drive or a flight to another city may be required. Highly skilled doctors, such as Dr. Paul Goldberg of Marietta, Georgia and Dr. George Petryk of Ft. Myers, Florida, often have patients who come from hundreds or thousands of miles away in order to see them. In many cases, patients come from foreign countries seeking health care from these doctors. For these patients, the long trip is well worth the time and expense. These doctors are highly skilled, highly regarded in the field, experts in the field of natural healing, and, most of all, obtain results using the methods they employ.

When contacting a practitioner, it is recommended that a brief description of the problem be given to the staff. If they feel that they can help, they will recommend that an appointment be scheduled. Prior to making an appointment, it is recommended that a brief description of the problem be prepared, including any medications, herbs, or natural remedies that may be currently taken. Any medications that have been taken in the previous five years should also be documented. The practitioner's staff may also request that other information, such as diet, activities, and work history be documented prior to the office visit. Some offices have forms that can be completed over the internet; take advantage of this option if possible. If any laboratory test results are available, please obtain copies of any reports and bring them to your consultation. These tests may include blood tests, imaging results, and other studies that may have been ordered. Even if the test results were reported to be negative, obtain them anyway, they still provide valuable information to the practitioner. Having this information prepared ahead of time will give the practitioner a better picture of your unique situation. Refrain, however, from including superfluous information and verbose detail. If additional information is required regarding any particular issue, the doctor will ask for further elaboration during the consultation.

Once a practitioner has been found, do not expect the practitioner to solve every problem during the first visit. The practitioner will schedule several follow-up visits. These visits are just as important as the initial visit. During follow-up visits, progress will be monitored, and adjustments to the plans will likely be made.

Following the practitioner's plan is of utmost importance. The fact that healing of the body takes time has been reiterated throughout this book. The point that certain changes in lifestyle, diet, employment, and attitude must be made has also been reiterated. The doctor is interested in getting the patient well in the fastest time possible and at the least expense to the patient. The best way to accomplish this is to follow the recommended advice. The doctor's favorite patients are those who follow their advice.

Glossary

Ad falsum
This term originates from philosophy, referring to that which is logically and mathematically false.

Ad ridiculum
This term originates from philosophy, referring to an implausibility or anomaly.

Allopathic Medicine
Allopathic medicine is the system of medical practice that treats disease by using synthetic pharmaceutical agents or performing surgery. Allopathic medicine is practiced by medical doctors.

Alternative Medicine
In the West, alternative medicine generally refers to any of the healing arts that are not included in allopathic medicine. Alternative medicine recognizes the innate healing ability of the body, and uses various modalities, herbs, or nutrition to maximize this ability. In the East, these alternative healing arts are considered mainstream, and not alternative in any sense of the word. Interestingly, allopathic medicine is considered alternative medicine in the East.

Applied Kinesiology
Developed in 1964 by Dr. George Goodheart, Applied Kinesiology is the study of muscles and the relationship of muscle strength to health. Applied Kinesiology is based on the theory organ dysfunction is accompanied by a specific muscular weakness. Diagnosis is performed through specific muscle testing procedures and treated through various means.

Chiropractic

Chiropractic is that art and science concerned with the preservation and restoration of health, focusing particular attention on a condition known as the vertebral subluxation. A vertebral subluxation is a complex of both functional and structural articular changes which results in compromised neural integrity, and, in advanced cases, pathology.

Chupacabra

Literally translated from Spanish to goat sucker, a chupacabra is a land dwelling animal indigenous to South America, Mexico, the Southern United States, and Puerto Rico. A chupacabra is reported to be approximately three feet in height and fifty pounds. A chupacabra is a purely fictitious animal.

Computer Aided Tomography (CAT) Scanner

Computer Aided Tomography is a medical imaging technique used for obtaining images of inside the body. Two-dimensional X-ray images are taken in numerous planes, the information subsequently fed into a computer that produces reconstructed three-dimensional images. CAT scans are often prescribed in cases when plain film radiography fails to deliver sufficient diagnostic information.

Dead End Diagnosis

A dead end diagnosis is a diagnosis for which no treatment can be offered.

Diagnosis of Absurdity

A diagnosis of absurdity is a diagnosis of a disease or disorder that, in all actuality, does not really exist. In other words, a diagnosis of absurdity refers to an invented disorder. Any diagnosis that simply renames the symptom is suspect of a diagnosis of absurdity. Whenever a diagnosis of absurdity is issued, the underlying cause has not been found.

Diagnosis of Exclusion

A diagnosis of exclusion is a diagnosis that is put forth when no other explanation for the signs and symptoms can be found. The diagnosis of exclusion is generally based upon subjective complaints found in the patient history.

Endocrine System Disruptor

An endocrine system disruptor is any chemical, whether ingested or absorbed, that, either in part or whole, disrupts the endocrine system. The mechanism of action of an endocrine system disruptor is found in the ability of the chemical to mimic an endocrine hormone or bind to a receptor site intended for a hormone.

Magnetic Resonance Imaging (MRI)

Magnetic resonance imaging (MRI) is a method of obtaining images inside the body. Magnetic resonance imaging employs radio frequency waves and an intense magnetic field to excite atoms. Information obtained from this excitation is fed into a computer, from which a three-dimensional view of organs, muscles, joints, or other structure is obtained.

Meridian

A meridian is a term originating from acupuncture, and refers to the system of energy channels and their collaterals that traverse the body. According to the traditional Chinese medicine, the body's vital energy, known as *qi*, circulates through the body along these specific interconnected channels. The concept of a meridian has also been incorporated into Applied Kinesiology and reflexology.

Natural Health Practitioner

A natural health practitioner typically practices one or more methods of alternative medicine. Chiropractic, Applied Kinesiology, naturopathy, homeopathy, massage therapy, Qi Gong, Reiki, and Oriental Meridian Therapy (acupuncture) are a few examples of what is practiced by a natural health practitioner.

Neuroplasticity

Neuroplasticity refers to the creation of new nerve endings of a neuron. Neuroplasticity generally is associated with pain nerves, and typically occurs as a result of a significant injury to an area of the body.

Neurotransmitter

A neurotransmitter is a chemical released from a nerve cell that subsequently transmits an impulse from that nerve cell to either another nerve cell, muscle, organ, immune system cell, or other tissue of the body.

Normal Variant

A condition is termed a normal variant when the condition is considered to be a normal condition, but occurs at a much decreased frequency than is found in the general population. Many so-called psychological disorders should fall into this category, but are instead categorized as a disorder, therefore requiring treatment and insurance reimbursement.

Off-label

A medication prescribed for a condition other than which it was intended is prescribed off-label. For example, methotrexate, an anti-cancer drug, is often prescribed off-label to terminate ectopic pregnancies.

Pathogen

A pathogen is any living organism that can cause disease of the body. Pathogens include, but are not limited to, bacteria, protozoa, viruses, fungi, mold, or parasites.

Positron Emission Tomography (PET) Scanner

A Positron Emission Tomography Scanner (PET scanner) is a nuclear medicine medical imaging device used to detect highly metabolic regions of the body. A PET scanner detects gamma rays emitted by a metabolically active molecule. The information is fed into a computer and three-dimensional images are subsequently created, displaying any regions of high metabolic activity. PET scanners are commonly used for early detection of cancer, but their use is not limited to this application.

Psychoneuroimmunology

Psychoneuroimmunology is the study of the interaction of psychological processes with the nervous and immune systems of the human body.

Qi

Qi is the life force energy that flows through the body's meridians. Qi is also known as Ki, bioplasma, Chi, Qi, Odic force, Orgone, vital energy, life force energy, or prana, depending on the culture originating the name.

Qi Gong

Qi Gong is an ancient Chinese healing art involving a combination of meditation, controlled breathing, and movement exercises. Medical Qi Gong specifically directs qi, or the life force energy, in a way to effect healing of the body.

Reductio ad absurdum

Reductio ad absurdum is a process of refutation on grounds that the premise is absurd. Accepting the premise would result in disastrous consequences.

Synaptogenesis

Synaptogenesis refers to the increase in efficiency of the transmission of nerve impulses. This increased efficiency is due to either the creation of new synaptic connections, or the activation of existing dormant synapses.

Yang

In Chinese medicine, Yang is classically representative of the energy of positive, bright, hot, dry, active, and masculine.

Yin

In Chinese medicine, Yin is classically representative of the energy of negative, darkness, cold, wetness, passiveness, and feminine.

Zen

Zen is a Japanese sect of Mahayana Buddhism in which the goal is to attain enlightenment through meditation.

References

Aftanas, L.I., Golocheikine, S.A. Human anterior and frontal midline theta and lower alpha reflect emotionally positive state and internalized attention: high-resolution EEG investigation of meditation. Neuroscience Letters 310: 57-60. 2001.

Ahn, Andrew C., Wu, Junru, Badger, Gary J., Hammerschlag, Richard, Langevin, Helene M. Electrical impedance along connective tissue planes associated with acupuncture meridians. Complement Altern Med. 2005; 5: 10.

Agency for Toxic Substances and Disease Registry. 2000a. Toxicological profile for arsenic. Atlanta: U.S. Department of Health and Human Services, 1825 Century Blvd, Atlanta, GA 30345.

Agency for Toxic Substances and Disease Registry. Case Studies in Environmental Medicine: Arsenic Toxicity. Atlanta: U.S. Department of Health and Human Services, 1825 Century Blvd, Atlanta, GA 30345.

Agency for Toxic Substances and Disease Registry. 2003. Toxicological Profile for Fluorine, Hydrogen Fluoride, and Fluorides. Atlanta, GA: U.S. Department of Health and Human Services, 1825 Century Blvd, Atlanta, GA 30345.

Agency for Toxic Substances and Disease Registry. 1999. Toxicological profile for Mercury. Atlanta, GA: U.S. Department of Health and Human Services, 1825 Century Blvd, Atlanta, GA 30345.

Agency for Toxic Substances and Disease Registry. 2003. Toxicological profile for Pyrethrins and Pyrethroids. Atlanta, GA: U.S. Department of Health and Human Services, 1825 Century Blvd, Atlanta, GA 30345.

Agostino, Jill. Once an Athletic Star, Now an Unheavenly Body. East Carolina University. 06-Jul-2006. Retrieved on 31-Oct-2007 from http://www.ecu.edu/cs-admin/news/inthenews/archives/2005/12/0706 2006nytimesathletics.cfm

American Cancer Society. Schneider, R. (Interview). Household Pets and Cancer. CA Cancer J Clinicians, Jul 1970; 20: 234-241.

American College of Sports Medicine. ACSM's Guidelines for Exercise Testing and Prescription. 5th Edition. Williams & Wilkins, Media, PA. 1995.

American Institute of Stress, The. Entire website. Retrieved 2007-Oct-22 from www.stress.org

Annunziata, Guy. Electrotherapy: Following Protocol. Chiropractic Products. Ascend Media; April, 2001.

Annunziata, Guy. Educational Seminar: Pain Management. University of Bridgeport. Atlanta, GA., December, 2007.

Annunziata, Guy. Educational Seminar: Physiological Therapeutics. New York Chiropractic College, Seneca Falls, New York. June, 1996.

Berkow, Robert, Fletcher, Andrew J., editors. The Merck Manual of Diagnosis and Therapy. 16th Ed. Merck Research Laboratories. Rahway, New Jersey. 1992.

Bööhme, Jakob. The Signature of All Things. Reprint. James Clarke & Co., Ltd., Cambridge. 1969.

Brenner, Hermann, Rothenbacher, Dietrich, Bode, Güünter, Adler, Guido. Relation of smoking and alcohol and coffee consumption to active *Helicobacter pylori* infection: cross sectional study. BMJ 1997;315:1489-1492. 6 Dec 1997.

Broughton, Alan. The diagnosis and effective treatment of candida overgrowth. Townsend Letter for Doctors and Patients. July, 2004.

Brudnak, Mark A. The role of probiotics in irritable bowel syndrome, food allergies, and detoxification of the bowel. Townsend Letter for Doctors and Patients. July, 2004.

Centers for Disease Control and Prevention. FACTS ABOUT STACHYBOTRYS CHARTARUM AND OTHER MOLDS. Centers for Disease Control and Prevention, 1600 Clifton Rd., Atlanta, GA 30333.

Cox, Caroline. DEET Repellent Fact Sheet. Journal of Pesticide Reform. 17 October 2005 25:3.

D'Amato, R.J., Lentzsch, S., Anderson, K.C., Rogers, M.S. Mechanism of action of thalidomide and 3-aminothalidomide in multiple myeloma. Semin Oncol. 2001 Dec; 28(6):597-601.

Diner, Barry MD. Toxicity, Mercury. October 18, 2005. eMedicine from WebMD. Retrieved 2007-Aug-25 from www.emedicine.com/EMERG/topic813.htm

Donohoe, Mark, ed. Proceedings of the Complementary Medicine in Chronic Fatigue Syndrome, National Consensus Conference. Sydney, Australia. February, 1995.

Dulcette Technologies, LLC. Material Safety Data Sheet. Sucralose. Dulcette Technologies, LLC, 707 Broadhollow Rd., Farmingdale, NY. 11735.

Fahy, T. Multiple personality disorder: where is the split? J R Soc Med. 1990 September; 83(9): 544-546.

Fleet Numerical Meteorology & Oceanography Center. Global Sea Surface Temperature and Sea Surface Temperature Anomaly Charts. U.S. Department of the Navy. Retrieved on various dates from www.fnmoc.navy.mil/public

Florida, State of. Department of Environmental Protection. CONSOLIDATED NOTICE OF DENIAL. WETLAND RESOURCE PERMIT AND AUTHORIZATION TO USE SOVEREIGN SUBMERGED LANDS. File No. 0129424-005-DF. Department of Environmental Protection, Marjory Stoneman Douglas Building, 3900 Commonwealth Boulevard, Tallahassee, Florida, 32399-3000.

Foote, B., Smolin, Y., Kaplan, M, Legatt, M.E., Lipschitz, D. Prevalence of dissociative disorders in psychiatric outpatients. The American journal of psychiatry. 2006 163 (4): 623-9.

Gaby, Alan R. Is aspartame safe? Townsend Letter for Doctors and Patients. May, 2005.

Gill, H.S., Rutherford, K.J., Cross, M.L. Dietary probiotic supplementation enhances natural killer cell activity in the elderly: an investigation of age-related immunological changes. J Clin Immunol. 2001; 21(4):264-271.

Goldberg, Paul A. Educational Seminar: A Foundational Approach to Allergies and Autoimmune Disorders. Georgia Chiropractic Association, Atlanta, GA. 2006.

Goldberg, Paul A. Infinite Variety: Exploring Biochemical Individuality Part I. Todays Chiropractic November/December 1999.

Goldberg, Paul A. Infinite Variety: Exploring Biochemical Individuality Part II. Todays Chiropractic May/June 2000.

Goldberg, Paul A. Infinite Variety: Exploring Biochemical Individuality Part III Todays Chiropractic September/October 2000.

Goldberg, Paul A. Fibromyalgia: Another Name For Impaired Health. Part I of II. Todays Chiropractic. October/November 1998.

Goldberg, Paul A. Fibromyalgia: Another Name For Impaired Health. Part II of II. Todays Chiropractic. December/January 1998.

Goldberg, Paul A. The Critical Role of the Gastrointestinal Tract in Systemic Illness. Part I; Todays Chiropractic. November/December 2002.

Goldberg, Paul A. The Critical Role of the Gastrointestinal Tract in Systemic Illness. Part II; Todays Chiropractic. January/February 2003.

Goldberg, Paul A. Rheumatoid Disease, Educational Series. Audio Disc. Original Medicine, 5500 Village Blvd., Suite 102, West Palm Beach, FL 33407. Undated.

Guyton, Arthur C., Hall, John E. Textbook of Medical Physiology, 11th Edition. W B Saunders Co, Philadelphia. July 2005.

Hach Company. Website. Retrieved 2008-Feb-20 from www.hach.com

Hill, Natasha J., Stotland, Aleksandr, Solomon, Michelle, Secrest, Patrick, Getzoff, Elizabeth, Sarvetnick, Nora. Resistance of the target islet tissue to autoimmune destruction contributes to genetic susceptibility in Type 1 diabetes. Biol Direct. 2007; 2: 5.

Holme, Ingar, Tonstad, Serena, Sogaard, Anne Johanne, Larsen, Per G Lund, Haheim, Lise Lund. Leisure time physical activity in middle age predicts the metabolic syndrome in old age: results of a 28-year follow-up of men in the Oslo study. BMC Public Health. 2007; 7: 154.

Holtmeier, Wolfgang, Caspary, Wolfgang F. Celiac disease. Orphanet J Rare Dis. 2006; 1.

Hughes, J.R., Kuhlman, D.T., Fichtner, C.G., Gruenfeld M.J. Brain mapping in a case of multiple personality. Clin Electroencephalogy. 1990 Oct; 21(4):200-9.

Hume, Anne L., PharmD. Letters to the Editor: Complementary and Alternative Medicine. Am J Pharm Educ. 2007 June 15; 71(3): 55.

IEEE C95.1-2005 Standard for Safety Levels with Respect to Human Exposure to Radio Frequency Electromagnetic Fields, 3 kHz to 300 GHz. Institute of Electrical and Electronics Engineers. 01-Jan-2006.

Itoh, Kazunori, Hirota, Satoko, Katsumi, Yasukazu, Ochi, Hideki, Hiroshi, Kitakoji. A pilot study on using acupuncture and transcutaneous electrical nerve stimulation (TENS) to treat knee osteoarthritis (OA). Chinese Medicine 2008, 3:2. 29-Feb-2008.

Jacobs, D.S., DeMott, W.R., Oxley, D.K., et al. Laboratory Test Handbook With Key Word Index, 5th ed, Hudson, OH: Lexi-Comp Inc, 2001.

Jahn, H.U., Ullrich, R., Schneider, T., et al. Immunological and trophical effects of *Saccharomyces boulardii* on the small intestine in healthy human volunteers. Digestion 1996; 57, pp. 95-104.

Jamieson, James, Dorman, L.E. Growth Hormone: Reversing Human Aging Naturally. Published by J. Jamieson, St. Louis, MO, 1997.

Jamieson, James, Dorman, L.E. Human Growth Hormone, The Methusaleh Factor: Reverse Aging Naturally. Safe Goods and Longevity News Network, E. Canaan, CT. 1997.

Jamieson, James, Dorman, L.E. The Role of Somatotroph-Specific Peptides and IGF-I Intermediates as an Alternative to HGH Injections. Presented for the American College for Advancement in Medicine, 30 Oct 1997.

Jean-Louis, Girardin, Kripke, Daniel F., Elliott, Jeffrey A., Zizi, Ferdinand, Wolintz, Arthur H., Lazzaro, Douglas R. Daily illumination exposure and melatonin: influence of ophthalmic dysfunction and sleep duration. J Circadian Rhythms. 2005; 3: 13.

Jin, Guanyuan, Xiang, Jia-Jia, Jin, Lei. Clinical Reflexology of Acupuncture and Moxibustion. Beijing Science and Technology Press, Beijing, 2004.

Jones, James F., Maloney, Elizabeth M., Boneva, Roumiana S., Jones, Ann-Britt, Reeves, William C. Complementary and alternative medical therapy utilization by people with chronic fatiguing illnesses in the United States. Complement Altern Med. 2007; 7: 12.

Jozwik, Marcin, Wolczynski, Slawomir, Jozwi, Michal, Szamatowicz, Marian. Oxidative stress markers in preovulatory follicular fluid in humans. Molecular Human Reproduction, Vol. 5, No. 5, 409-413, May 1999.

Kaufman, Stephen J. An appreciation of George Goodheart, DC, originator of applied kinesiology. Townsend Letter for Doctors and Patients. July, 2004.

Kilbourne, Amy M., Rofey, Dana L., McCarthy, John F., Post, Edward P., Welsh, Deborah, Blow, Frederic C. Nutrition and exercise behavior among patients with bipolar disorder. Bipolar Disorders 9 (5), 443-452. 2007.

Ko, Kam Ming, Leung, Hoi Yan. Enhancement of ATP generation capacity, antioxidant activity and immunomodulatory activities by Chinese Yang and Yin tonifying herbs. Chin Med. 2007; 2: 3.

Kraja, Aldi T., Borecki, Ingrid B., North, Kari, Tang, Weihong, Myers, Richard H., Hopkins, Paul N., Arnett, Donna, Corbett, Jonathan, Adelman, Avril, Province, Michael A. Longitudinal and age trends of metabolic syndrome and its risk factors: The Family Heart Study. Nutr Metab (Lond). 2006; 3: 41.

Larsson, Henrik, Lichtenstein, Paul, Larsson, Jan-Olov. Genetic contributions to the development of ADHD subtypes from childhood to adolescence. Journal of the American Academy of Child and Adolescent Psychiatry, August, 2006.

Lehninger, A. Principles of Biochemistry. Worth Publishers, Inc., New York, NY. 1982.

Lenon, George B., Xue, Charlie C.L., Story, David F., Thien, Frank C.K., McPhee, Sarah, Li, Chun G. Inhibition of release of inflammatory mediators in primary and cultured cells by a Chinese herbal medicine formula for allergic rhinitis. Chin Med. 2007; 2: 2.

Loving, Richard T., Kripke, Daniel F., Elliott, Jeffrey A., Knickerbocker, Nancy C., Grandner, Michael A. Bright light treatment of depression for older adults. BMC Psychiatry. 2005; 5: 41.

Luzza, Francesco, Imeneo, Maria, Maletta, Maria, Pallone, Francesco. Smoking, alcohol and coffee consumption, and *H. pylori* infection. BMJ. 1998 March 28; 316 (7136): 1019.

Mackin, Paul, Bishop, David R., Watkinson, Helen M.O. A prospective study of monitoring practices for metabolic disease in antipsychotic-treated community psychiatric patients. BMC Psychiatry. 2007; 7: 28.

Majowicz, Shannon E., Horrocks, Julie, Bocking, Kathryn. Demographic determinants of acute gastrointestinal illness in Canada: a population study. BMC Public Health. 2007; 7: 162.

Mamdani, Firoza, Sequeira, Adolfo, Alda, Martin, Grof, Paul, Rouleau, Guy, Turecki, Gustavo. No association between the *PREP* gene and lithium responsive bipolar disorder. BMC Psychiatry. 2007; 7: 9.

Manson, Jessica J., Rahman, Anisur. Systemic lupus erythematosus. Orphanet J Rare Dis. 2006; 1: 6.

Margolese, Howard C., Ferreri, Florian. Management of conventional antipsychotic-induced tardive dyskinesia. J Psychiatry Neurosci. 2007 January; 32(1): 72.

Maris, Charles H., Chappell, Craig P., Jacob, Joshy. Interleukin-10 plays an early role in generating virus-specific T cell anergy. Immunol. 2007; 8: 8.

Meschino, James. Growth Hormone Secretagogue Supplements: Do They Reverse Aging in Patients Over Age 40? Dynamic Chiropractic. 15 Jan 2005.

Moffet, Howard H. How might acupuncture work? A systematic review of physiologic rationales from clinical trials. Complement Altern Med. 2006, 6: 25.

Office of Dietary Supplements. Dietary Supplement Fact Sheet: Vitamin D. National Institutes of Health, Office of Dietary Supplements, Bethesda, Maryland 20892 USA. 2007-Aug-30.

Ibid : Dietary Supplement Fact Sheet: Vitamin A and Carotenoids. 2006-Apr-23

Ibid : Vitamin E. 2007-Jan-23.

National Institute of Mental Health. Attention Deficit Hyperactivity Disorder. Atlanta: U.S. Department of Health and Human Services, 200 Independence Avenue, S.W., Washington, D.C. 20201. 9-Nov-2007.

National Oceanographic and Atmospheric Administration. Real Time POES Imagery. United States Department of Commerce. Retrieved on various dates from
www.ssd.noaa.gov/PS/TROP/DATA/RT/sst-atl-loop.html

National Oceanographic and Atmospheric Administration. Real Time POES Imagery. United States Department of Commerce. Retrieved on various dates from
www.ssd.noaa.gov/PS/TROP/DATA/RT/sst-pac-loop.html

National Oceanographic and Atmospheric Administration. Current Operational SST Anomaly Charts. United States Department of Commerce. Retrieved on various dates from
www.osdpd.noaa.gov/PSB/EPS/SST/climo.html

National Oceanographic and Atmospheric Administration. Photo Library. United States Department of Commerce. Retrieved on 2008-March-4 from www.photolib.noaa.gov

Nochimson, Geofrey MD. Toxicity, Fluoride. January 8, 2007. eMedicine from WebMD. Retrieved 2007-July-14 from
www.emedicine.com/EMERG/topic181.htm

Nguyena, D.T., Kang, J.H., Lee, M.S. Characterization of *Lactobacillus plantarum* PH04, a potential probiotic bacterium with cholesterol-lowering effects, International Journal of Food Microbiology, Volume 113, Issue 3, 15 February 2007, pp. 358-361.

O'Hara, Ann M., O'Regan, Padraig, Fanning, Áine, O'Mahony, Caitlin, MacSharry, John, Lyons, Anne, Bienenstock, John, O'Mahony, Liam, Shanahan, Fergus. Functional modulation of human intestinal epithelial cell responses by *Bifidobacterium infantis* and *Lactobacillus salivarius*. Immunology. 2006 June; 118(2): 202-215.

O'Reilly, Denis St.J., Director, et al. Entire Website. Scottish Trace Element and Micronutrient Reference Laboratory. NHS Scotland. Retrieved 2007-Sept-15 from www.trace-elements.org.uk

Panjwani, U., Selvanurthy, W., Singh, S.H., Gupta, H.L., Thakur, L, Rai, U.C. Effect of Sahaja Yoga practice on seizure control & EEG changes in patients of epilepsy. Indian Journal of Medical Research 103(3): 165-172. 1996.

Penfold, P.S. The repressed memory controversy: is there middle ground? CMAJ. 1996 September 15; 155(6): 647-653.

Petryk, George. Personal conversations. 2000-2007.

Pothoulakis, C., Kelly, C.P., Joshi, M.A., Gao, N., O'Keane, C.J., Castagliuolo, I., Lamont, J.T. Saccharomyces boulardii inhibits Clostridium difficile toxin A binding and enterotoxicity in rat ileum. Gastroenterology. 1993 Apr;104(4):1108-1115.

Pynnöönen, Pääivi A., Isometsää, Erkki T., Verkasalo, Matti A., Käähköönen, Seppo A., Sipilää, Ilkka, Savilahti, Erkki, Aalberg, Veikko A. Gluten-free diet may alleviate depressive and behavioural symptoms in adolescents with coeliac disease: a prospective follow-up case-series study. BMC Psychiatry. 2005; 5: 14.

Rai U.C., Setji S., Singh, S.H. Some effects on Sahaja Yoga and its role in the prevention of stress disorders. Journal of International Medical Sciences:19-23. 1988.

Rajendra, P., Sujatha, H.N., Devendranath, D., Gunasekaran, B., Sashidhar, R.B., Subramanyam, C., Channakeshava. Biological effects of power frequency magnetic fields: Neurochemical and toxicological changes in developing chick embryos. Biomagn Res Technol. 2004; 2: 1.

Rautava, S., Kalliomääki, M., Isolauri, E. New therapeutic strategy for combating the increasing burden of allergic disease: Probiotics – A Nutrition, Allergy, Mucosal Immunology and Intestinal Microbiota (NAMI). Journal of Allergy and Clinical Immunology, Volume 116, Issue 1, pp. 31-37, 2005.

Rautava, Samuli, Ruuskanen, Olli, Ouwehand, Arthur, Salminen, Seppo, Isolauri, Erika. The Hygiene Hypothesis of Atopic Disease-An Extended Version. Journal of Pediatric Gastroenterology and Nutrition: Volume 38 (4) April 2004, pp. 378-388.

Rosenthal, N.E. Winter Blues: Seasonal Affective Disorder – What It Is and How to Overcome It. (rev. ed.) New York: Guilford Press, 1998.

Ross, C. A. DSM-III: problems in diagnosing partial forms of multiple personality disorder: discussion paper. J R Soc Med. 1985 November; 78(11): 933-936.

Sagar M.D., S.M., Dryden M.Ed., RMT, T., Wong MD, R.K. Massage therapy for cancer patients: a reciprocal relationship between body and mind. Curr Oncol. 2007 April; 14(2): 45-56.

Sagduyu, Kemal, Dokucu, Mehmet E., Eddy, Bruce A., Craigen, Gerald, Baldassano, Claudia F., Yıildıiz, Ayşsegüül. Omega-3 fatty acids decreased irritability of patients with bipolar disorder in an add-on, open label study. Nutr J. 2005; 4: 6.

Selye, Hans. A Syndrome Produced by Diverse Nocuous Agents. Nature, vol. 138, July 4, 1936, p. 32. Reprint available in public domain.

Shaw, P. Proceedings of the National Academy of Sciences, week of Nov. 12-16, 2007. News release, National Institute of Mental Health. Summary retrieved on 12-Nov-2007 from www.nih.gov/news/pr/nov2007/nimh-12.htm

Soghoian, Samara. Toxicity, Heavy Metals. June 28, 2006. eMedicine from WebMD. Retrieved 2007-Sept-16 from www.emedicine.com/EMERG/topic237.htm

Strachan, David P. Hay fever, hygiene, and household size. British Medical Journal 299: 1259-1260, 1989.

Sigma Chemical Co. Sodium fluoride. Material Safety Data Sheet. Sigma Chemical Co., P.O. Box 14508, St. Louis, MO 63178 USA.

Silverstone, Peter H., Bell, Emily C., Willson, Morgan C., Dave, Sanjay, Wilman, Alan H. Lithium alters brain activation in bipolar disorder in a task- and state-dependent manner: an fMRI study. Ann Gen Psychiatry. 2005; 4: 14.

Sloka, J.S., Phillips, Pryse-WEM, Stefanelli, M.l, Joyce, C. Co-occurrence of autoimmune thyroid disease in a multiple sclerosis cohort. J Autoimmune Dis. 2005; 2: 9.

Smith, Wayne R., White, Peter D., Buchwald, Dedra. A case control study of premorbid and currently reported physical activity levels in chronic fatigue syndrome. BMC Psychiatry. 2006; 6: 53.

Steinman, M.A., Gonzales, R., Linder, J.A., et al. Changing use of antibiotics in community-based outpatient practice. Ann Intern Med 138, pp525-33. 2003.

Suzuki, D.T. Essays in Zen Buddhism, New York: Grove Press. 1949.

Swan, Euan. Dietary Fluoride Supplement Protocol for the New Millennium. J Can Dent Assoc 66 (2000): 362-363.

Tanahashi, Kazuaki, Chayat, Roko Sherry, Editors. Endless Vow: The Zen Path of Soen Nakagawa. Boston: Shambhala Publications, Inc. 1996.

Tarricone, Ilaria, Casoria, Michela, Gozzi, Beatrice Ferrari, Grieco, Daniela, Menchetti, Marco, Serretti, Alessandro, Ujkaj, Manjola, Pastorelli, Francesca, Berardi, Domenico. Metabolic risk factor profile associated with use of second generation antipsychotics: a cross sectional study in a community mental health centre. BMC Psychiatry. 2006; 6: 11.

Tarrington, Jenilee. Kasiya Gateway. Entire website, including links. Retrieved 2007-Jul-24 through 2007-Sept-28 from www.kasiya.net

te Velde, Saskia J., van Rossum, Elisabeth F.C., Voorhoeve, Paul G., Twisk, Jos W.R., van de Waal, Henriette A., Delemarre, Stehouwer, Coen D.A., van Mechelen, Willem, Lamberts, Steven W.J., Kemper, Han C.G. An IGF-I promoter polymorphism modifies the relationships between birth weight and risk factors for cardiovascular disease and diabetes at age 36. Endocr Disord. 2005; 5: 5.

U.S. Army Corps of Engineers. ENVIRONMENTAL ASSESSMENT INTERIM OPERATIONS PLAN FOR SUPPORT OF ENDANGERED AND THREATENED SPECIES JIM WOODRUFF DAM GADSDEN AND JACKSON COUNTIES, FLORIDA AND DECATUR COUNTY, GEORGIA. U.S. Army Corps of Engineers, Mobile District, Planning and Environmental Division, Environment and Resources Branch, Inland Environment Team. October 2006.

U.S. Army Corps of Engineers. Mobile District, Water Management Section. Website. Retrieved 2007-Jul-30 to 2007-Nov-28 from http://water.sam.usace.army.mil/enhw.htm

U.S. Department of Labor, Occupational Safety & Health Administration. Regulations (Standards-29 CFR). Lead: Standard Number 1910.1025. U.S. Department of Labor, Occupational Safety & Health Administration. 200 Constitution Avenue, NW, Washington, DC 20210.

U.S. Department of Labor, Occupational Safety & Health Administration. OCCUPATIONAL SAFETY AND HEALTH GUIDELINE FOR ALUMINUM. U.S. Department of Labor, Occupational Safety & Health Administration. 200 Constitution Avenue, NW, Washington, DC 20210.

U.S. Department of Labor, Occupational Safety & Health Administration. OCCUPATIONAL SAFETY AND HEALTH GUIDELINE FOR MERCURY VAPOR. U.S. Department of Labor, Occupational Safety & Health Administration. 200 Constitution Avenue, NW, Washington, DC 20210.

U. S. Food and Drug Administration. Overview of Dietary Supplements. Center for Food Safety and Applied Nutrition. January 3, 2001.

U.S. Geological Survey. Arsenic in ground water in the United States. Retrieved 2008-Feb-09 from water.usgs.gov/nawqa/trace/arsenic van Roon, J.A., Lafeber, F.P., Bijlsma J.W. Synergistic activity of interleukin-4 and interleukin-10 in suppression of inflammation and joint destruction in rheumatoid arthritis. Arthritis Rheum. Jan 2001; 44(1):3-12.

Veldhoen, N., Skirrow, R.C., Osachoff, H., Wigmore, H., Clapson, D.J., Gunderson, M.P., Van Aggelen, G., Helbing C.C. The bactericidal agent triclosan modulates thyroid hormone-associated gene expression and disrupts postembryonic anuran development. Aquat Toxicol. 2006 Dec 1;80 (3):217-27.

Watts, Alan. Psychotherapy East and West. New York: Random House, Pantheon Books, 1961.

Watts, Alan. The Book – On the Taboo Against Knowing Who You Are. New York: Random House, Pantheon Books, 1966.

Watts, Alan. The Way of Zen. New York: Pantheon Books, Inc., 1957.

Wikipedia, the free encyclopedia. Dissociative Identity Disorder. Retrieved 2007-Sept-26 from http://en.wikipedia.org/wiki/Dissociative_identity_disorder

Wilk Case, The. Wilk et. al. v. American Medical Association. Summary provided by www.chiro.org. Retrieved 2007-12-11 from www.chiro.org/abstracts/amavschiro.pdf

WIRUD Co.Ltd, MATERIAL SAFETY DATA SHEET – TRICLOSAN, WIRUD Co. Ltd, China. Undated.

Wongpakaran, Nahathai, van Reekum, Robert, Wongpakaran, Tinakon, Clarke, Diana. Selective serotonin reuptake inhibitor use associates with apathy among depressed elderly: a case-control study Ann Gen Psychiatry. 2007; 6: 7.

World Health Organization. Undated. Data sheet, No. 80: DEET.

World Health Organization. Publications and documents. Standard acupuncture nomenclature. Second edition. 1993.

Yue, Patrick Ying Kit, Mak, Nai Ki, Cheng, Yuen Kit, Leung, Kar Wah, Ng, Tzi Bun, Fan, David Tai Ping, Yeung, Hin Wing, Wong, Ricky Ngok Shun. Pharmacogenomics and the Yin/Yang actions of ginseng: anti-tumor, angiomodulating and steroid-like activities of ginsenosides. Chin Med. 2007; 2: 6.

Zacharias, Ravi. Ravi Zacharias International Ministries. Retrieved 2007-Nov-02 from www.rzim.org

Why Am I Sick? And What To Do About It

Index

in the General Adaption
    Syndrome, 142
Appetizers, 91
Applied Kinesiology
    meridians and, 56, 60, 61, 211
    muscle testing, 59, 60
    neurological switching, 29,
        210, 211
    neurolymphatic reflex, 60
    therapy localization, 60, 61
Arsenic
    in pressure treated wood, 228
    presence in water, 220, 229
    removal through chelation,
        229
    toxicity, 217, 228
Artificial Sweeteners
    aspartame, 162, 163, 170,
        175, 230
    Saccharin, 231, 232
    Stevia, 232
    sucralose, 231
Aura, 61
Autoimmune disease
    Addison's disease, 124
    Alopecia Areata, 124
    Ankylosing Spondylitis, 124
    Antiphospholipid syndrome,
        124
    Aplastic Anemia, 124
    Autoimmune Hemolytic
        Anemia, 124
    Bursitis, 124
    Celiac disease, 118, 124, 126
    Chronic active hepatitis, 124
    Crohn's disease, 124
    Diabetes Mellitus Type 1, 124
    Eczema, 124
    Goodpasture's Syndrome, 124,
        126
    Graves's disease, 124, 126
    Guillain-Barré Syndrome, 124
    Hashimoto's Thyroiditis, 124,
        126
    Hypoparathyroidism, 124
    Iritis, 124
    Kawasaki's disease, 124
    Multiple Sclerosis, 47, 124,
        127
    Myasthenia Gravis, 124, 126
    Pemphigus, 124, 126

Pernicious Anemia, 124
Polymyalgia Rheumatica, 124
Psoriatic Arthritis, 124
Rheumatoid arthritis, 124-126
Rheumatoid fever, 124
Sjögren's Syndrome, 124
Systemic Lupus Erythematosus,
    124, 126
Ulcerative Colitis, 115, 124
Wegener's granulomatosis, 124
Ayurveda, 300
Bacteria
    antibiotic resistant, 111, 243
    beneficial, 33, 90, 92, 98, 109,
        110, 114, 116, 117, 129,
        243, 246
    Bifidobacteria sp., 112, 117
    Bifidobacterium lactis, 117,
        129
    Clostridium difficile, 244
    cyanobacteria, 213, 221
    disruption of flora, 34, 90,
        110-112, 114, 243, 244
    Helicobacter pylori, 15, 99
    Lactobacillus acidophilus, 117
    Lactobacillus paracasei, 117
    Lactobacillus plantarum, 34,
        117
    Lactobacillus salivarius, 117,
        129
    Lactobacillus sp., 112, 116
    pathogenic, 109, 111, 226
    Staphylococcal aureus, 98,
        102, 103
Basal Metabolic Rate (BMR)
    change with age, 199
    effect of exercise on, 199, 290
Beef, 91, 111, 119
Biochemistry, as related to
    bipolar disorder, 157
    definition of, 44
    depression, 173, 175
    diet, 64, 65
    hung biochemical reactions,
        79, 86, 87, 230
    pharmacology, 246
    stress, 143
    toxic substances, 214, 215,
        218, 219, 228, 229
Biological Value
    definition of, 68

of foods, 69
Bipolar Disorder
    discussion of, 153
    types of, 160
Bisphenol-A
    dental, 224
    environmental, 224
    mechanism of toxicity, 224
Blood donation
    apheresis, 270
    risks of, 269
Blood-brain barrier
    and Gamma-aminobutyric acid,
        161, 305, 306
Body piercing
    infections, 245
    safety of, 245
Body-Mind-Spirit
    discussion of, 41
    enlightenment, 44, 276, 280,
        282
    harmony of, 27, 38, 44, 280,
        282
Brain
    development, 262-264, 310
    disease of, 217, 221, 227,
        259, 263
    left vs. right, 36, 264, 275
    Limbic system, 49, 161
    neurotransmitters, 69, 70,
        144, 156-158, 163, 172,
        175, 182, 190, 191, 230,
        257, 259, 309
    organ, 46, 49, 162, 191
    reward centers, 157, 159, 161
    sensory overload of, 51, 135
Bread
    desirable, 91
    served with meals, 91
    undesirable, 18, 91, 200
Carbohydrate
    discussion of, 70
    importance in exercise, 290,
        292
    refined, 19, 71, 292
    unrefined, 71
Carbonic acid
    interference with digestion, 66,
        92
    osteoporosis and, 265
Celiac disease

genetic basis, 118, 169
    in depression, 169
    Type IV hypersensitivity, 126
Chakra
    blocked, 52, 53
    definition of, 52
    discussion of, 52
    emotional associations, 54, 55
    locations of, 54
    normal, 52, 53
Chi, 52, 55
Chicken, 91, 119
Chiropractic
    and fibromyalgia, 194, 195
    and low back pain, 267
    Applied Kinesiology, 59
    definition of, 194
    Wilk v. AMA, 13
Chlorine
    in sucralose, 231
    in water, 112, 222, 223
Cholesterol
    and Metabolic Syndrome, 246,
        247
    effect of exercise on, 286
    effect of fiber on, 83, 84
    probiotics and, 33, 34
Chronic Fatigue Syndrome
    and General Adaption
        Syndrome, 192
    discussion of, 188
Complement system
    pathways, 100
    purpose of, 100
    Type III hypersensitivity and,
        126
Connective tissue
    autoimmunity and, 123
    inflammation of, 139
Contents, xi
Controversial treatments, 12
Cooking, 92
Cosmetics
    perfumes, 234
    toxicity, 234
DEET
    absorption, 232
    alternatives, 233
    toxicity, 232
Depression

and Th1/Th2 balance, 129
in allergies, 103
in autoimmune disease, 125,
    130, 131
in bipolar disorder, 155, 160
in depression, 170, 173
in immunodeficiency, 105
in obsessive-compulsive
    disorder, 182
Enzyme
    amino acid oxidase, 66
    amylase, 93, 116
    cellulase, 116, 244
    cyclooxygenase, 75, 246
    denatured, 92, 220
    genetically defective, 65, 118
    glucoamylase, 116
    hemicellulase, 116, 244
    invertase, 116
    lactase, 118
    lactate dehydrogenase, 287
    lipase, 93
    malt diastase, 116
    pepsin, 66
    protease, 66, 93
    pyruvate dehydrogenase, 228
    role in digestion, 66, 90, 91,
        93
    tissue transglutaminase, 118
    tryptophan pyrrolase, 88, 170,
        196, 242
Essential fatty acid
    deficiencies, 75, 87, 168
    in depression, 168
    Omega-3, 75, 162, 168
    Omega-6, 75
    proper balance of, 75
    sources of, 75
Exercise
    aerobic, 89, 287-290, 296,
        297
    agility training, 287, 288, 297
    anaerobic, 287-289, 296, 297
    benefits, 196, 286
    endurance training, 287, 288,
        296
    flexibility training, 287, 288,
        295, 297
    schedule, 295
    setting goals, 297

strength training, 197,
    287-289, 297
training partners and, 297
Fat
    as a nutrient, 65, 74
    blocking of absorption, 76
    ideal body, 292
    substitutes, 65, 76
    tissue, 19, 70, 71, 74, 88, 91,
        92, 199, 200, 230, 234,
        268, 292
Fatigue
    adrenal, 142
    muscular, 139, 199, 267
    neuronal, 156, 158, 190, 191
    physical, 37, 88, 102, 145,
        156, 169, 187, 188, 190,
        191
Fiber
    appropriate amounts, 84
    discussion of, 83
    insoluble, 83, 84, 120
    natural sources, 84
    soluble, 83, 84, 120
Fibromyalgia
    discussion of, 187
Fish
    dietary consumption of, 67, 91
    oil supplements, 75
    toxins in, 217, 221
Fluoride
    as a toxin, 216
    in drinking water, 222
Food Allergy
    causes, 64, 90, 118
    definition of, 118
    immunological response, 118
    tests for, 113, 118, 119
    treatment, 31, 113
    types of, 118
Food hypersensitivity
    causes, 90
    treatment, 113
Food poisoning, 109, 110
Fruit
    dietary consumption of, 67,
        71, 84, 93, 200
    dried, 73, 93
    glycemic index and ripeness,
        73
    natural, 89, 90

Iron, 80, 82
macrominerals, 79
Magnesium, 79–82, 114, 216,
    227, 265
Manganese, 79, 82
Molybdenum, 82
Phosphorus, 79, 82
Potassium, 79–82, 216, 265
Selenium, 82
Sodium, 79, 81–83
trace minerals, 79, 219, 229,
    265
Zinc, 82
Mold
    black (Stachybotrys
        chartarum), 219
    eradicating, 219
    Penicillium notatum, 219
Mood
    artificial sweeteners and, 231
    component of the mind, 49
    neurotransmitters and, 146,
        163, 187, 196, 231
    sunlight and, 197, 198
    swings in bipolar disorder,
        153, 154, 156, 159
Multiple Personality Disorder
    response to stress, 148
Multiplicity
    acquired, 209
    discussion of, 203
    normal variant, 204, 207, 210,
        211
    preserving inborn mechanism,
        207, 208
    stress and, 150, 151, 207–209
    switching mechanism, 210,
        211
Muscle
    spasms, 252, 253
    strain, 250, 251
Naturopathy, 7
Nervous system
    autonomic, 46, 49
    heart, 50
    parasympathetic, 46, 161
    somatic, 46, 49
    sympathetic, 46, 141, 143,
        144
Neurons
    communication, 49

sensitivity to electrical fields,
    225
Neurotransmission
    electrolytes and, 258
    neurotransmitters involved in,
        258
    process of, 49
Neurotransmitter
    acetylcholine, 174, 258
    aspartic acid, 162, 163, 175,
        230, 258
    dopamine, 50, 70, 155, 157,
        159, 162, 163, 171–175,
        187, 188, 230, 258, 259
    dynorphin, 258
    endorphin, 66, 159, 160, 254,
        258
    enkephalins, 258
    Gamma-aminobutyric acid,
        156–159, 161, 164, 172,
        173, 182, 205, 258, 259,
        305, 306, 309
    glutamic acid, 258
    glycine, 69, 173, 174, 258
    histamine, 103, 104, 258
    norepinephrine, 50, 70, 140,
        141, 143, 144, 147,
        157–159, 162, 163,
        171–175, 187, 188, 230,
        241, 242, 258
    phenylethylamine, 70,
        172–174
    purine, 258
    serotonin, 70, 86, 87, 95, 144,
        155, 157, 163, 168–175,
        182, 187, 188, 196, 198,
        230, 242, 258, 259, 309
    substance P, 50, 188, 258
Nutrition
    bipolar disorder and, 160–162
    chronic fatigue syndrome and,
        197, 200
    definition of, 63
    depression and, 172, 174
    discussion of, 63
    fibromyalgia and, 197, 200
Nuts
    as a snack, 93
    peanuts, 118
    source of essential fatty acids,
        93, 94

Why Am I Sick? And What To Do About It

About the Author

Dr. Robert Zee is in private practice in Cumming, Georgia. The practice offers Chiropractic care, Applied Kinesiology, Massage Therapy, Reiki, and other forms of energy healing, Medical Qi Gong, Reflexology, Yoga and Pilates classes. Dr. Zee holds a degree in Engineering from the Georgia Institute of Technology and a Doctorate of Chiropractic from Life University in Marietta, Georgia. The doctor is fully board certified in both Chiropractic and Physiological Therapeutics.

Please visit the doctor's website at www.rue309.com for information about classes, announcements, and upcoming publications. Information regarding how to find qualified practitioners can also be found on the site. To order this publication online, go to www.rue309.com and click on the **Publications** button.

Crííost an Sláánaitheoir Fééin

Why Am I Sick? And What To Do About It